Clinical Neuroscience for Communication Disorders

Neuroanatomy and Neurophysiology

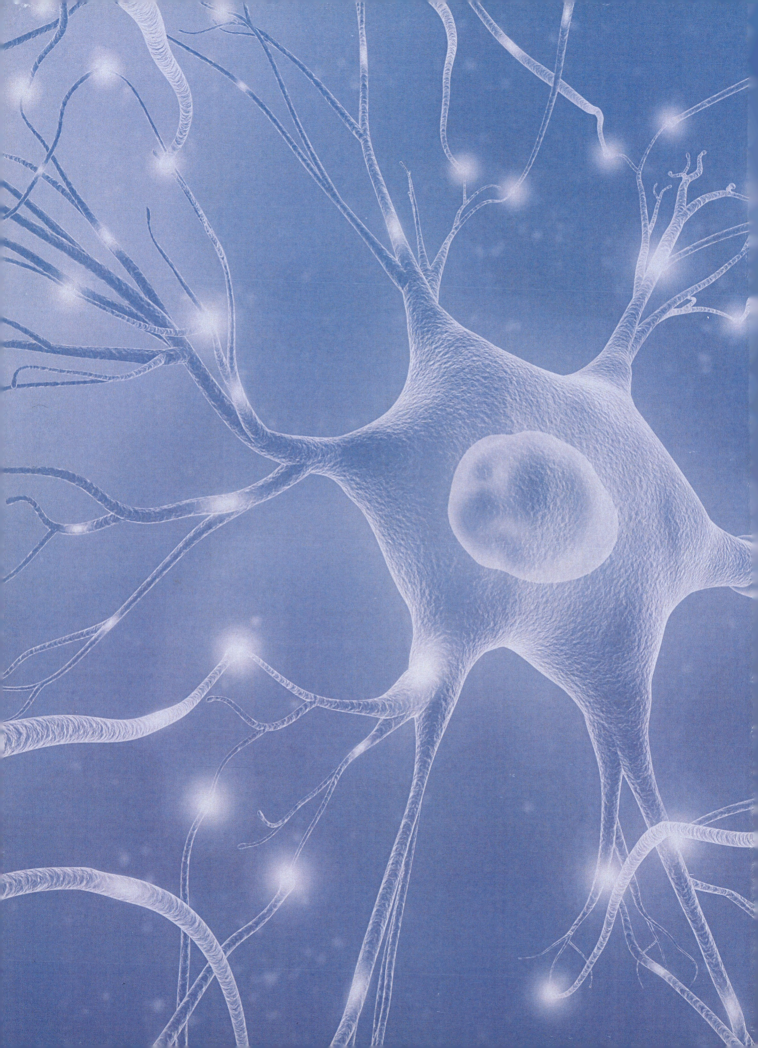

Clinical Neuroscience *for* Communication Disorders

Neuroanatomy and Neurophysiology

Margaret Lehman Blake, PhD, CCC-SLP
Jerry K. Hoepner, PhD, CCC-SLP

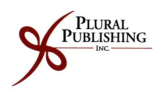

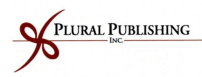

5521 Ruffin Road
San Diego, CA 92123

e-mail: information@pluralpublishing.com
Website: https://www.pluralpublishing.com

Copyright © 2023 by Plural Publishing, Inc.

Typeset in 10.5/13 Adobe Garamond by Flanagan's Publishing Services, Inc.
Printed in China by Regent Publishing Services Ltd.

All rights, including that of translation, reserved. No part of this publication may be reproduced, stored in a retrieval system, or transmitted in any form or by any means, electronic, mechanical, recording, or otherwise, including photocopying, recording, taping, Web distribution, or information storage and retrieval systems without the prior written consent of the publisher.

For permission to use material from this text, contact us by
Telephone: (866) 758-7251
Fax: (888) 758-7255
e-mail: permissions@pluralpublishing.com

Every attempt has been made to contact the copyright holders for material originally printed in another source. If any have been inadvertently overlooked, the publisher will gladly make the necessary arrangements at the first opportunity.

Library of Congress Cataloging-in-Publication Data

Names: Blake, Margaret Lehman, author. | Hoepner, Jerry K., author.
Title: Clinical neuroscience for communication disorders : neuroanatomy and neurophysiology / Margaret Lehman Blake, Jerry K. Hoepner.
Description: San Diego, CA : Plural Publishing, Inc., [2023] | Includes bibliographical references and index.
Identifiers: LCCN 2021029583 (print) | LCCN 2021029584 (ebook) | ISBN 9781635503654 (hardcover) | ISBN 1635503655 (hardcover) | ISBN 9781635503661 (ebook)
Subjects: MESH: Communication Disorders | Nervous System Physiological Phenomena | Nervous System—anatomy & histology | Neurosciences
Classification: LCC QP360 (print) | LCC QP360 (ebook) | NLM WL 340.2 | DDC 612.8—dc23
LC record available at https://lccn.loc.gov/2021029583
LC ebook record available at https://lccn.loc.gov/2021029584

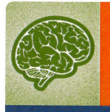

Contents

Preface: How to Use This Textbook — xiii
Acknowledgments — xv
Reviewers — xvii

Chapter 1. Overview of the Nervous System — 1

Overview — 1
Major Components — 1
Organization of the Nervous System — 5
    Organizational Systems — 6
        Cytoarchitecture Organization — 6
        Organization by Function — 7
Terminology — 10
Nervous System Cells — 12
    Neurons — 14
    Glial Cells — 15
Structures and Landmarks — 18
    Lobes — 21
        Frontal Lobes — 21
        Parietal Lobes — 21
        Temporal Lobes — 24
        Occipital Lobes — 24
    Subcortical Structures — 26
        Basal Ganglia — 26
        Thalamus — 28
    Cerebellum — 28
    Brainstem — 28
Summary — 29
References — 29

Chapter 2. Ventricular System: Cranium, Ventricles, and Meninges — 31

Overview — 31
Cranium, Cranial Vault, and Its Contents — 31
Meningeal Layers — 34
    Dura Mater — 34
    Arachnoid Layer and Pia Mater — 36
Ventricles — 37
    Cerebrospinal Fluid Path and Functions — 37

Communication Through the Ventricular System 39
Disruptions to the Ventricular and Meningeal Systems 40
    Hydrocephalus 40
    Meningeal Damage 42
Summary 42
Additional Resources 43

Chapter 3. Neuron Anatomy and Physiology — 45

Overview 45
Classification of Neurons 45
Neuronal Communication 46
    Big Picture Overview 47
    Membrane Potentials 47
Synaptic Transmission 49
    Action Potentials 51
    Myelinated Versus Unmyelinated Axons 54
    Synaptic Transmission 54
        Types of Neurotransmitters 57
        Neurotransmitter Recovery and Degradation 59
Creating Meaning from Binary Signals 59
    Patterns of Signals 59
    Source of Signals 61
    Region or Location 61
Conditions That Alter Synaptic Transmission 61
    Neurologic Disorders and Diseases That Affect Synaptic Transmission 61
        Parkinson Disease 61
        Multiple Sclerosis 62
        Myasthenia Gravis 62
    Pharmacological Effects on Synaptic Transmission 63
        Blocking Effects 63
        Prolonging Effects 63
        Mimicking Effect 64
Summary 64
Reference and Additional Resources 65

Chapter 4. Neuroembryology — 67

Overview 67
The Neural Tube 70
    Developmental (Embryologic) Precursors 70
    Sulcus Limitans 72
    Lamina Terminalis (Precursor to the Corpus Callosum) 72
    Vesicles of the Neural Tube (CNS Precursors) 72
    Landmark Timelines 74
Telencephalon and C-Shaped Development 76
Disruptions to Development and Consequences 78
Summary 79
References and Additional Resources 79

Chapter 5. Diencephalon — 83

- Overview — 83
- Diencephalic Structures — 83
  - Thalamus — 83
    - Thalamic Nuclei — 84
  - Epithalamus — 86
  - Subthalamus — 87
  - Hypothalamus — 87
  - Pituitary Gland — 87
- Damage to the Diencephalon — 88
- Summary — 88

Chapter 6. Somatosensory Systems — 91

- Overview — 91
- Somatosensory System Structures — 91
  - Sensory Receptors — 91
    - Mechanoreceptors — 94
    - Nociceptors — 94
    - Proprioceptive Sensory Receptors — 94
  - Thalamic Nuclei — 95
  - Primary Somatosensory Cortex — 95
  - Cortical Association Areas — 95
- Sensory Pathways — 97
  - Dorsal Column–Medial Lemniscal Pathway — 97
  - Spinothalamic Tracts — 98
  - Spinocerebellar Tracts — 101
- Sensory Innervation — 102
- Damage to Somatosensory System Components — 102
  - Spinal Cord Damage — 102
  - Thalamic Damage — 103
  - Cortical Damage — 104
- Summary — 105

Chapter 7. Visual System — 107

- Overview — 107
- The Eye — 107
  - Anterior Structures — 107
  - Posterior Structures: The Retina — 108
  - Visual Fields — 109
- Visual Pathway — 111
- Visual Cortex — 113
  - Dorsal Pathway — 114
  - Ventral Pathway — 114
- Damage to the Visual System — 115
  - Visual Field Cuts — 115
  - Cortical Damage — 116
- Summary — 118

Chapter 8. Auditory and Vestibular Systems — 121

- Overview — 121
- Auditory System — 121
  - The Cochlea — 123
    - Converting Sound Waves Into Neural Signals — 125
  - Auditory Pathway — 127
  - Frequency and Intensity Coding in the Auditory System — 128
  - Localization of Sound — 129
  - Auditory Processing in the Cortex — 131
  - Hearing Impairment and Damage to the Auditory System — 132
    - Conductive Hearing Loss — 132
    - Sensorineural Hearing Loss — 132
- Vestibular System — 133
  - Vestibular Pathways — 134
- Summary — 135
- Reference — 136

Chapter 9. Chemical Senses: Smell and Taste — 139

- Olfaction — 139
- Olfaction: The Sense of Smell — 139
  - Olfactory Pathway — 139
  - Impairments of Olfaction — 142
- Gustation: The Sense of Taste — 144
  - Gustatory Pathway — 144
  - Factors Influencing Taste Perception — 146
  - Impairments of Gustation — 146
- Summary — 147
- Reference — 147

Chapter 10. Motor Systems — 149

- Overview — 149
- Motor System Structures — 150
  - Primary Motor Strip — 150
  - Premotor and Supplementary Motor Areas — 150
  - Basal Ganglia — 151
  - Cerebellum — 155
- Motor Pathways — 158
  - Pyramidal Tracts — 158
    - Cranial and Spinal Nerves — 158
    - Corticospinal Tracts — 159
    - Corticobulbar Tract — 162
  - Extrapyramidal Tracts — 162
    - Rubrospinal Tract — 162
    - Tectospinal Tract — 162
    - Vestibulospinal Tract — 162
    - Reticulospinal Tract — 163

Motor Units and Muscle Innervation	163
Clinical Implications	165
Motor Cortex	166
Motor Pathways	166
Neuromuscular Junction	167
Basal Ganglia	168
Cerebellum	169
Summary	169

Chapter 11. Cranial Nerves — 173

Overview	173
General Functions	175
Cranial Nerve Pathways	179
Motor Pathways: Corticobulbar Tract	179
Sensory Pathways	179
Cranial Nerves III, IV, and VI: Oculomotor, Trochlear, and Abducens	179
Muscles of the Eye	179
Oculomotor Nerve	181
Trochlear Nerve	181
Abducens Nerve	181
Cranial Nerve V: Trigeminal Nerve	182
Cranial Nerve VII: Facial Nerve	185
Cranial Nerve IX: Glossopharyngeal	187
Cranial Nerve X: Vagus Nerve	187
Pharyngeal Branch of the Vagus	187
Superior Laryngeal Nerve of the Vagus	188
Recurrent Laryngeal Nerve of the Vagus	188
Pharyngeal Plexus	189
Cranial Nerve XI: Spinal Accessory Nerve	189
Cranial Nerve XII: Hypoglossal Nerve	190
Integration of Cranial Nerve Functions	190
Speech Production	190
Swallowing	192
Clinical Implications: Examinations of Speech and Swallowing Mechanisms	192
Cranial Nerve/Oral Mechanism Examination	192
Smell and Taste	192
Vision	193
Extraocular Movements (CNs III, IV, and VI)	193
Jaw Movements and Mastication (CN V)	193
Facial Sensation (CN V)	193
Muscles of Facial Expression and Oral Preparation (CN VII)	193
Hearing (CN VIII)	194
Velar Functions—Motor and Sensory (CNs V, IX, and X)	194
Laryngeal Functions—Motor and Sensory (CN X)	194
Spinal Accessory (CN XI)	194
Lingual Motor Functions (CN XII with a Little Help from CN X)	194
Lingual Sensation (CNs V and IX)	196
Oral and Laryngeal Diadochokinetic Rate	196

Evidence for the Oral Mechanism Examination	196
Clinical Bedside Swallow Examination and Instrumental Assessment	196
Summary	197
Additional Resources	197

Chapter 12. Limbic System and Reticular Formation — 199

Limbic System Structures and Functions	199
Homeostasis	200
Olfaction	202
Memory	204
Emotions	206
Integrating Limbic Information	209
Reticular Formation and Reticular Activating System	209
Summary	213
References and Additional Resources	214

Chapter 13. Cerebrovascular System — 217

Overview	217
Blood Supply and Functional Organization	217
Circle of Willis	218
Cerebral Blood Supply Distributions	222
Blood Supply to the Thalamus and Basal Ganglia	226
Blood Supply to the Cerebellum	226
Brainstem and Spinal Cord Distributions	228
Midbrain	228
Pons	229
Medulla	229
Spinal Cord	229
Blood–Brain Barrier	230
Disruptions to Blood Supply	231
Summary	234
References and Additional Resources	234

Chapter 14. Communication and Cognition — 237

Overview	237
Common Developmental Disruptions	238
Developmental Language Disorders	238
Autism Spectrum Disorder	238
Down Syndrome	239
Fragile X Syndrome	239
Common Neurologic Insults and Diseases	240
Traumatic Brain Injury	240
Degenerative Diseases and Tumors	240
Communication	241
Language	243
Networks	243

Development	245
Lesions and Disorders	246
Pragmatics and Social Cognition	248
Networks	248
Development	249
Lesions and Disorders	250
Cognition	251
Executive Functions	251
Networks	251
Development	252
Lesions and Disorders	252
Memory	252
Networks	253
Development	253
Lesions and Disorders	254
Attention	255
Networks	255
Development	255
Lesions and Disorders	257
Summary	257
References and Additional Resources	258

Chapter 15. Neuroplasticity — 263

Overview	263
Neural (Cellular) Plasticity	263
Behavioral Plasticity	265
Intensity and Dosage	269
Factors That Contribute to Participation	270
Functional Reactivation Versus Functional Reorganization	271
Summary	271
References and Additional Resources	272

Chapter 16. Clinical Cases — 275

Overview	276
Approach to Solving (Thinking Through) Cases	276
Section 1: Acquired Cases	277
Case 16–1: 48-Year-Old Female With Traumatic Brain Injury	277
Case 16–2: 32-Year-Old Male With Postural Headaches and Mixed Upper/Lower Motor Neuron Signs	277
Case 16–3: 56-Year-Old Female With Progressive Onset of Dysphagia and Speech Impairments	278
Case 16–4: 17-Year-Old Female with Traumatic Brain Injury	279
Case 16–5: 63-Year-Old Male With Aphasia and Right Hemiparesis	279
Case 16–6: 86-Year-Old Male With Insidious Onset of Cognitive–Communication Changes	280
Case 16–7: 45-Year-Old Female With Acute Onset of Confusion and Language Impairment	281

Case 16–8: 62-Year-Old Male With Acute Onset of Lethargy and Impaired Attention	282
Case 16–9: 52-Year-Old With Acute Onset of "Slurred" Speech and "Drunken" Gait	283
Case 16–10: 70-Year-Old Male With Acute Onset of Dysarthria, Vertigo, Nausea, and Double Vision	283
Case 16–11: 22-Year-Old Male With Acute Onset of Weakness and Respiratory Distress	284
Case 16–12: 62-Year-Old Female With Gradual Onset of Speech and Swallowing Impairments	285
Case 16–13: 78-Year-Old Female With Gradual Onset of Speech and Gait Disturbances	285
Case 16–14: 52-Year-Old Female With Declining Cognition, Speech, and Swallowing Function	286
Case 16–15: 86-Year-Old Female With Memory and Swallowing Difficulties	288
Case 16–16: 73-Year-Old Male With Right Facial and Tongue Atrophy	290
Section 2: Pediatric and Developmental Cases	291
Case 16–17: 5-Year-Old Male With Shunt Malfunction	291
Case 16–18: 4-Year-Old Male With Fetal Alcohol Syndrome	293
Case 16–19: 30-Year-Old Female With Agenesis of the Corpus Callosum	294
Case 16–20: 11-Year-Old Male With Brainstem Tumor	296
Case 16–21: 11-Year-Old Female with Traumatic Brain Injury	296
Case Question Answers	298
Reference	310

Appendix Review of Head and Neck Anatomy — 313

Review	313
Face	313
Facial Skeleton and Cranium	313
Facial Muscles	315
Velum	317
Tongue	319
Pharynx	319
Larynx	319
Neck	322

Index 325

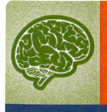

Preface: How to Use This Textbook

Thank you for choosing *Clinical Neuroscience for Communication Disorders: Neuroanatomy and Neurophysiology*. The intent of this tutorial is to briefly describe and demonstrate the organization of chapters, which follow the format below with a few exceptions [e.g., the cases chapter (Chapter 16)]. Understanding the organization may help both course instructors and students to best utilize the resources.

Initial paragraph ties content to clinical applications. Each chapter begins, like this, with an application to everyday clinical practice for speech-language pathologists, audiologists, and related professionals. Clinical applications are intuitive for many of the chapters/topics, but we do our best to connect the dots in those chapters and with content where the connection might not be as obvious.

Our **customized illustrations** help solidify connections between anatomy and physiology. This is accomplished through

- a variety of views and perspectives (superior/inferior, dorsal/ventral, sections—coronal/transverse/sagittal, frontal/lateral/posterior);
- resections/cutaway illustrations to visualize deep, difficult to see/visualize structures;
- close-up (magnified) pull-out illustrations of small sections of a structure along with the broader view of the structure itself for context;
- structures in situ (within the larger structure, which is transparent to allow you to see the deeper structure); and
- schematics, depicting sequences or processes, systems or networks.

In addition, we intentionally use both left and right hemisphere views throughout the book. This is done to implicitly support the message made explicit in Chapter 14 that both hemispheres play critical roles in communication.

We have highlighted foundational concepts and terminology by **bolding keywords** throughout, as well as including Latin and Greek word origins and meanings.

Tables. Help sort out complex, multicomponent anatomy, physiology, and networks.

Examples		
Structure		
Blood supply		
Innervation		

Boxes. A place for applying learning.

Applications—These include everyday examples such as hitting your funny bone, which help tie anatomy and physiology with practical experiences.

Key terminology and concepts—Whenever there are numerous key terms necessary to understand broader concepts, a mini-glossary is included to define terms and concepts.

Exercises—Some applications include mini-labs or experiments you can conduct on yourself or a friend. These include things such as mapping your sensory receptor fields.

Clinical cases—Those embedded within each chapter are typically abridged to highlight the concepts of the chapter (e.g., hemorrhagic stroke, consequences of cerebellar damage). Expanded versions of key cases are included in the clinical cases chapter (Chapter 16) to provide more opportunities to interact with foundational concepts. Expanded cases also include guiding questions and an answer key for instructors/students. The broad intent of cases is to solidify understanding of content knowledge and make direct applications to clinical practice. This is intended to provide an initial exposure to the process of localization and differential diagnosis, preparing learners for much deeper learning about diagnostics and interventions within their future disorder-based coursework.

The appendix: This provides a review of anatomical foundations typically covered in-depth in courses and texts on anatomy and physiology of the speech and hearing mechanism. This is particularly helpful to use in combination with Chapter 11: Cranial Nerves to remind students of the head and neck musculature.

The oral mechanism examination: Although not intended to be a replacement for a fully comprehensive and exhaustive oral mechanism exam for all types of clients and situations, this element of Chapter 11 ties anatomy directly to an application for our profession. Ties to clinical assessment of swallowing are also presented briefly here.

The neuroplasticity chapter (Chapter 15): This chapter connects readers to key principles of contemporary neuroscience, particularly extensions to everyday practice and broad support for habilitation and rehabilitation.

The communication and cognition chapter (Chapter 14): This chapter is broader than the typical language application chapter found in neuroscience books for communication disorders. Not only are the left and right hemisphere contributions to communication covered equally but also developmental cognitive communication disorders are discussed as well as acquired neurological disorders. Motor speech disorders are covered in Chapter 10: Motor Systems and Chapter 11: Cranial Nerves.

The cases chapter (Chapter 16): Mentioned previously, this is cross-referenced within and across chapters.

Summary: At the end of each chapter, there is a plain-language summary that highlights key concepts within the chapter. Some learners may wish to begin there by reading the summary and key concepts before delving into the content, returning to it at the end of the chapter.

Key concepts:
1. A bulleted list is included at the end of each chapter to highlight key concepts and learning outcomes.
2. For students: at minimum, you should be sure to understand these key concepts. If you don't, we suggest that you return to the chapter resources provided by your instructor (recorded lectures/screencasts, animations, supplementary readings), and ask your peers/instructors clarifying questions.

References and additional resources: In some cases, these items are referenced directly in the text, whereas others are useful resources to augment your learning.

Final note: The order of the chapters is based on how we teach neuroanatomy and physiology, but in some cases the order is a bit arbitrary. Instructors can choose to assign chapters in the order that best fits their conceptualization and teaching style. Each chapter has references to others for more information, so you can easily find background or in-depth information if you teach the chapters in a different order.

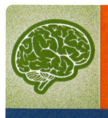
Acknowledgments

JKH: I acknowledge my mentor, Lyn Turkstra, for instilling a passion for teaching neuroanatomy and neurophysiology. The phrase, "You've come a long way . . ." seems fitting.

We thank Tatiana Gandlin, who created most of the artwork for this book. We were thrilled with each new set of illustrations she sent, and we hope that they aid in learning the structures and concepts of the human nervous system. We are fortunate to have additional illustrations from Jerry's oldest daughter, Mariah Hoepner. Mariah is a student at the University of Wisconsin–Madison studying communication sciences and disorders, hoping to attend graduate school in medical illustration. Thanks as well to Rob Mattison, videographer from the University of Wisconsin–Eau Claire, who filmed and edited videos for the Oral Mechanism Examination and Clinical Bedside Swallowing Evaluation. We are also grateful to Diana Cataldi, a graduate student, who shared her talents in these two video series.

In this book, we were very intentional about providing broad clinical applications. This includes equally emphasizing left and right hemisphere contributions to communication, discussion of both developmental and acquired neurologic disorders, and consideration of pediatric and adult clients. We thank Angela Ciccia and Jenny Lundine for providing pediatric clinical cases to help us achieve this goal. Thank you as well to all of the other clients and families who have inspired the remaining clinical cases. It is important for readers to know that these are real cases (albeit with names changed), and we owe those individuals a debt of gratitude for shaping our knowledge on these topics.

Thanks to our colleagues who have supported this effort. Their initial excitement when we told them about the book, continued encouragement along the way, feedback on content, and support of our need for more time to write made this gigantic task doable. We also appreciate the time and effort of the reviewers, who pointed out areas that were lacking and made thoughtful suggestions for improvements.

Finally, we extend our thanks to the hundreds of students we have taught throughout the years. Their curiosity and questions drive us to learn more, and seeing them grasp the complexities of the nervous system and the importance of understanding neuroanatomy and neurophysiology to fully understand communication was our inspiration to extend our teaching beyond our individual classes. A special thanks to students at the University of Houston who provided feedback on the clinical cases: Amanda, Anna, Arden, Carson, Daisy, Saige, and Samantha.

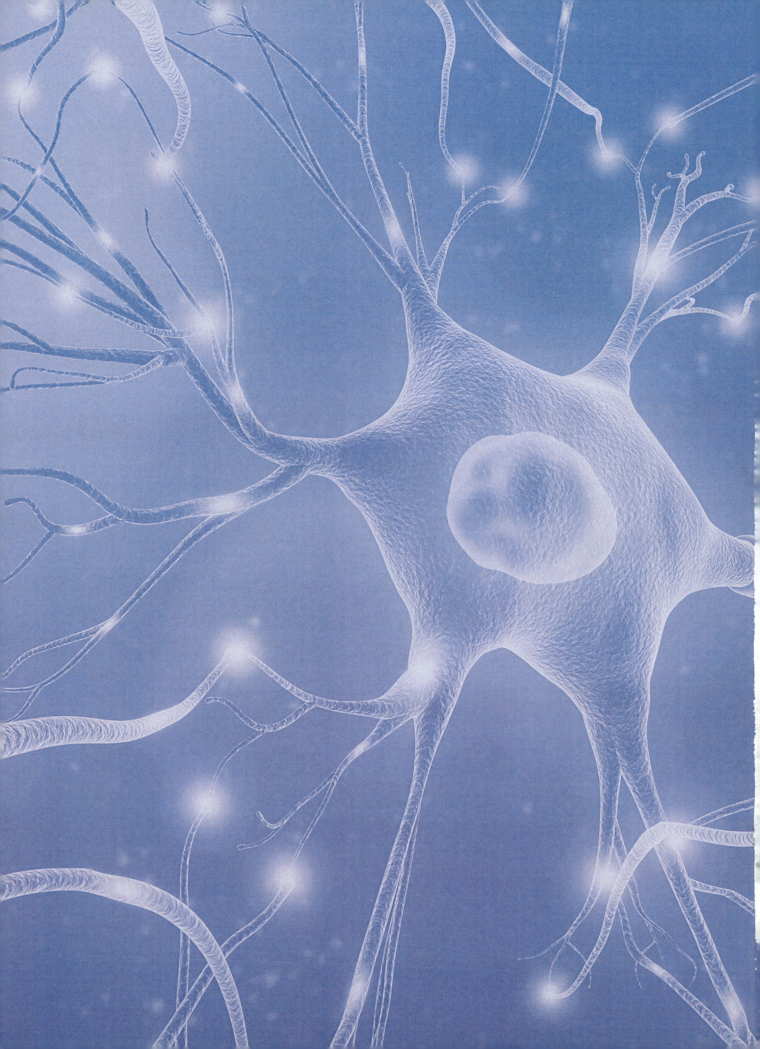

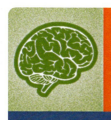

Reviewers

Plural Publishing and the authors thank the following reviewers for taking the time to provide their valuable feedback during the manuscript development process. Additional anonymous feedback was provided by other expert reviewers.

Jamie H. Azios, PhD, CCC-SLP
Assistant Professor
Lamar University
Beaumont, Texas

Audrey A. Hazamy, PhD, CCC-SLP
Assistant Professor
Brooklyn College–City University of New York
Brooklyn, New York

Kelly Knollman-Porter, PhD, CCC-SLP
Associate Professor
Miami University
Oxford, Ohio

Amy Shollenbarger, PhD, CCC-SLP
Department Chair and Associate Professor
Arkansas State University
Jonesboro, Arkansas

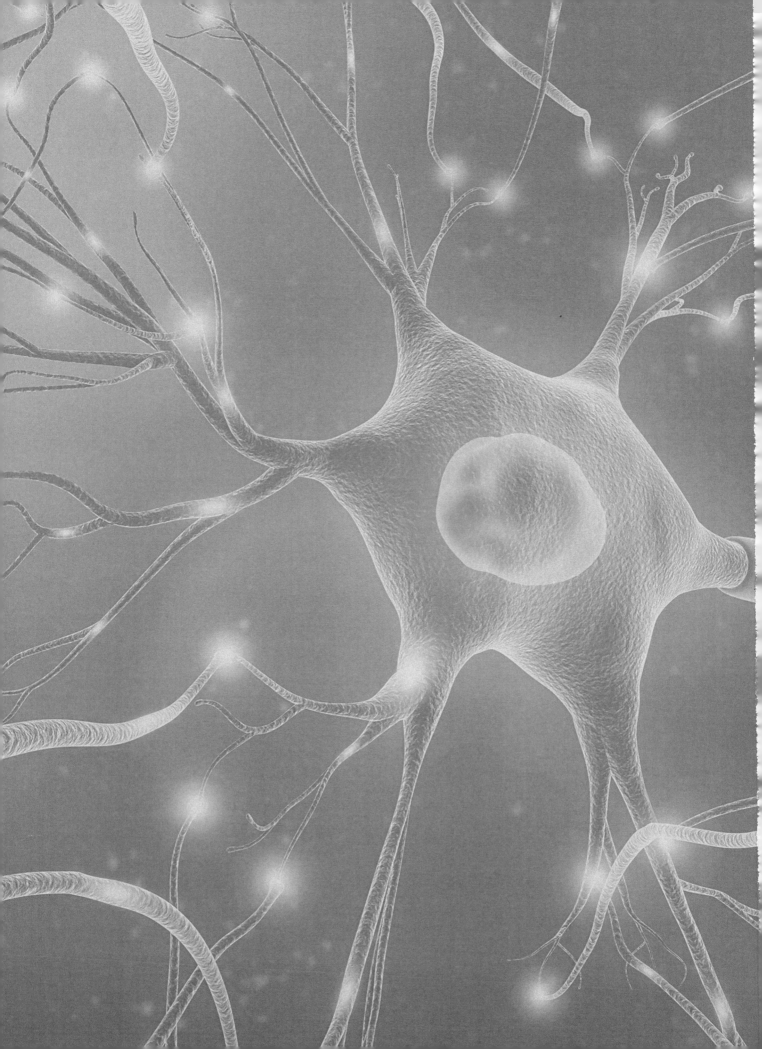

I dedicate this book to my family. Without their support, I would not be in a position to write this textbook. Thank you to my wife, Carol, for always being there to support me and for patiently listening to too many discussions about neuroanatomy and neurophysiology. Thank you to my daughters, Mariah and Madelyn, for the coffee, hugs, and encouragement necessary to complete this book. I can honestly say that having both of you alongside of me almost every day as a result of the pandemic made this an exceptional year to write, knowing that we could have a cup of coffee, go for a walk, or take a break together when needed.

J. K. Hoepner

I dedicate this book to my Dad, Chuck Lehman, who gave each of his kids what he had to give: acceptance of who we are, resources to pursue our goals (within reason!), strong and steady love, a solid base on which to fall when we needed, and humor to make sure we didn't take ourselves too seriously.

M. Lehman Blake

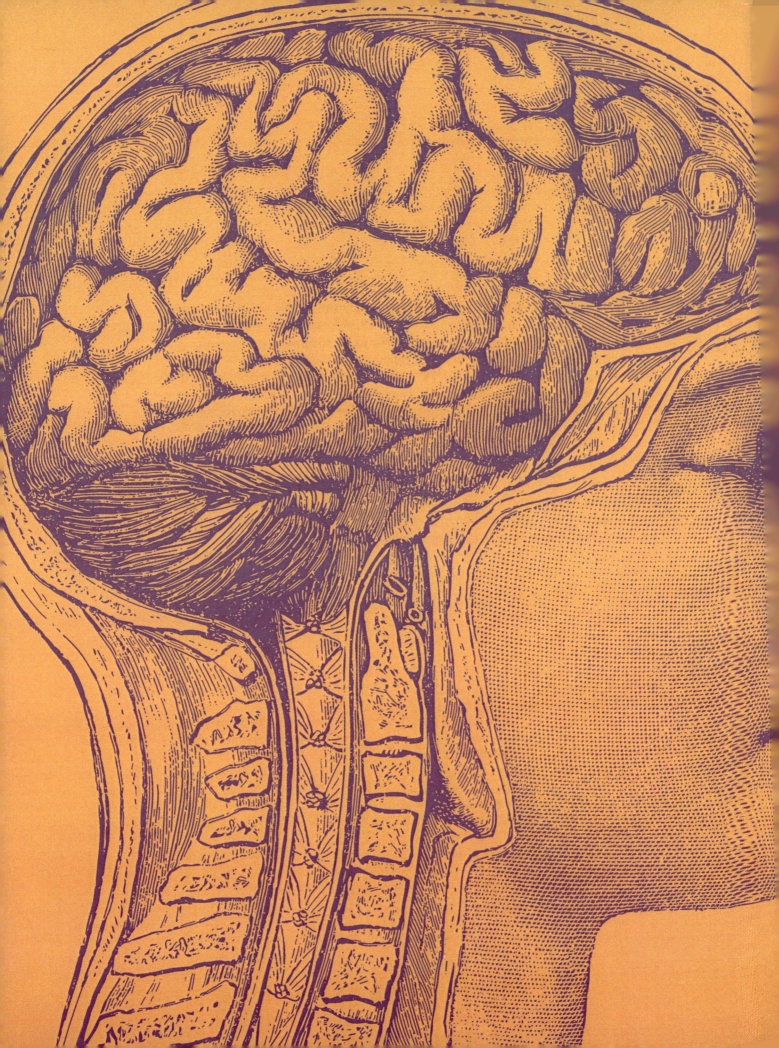

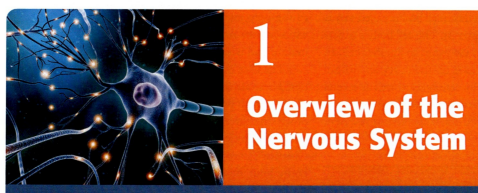

1
Overview of the Nervous System

CHAPTER OUTLINE

Overview
Major Components
Organization of the Nervous System
  Organizational Systems
    Cytoarchitecture Organization
    Organization by Function
Terminology
Nervous System Cells
  Neurons
  Glial Cells
Structures and Landmarks
  Lobes

  Frontal Lobes
  Parietal Lobes
  Temporal Lobes
  Occipital Lobes
  Subcortical Structures
    Basal Ganglia
    Thalamus
  Cerebellum
  Brainstem
Summary
References

Overview

Welcome to *Clinical Neuroscience for Communication Disorders*. We are excited to share foundations in neuroanatomy, physiology, and contemporary neuroscience, while making connections to the everyday practices of speech–language pathologists and audiologists. Throughout this textbook, you will find clinical cases and everyday applications that connect neuroanatomy and physiology to development (both typical and disrupted), aging (both typical and disrupted), and acquired neurological disorders.

The nervous system can be divided into structures and regions that are anatomically or functionally distinct. This chapter provides an overview of the major components and their functions as well as common terminology. Everything that is mentioned here will be discussed in more detail in later chapters of the book. You can think of this as a quick tour so you know your way around the nervous system to prepare you to dive in deeper.

Major Components

The human nervous system can be broken down into two major components: the central nervous system (CNS) and the peripheral nervous system (PNS). The **central nervous system** includes the brain and spinal cord. The word "brain" commonly is used to refer to a collection of several major structures: the right and left cerebra (cerebrum), otherwise known as the two hemispheres; the brainstem; and the cerebellum. All are encased within the **cranium** (Figure 1–1). At the point at which the brainstem exits the skull through the **foramen magnum**, the structure becomes the spinal cord. The spinal cord extends down through the spinal canal, the protective "tunnel" created by the stacked vertebrae.

A slice through the CNS—whether in the brain or spinal cord—will show dark and light areas, referred to as **gray matter** and **white matter**, respectively (Figure 1–2). The gray matter is made up of **cell bodies**. The white matter

2   Clinical Neuroscience for Communication Disorders: Neuroanatomy and Neurophysiology

is made up of extensions from those cell bodies called **axons** (discussed later; see also Chapter 3). The cell bodies generate signals that are sent down the axons to another cell. In the brain, the gray matter makes up the outer, superficial surface called the cortex (Latin: *tree bark*) as well as several collections of cell bodies (called **nuclei** or ganglia) deep in the brain. In the spinal cord, the arrangement is reversed, so the gray matter is deep (internal) and surrounded by white matter. As a general rule, gray matter processes information and white matter transmits signals.

The slice through the CNS also will reveal some cavities. These are the ventricles, filled with cerebrospinal fluid (CSF), which provides nutrients as well as protection. Two other structures that provide protection are the meninges and the bony encasing (Figure 1–3). The meninges (see Chapter 2) are a set of three tissue layers that cover the entire brain and spinal cord and provide a space for CSF to surround the CNS structures. The combination of the tissues and the fluid limits the movement of the brain and spinal cord. Superficial to the meninges is the bony structure. The cranium encases the brain, and the vertebral column surrounds and protects the spinal cord.

The PNS consists of all of the nerves that exit from the brainstem or spinal cord that extend out into the body (the periphery) to innervate muscles, organs, and tissues of the body (Figures 1–4 and 1–5). Twelve pairs of cranial nerves exit from the brainstem and innervate structures of the head and neck. An additional 31 pairs of spinal nerves exit from the spinal cord and innervate the structures below the neck.

The PNS can be further divided into functional subsystems. The somatic nervous system innervates skeletal muscles and is primarily responsible for conducting signals regarding body sensation and movement. The autonomic nervous system is responsible for unconscious control of body systems. It can be subdivided into the sympathetic

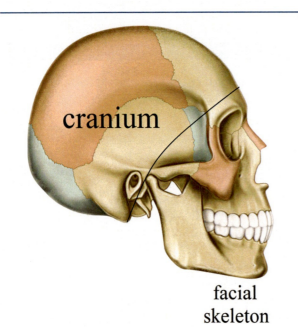

FIGURE 1–1. Cranium and facial skeleton.

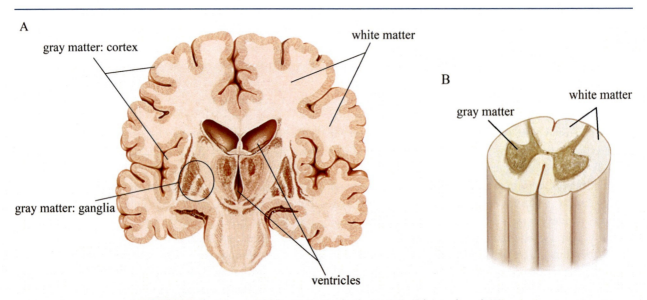

FIGURE 1–2. Gray and white matter in the brain (**A**) and spinal cord (**B**).

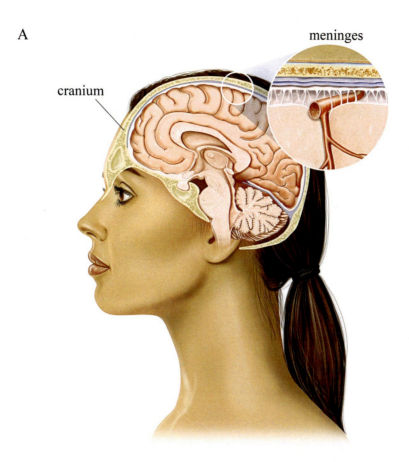
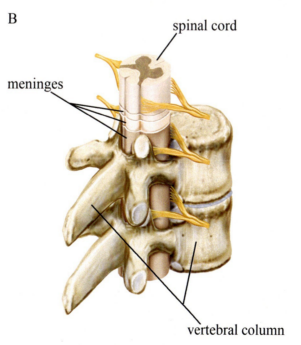

FIGURE 1–3. Meninges and bony casing for brain (**A**) and spinal cord (**B**).

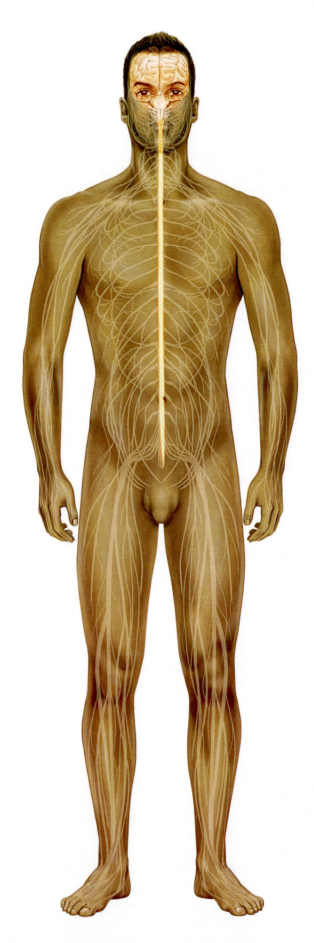

FIGURE 1-4. Peripheral nervous system. The central nervous system (brain and spinal cord) is highlighted. All nerves exiting from the brainstem and spinal cord make up the peripheral nervous system.

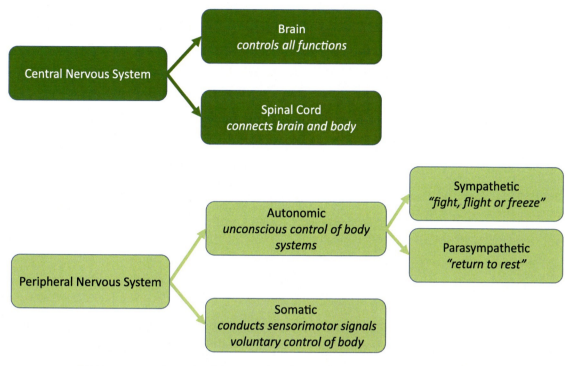

FIGURE 1–5. Schematic of the central and peripheral nervous system components.

and parasympathetic nervous systems. The sympathetic system prepares the body for "fight, flight, or freeze": When encountered with an emergency or crisis situation, the sympathetic nervous system will divert blood flow from unnecessary regions (e.g., the digestive system) to muscles and to the CNS to heighten perception, speed up response times, and facilitate muscle movements. The parasympathetic system returns the body to homeostasis (Greek: *same*, *steady*) or to baseline levels once the crisis has passed.

 Box 1–1. That's Not So Funny

When you "hit your funny bone," you actually are hitting a nerve of the PNS. The ulnar nerve extends from the spinal cord and travels along the arm out to the medial arm, including the pinky and ring fingers. When you hit your elbow just right, you compress the ulnar nerve, resulting in a painful tingling sensation. Because the PNS is not protected by a bony structure, the nerves can be impacted by everyday actions.

Unlike the CNS, the PNS is not protected by either a layer of tissue or a bony structure. The nerves exit from the spinal cord and extend out to the organs, tissues, and muscles of the body.

Organization of the Nervous System

The nervous system is organized in several different ways. Along the vertical (superior–inferior) axis, there are both structurally and functionally distinct sections. In addition, there are functional differences along the horizontal (right–left) axis.

There is a hierarchy of complexity along the vertical axis. Beginning from the bottom and moving superiorly, the spinal cord primarily serves as a conduit for signals and controls only the most basic functions—reflexes. The brainstem controls autonomic and visceral systems. These are of the utmost importance for keeping your body alive, such as by regulating heart rate and respiration, but they are not part of the "thinking brain." Integration of signals begins in the brainstem, such as integration of auditory signals from the left and right ear and integration of auditory and visual signals. The diencephalon extends superiorly from the brainstem and is involved in not only relaying signals coming up from the spinal cord but also integration of signals from multiple sources (see Chapter 5). Some cognitive processing occurs in the diencephalon, although this is not well understood. Finally, the cerebrum is responsible for complex sensory and motor integration, perception, and cognitive functions such as planning, organization, reasoning, language processing, and emotions (see Chapter 14).

Organizational Systems

The hemispheres of the brain have been subdivided in multiple ways. Broadly, they are divided into lobes (frontal, parietal, occipital, and temporal; Figure 1–6), each with a variety of functions, many of which (e.g., reading, social interacting) require input and integration from multiple lobes.

Cytoarchitecture Organization

The cortex (outer gray matter of the brain) is made up of six layers of cells. The thickness of these six layers varies across regions of the brain. Layers III (cortex-to-cortex connections) and IV (thalamus-to-cortex connections) are particularly important for signaling within the cerebrum (Blumenfeld, 2010; Shipp, 2007; Figure 1–7). In 1909, Korbinian Brodmann published a numbered map of the cortex based on the cellular organization (Figure 1–8). The

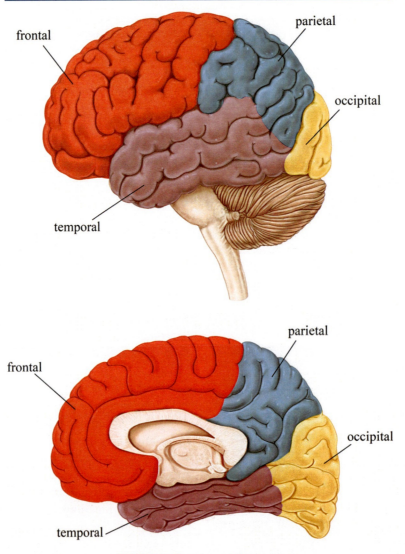

FIGURE 1–6. Lobes of the brain.

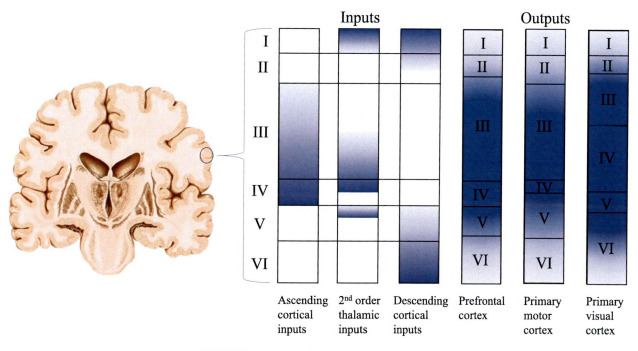

FIGURE 1–7. Cortical layers and connections.

implication of the map was that cellular organization was linked to function: Each numbered area had a different function. Although the map is not perfect, functional differences are related to cellular structures. Throughout this book, Brodmann areas are noted for areas commonly identified by the numbers.

Organization by Function

Another way to describe organization of the CNS is by function. CNS regions can be subdivided into those that control movement (motor) and body sensation (somatosensory), special senses such as visual and auditory functions, language, and higher level cognition. There are several principles that govern functional organization. First, throughout the CNS, motor areas tend to be located more anteriorly and sensory areas are located more posteriorly (see Chapter 4). Second, sensory and motor functions are controlled contralaterally. This means that the right side of the brain controls the left side of the body and vice versa. Third, the cortex contains **primary**, **secondary (association)**, and **tertiary (heteromodal)** areas. **Primary regions** are the core and initial location of processing. For example, in the auditory system, all input is processed initially in the primary auditory area in the superior temporal lobe. Further processing then occurs in **association areas** where there is integration of multiple aspects of signals (e.g., pitch and intensity and duration) as well as integration across modalities (e.g., linking visual with auditory signals to determine what object is creating a sound). The heteromodal areas are characterized by multimodal inputs and functions. The highest order areas of the brain are heteromodal, such as the prefrontal cortex.

Primary processing areas are precisely organized based on a relevant principle. The organizing principle for motor and sensory areas is **somatotopy**. This means that they are arranged in reference to the body (soma). As shown in Figure 1–9, regions of the body are controlled by different areas within the primary motor and sensory areas. The resulting map, shown in Figure 1–10, is called a homunculus (Latin: *little human*). As you can see, the representation is oddly distorted, with overly large areas for the hands, lips, and tongue. This means that there are more brain cells controlling these body areas. The reason for this is discussed in more detail in Chapters 6 and 10, but it is related to the level of fine motor control and sensitivity.

Within the auditory system, regions are organized **tonotopically**, or in relation to the pitch of a sound. Low-pitched sounds are processed more anteriorly and high-pitched sounds more posteriorly. For vision, the organizing

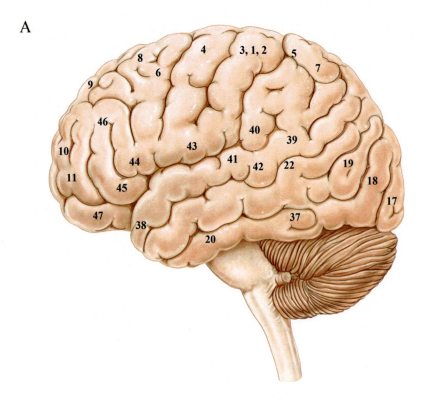

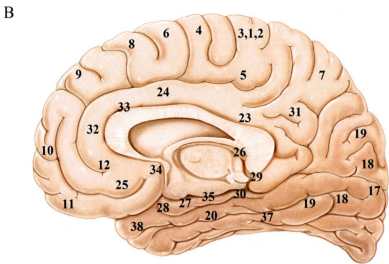

FIGURE 1–8. A. Brodmann areas shown on the lateral surface of the left hemisphere. **B.** Brodmann areas shown on the medial surface of the right hemisphere.

principle is location, called **retinotopy**. Neurons in the visual cortex are arranged based on where an image hits the retina.

Primary motor and sensory areas are relatively circumscribed, and the specific organizing principle can be mapped fairly directly onto the brain area. Thus, there are clear, reproducible maps of visual, auditory, and primary motor and somatosensory cortices. The more complex the processing, however, the less specific the maps become and the more variation there is across individuals. For example,

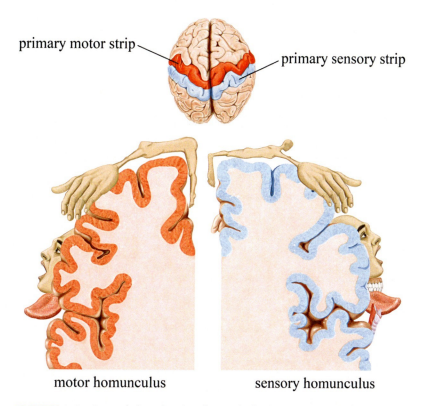

FIGURE 1–9. Coronal slice showing the cortical primary motor (*red*) and sensory (*blue*) strips.

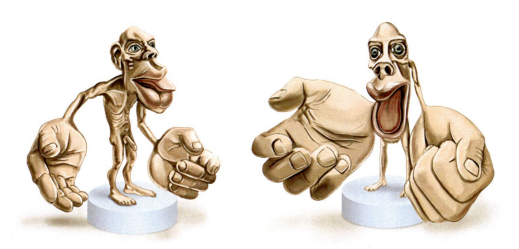

FIGURE 1–10. Sensory (*left*) and motor (*right*) homunculi.

the majority of basic language processing occurs in the left hemisphere, but it is distributed through frontal, parietal, and temporal lobes. Generally speaking, comprehension occurs more posteriorly (parietal/temporal regions) and production is controlled anteriorly (frontal lobe), but there are many connections between the areas. In addition, connections to the right hemisphere are needed to go beyond basic word and sentence-level comprehension, to understand communication that includes facial expressions, gestures, and tone of voice. Higher level cognition, such as reasoning, judgment, and insight, is controlled by the frontal lobes bilaterally, which have extensive connections to many other areas of the brain. Thus, the more complex the task, the less likely it is that there is a single area of the brain with primary control, and the more interconnectivity is needed for adequate function.

Gross organization is very similar across people, such that the functions of the lobes described previously hold for all humans without significant disruption to neural development. The organization of the motor and sensory homunculi is also consistent from person to person. Delving deeper, though, differences can occur. As explained in Chapter 10, fine motor movement practice will lead to increased space allotted to control those movements. Thus, concert pianists will have larger representations of the hand and fingers compared to an Olympic runner, who does not spend hours a day carrying out fine movements of the hands.

Terminology

Anatomical terminology is essential for establishing a common frame of reference. Learning neuroanatomy will be much easier if you have a solid understanding of a basic vocabulary. This terminology will be used to clearly indicate location and prevent misunderstandings (e.g., your left or my left?).

The terminology is used in reference to a human body in anatomical position (Figure 1–11): standing upright,

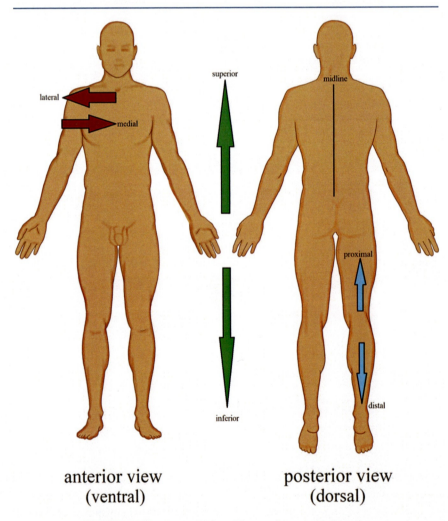

FIGURE 1–11. Anatomical position and terms of direction.

viewed from the front, with the palms facing the front. Definitions are provided in Box 1–2, and exercises are provided in the supplementary material to give you a chance to practice until you feel completely comfortable with the terms. The following terms deserve a little extra explanation to ensure clear understanding (Table 1–1):

Box 1–2. Additional Neuroanatomical Terminology

- **Gray matter:** Central nervous system tissue made up of cell bodies; appears dark in dissections
- **White matter:** Central nervous system tissue made up of axons; appears light in dissections due to the white, fatty covering called myelin that surrounds axons
- **Gyrus** (Latin: *ring*; pl. gyri): A hill or ridge; also called a convolution
- **Sulcus** (Latin: *furrow, wrinkle*; pl. sluci): A valley or enfolding
- **Fissure:** A valley or enfolding; usually deeper than a sulcus (but not always)
- **Cortex:** The outer layer of gray matter in the cerebral hemispheres
- **Nucleus** (pl. nuclei): A group of cell bodies—usually used to refer to structures in the central nervous system
- **Ganglion** (Greek: *tumor on a tendon* or *tissue that resembled such tumor*; pl. ganglia): A group of cell bodies—usually used to refer to structures in the peripheral nervous system
- **Fasciculus** (Latin: *little bundle*)/funiculus (Latin: *little rope*)/tract: A group of axons
- **Commissure** (Latin: *juncture*): Band of fibers/axons connecting the two sides of the nervous system
- **Projection tract:** Groups of axons that begin in the brain and extend out of the brain (i.e., to the spinal cord)
- **Association tract:** Groups of axons that lie within a hemisphere. These connect one lobe to another or one gyrus to another within a lobe.
- **Commissural tract:** Groups of axons that extend from one hemisphere to the other

Table 1–1. Terms of Position and Orientation

Superior: toward the top	**Inferior:** toward the bottom
Superficial: toward the surface	**Deep:** away from the surface
External: toward the surface	**Internal:** away from the surface
Medial: toward the midline (mesial, median)	**Lateral:** away from the midline; toward the side
Proximal: toward the point of attachment	**Distal:** away from the point of attachment
Dorsal (brain): top of head (superior) **Dorsal (body):** toward the backbone from the neck down (posterior)	**Ventral (brain):** bottom of head (inferior) **Ventral (body):** toward the belly from the neck down (anterior)
Rostral: toward the nose	**Caudal:** toward the tail
Central: toward the center	**Peripheral:** away from the center
Afferent: conducting inward or toward the central nervous system; sensory	**Efferent:** conducting outward or away from the central nervous system; motor
Ipsi-: same (ipsilateral = same side)	**Contra-:** opposite (contralateral = opposite side)

12 Clinical Neuroscience for Communication Disorders: Neuroanatomy and Neurophysiology

- Anterior: toward the front of the body
- Posterior: toward the back or rear of the body
- Ventral: toward the belly
- Dorsal: toward the backbone

In quadrupedal animals (think dogs, cats, elephants, etc.), these four terms have four different meanings. Anterior is toward the head, posterior is toward the tail, ventral is toward the underside/belly, and dorsal is toward the top/backbone. In humans, from the neck down, anterior and ventral can be used interchangeably because the belly is toward the front of the body. The same holds for posterior and dorsal, which both refer to the back of the body. When it comes to the head, the axis of reference shifts along with the curve of the CNS (from the front of the brain to the brainstem), and the terms mirror those used for quadrupeds. Thus, anterior means toward the front of the head (face); posterior is toward the back of the head; but dorsal refers to the top of the head/brain, and ventral refers to the bottom. In the brain, dorsal can be used interchangeably with superior, and ventral can be used interchangeably with inferior (Figure 1–12).

Another set of terminology refers to planes of section, or slices through the body (Figure 1–13). Slices also let you see deep structures.

A sagittal slice divides the body into right and left portions. A midsagittal slice goes through the midline of the body, creating equal right and left sections. All other sagittal slices are parallel to the midline. A frontal or coronal slice creates front and back sections. Horizontal slices, as the name suggests, are aligned horizontally, creating top and bottom sections. A transverse section cuts across the vertical axis. In the brain, horizontal and transverse sections are the same thing. But the brainstem sits at an angle, sloping posteriorly down to the spinal cord. Transverse slices cut the brainstem perpendicular to the structure itself (Figure 1–14).

Nervous System Cells

The nervous system is made up of two categories of cells: **neurons** and **glial cells.** Neurons are the specialized brain cells that send signals to create all of our experiences. Glial cells are support cells that provide structure, protection, and waste management. Approximately 90% of the cells in the nervous system are glial cells. One of my early neuroscience textbooks described the nervous system as a chocolate chip cookie: The neurons are the chocolate chips, and the glial cells are the dough that supports them.

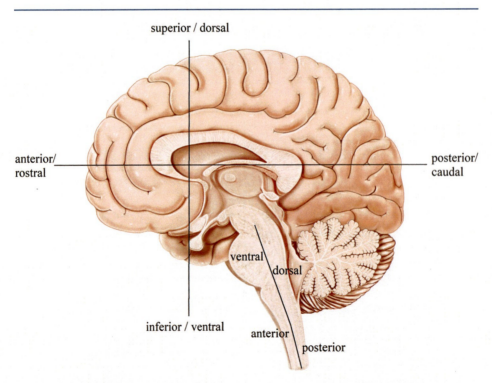

FIGURE 1–12. Anatomical terminology for the brain and brainstem.

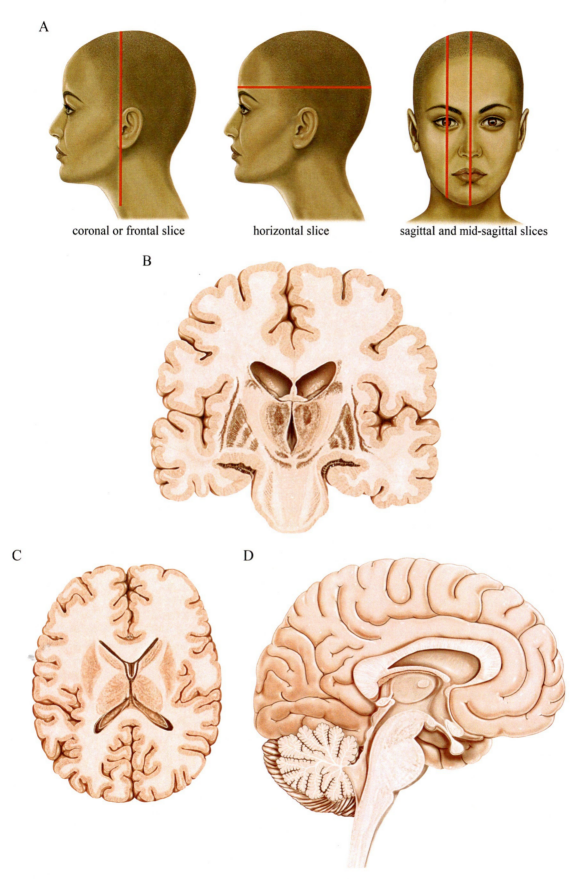

FIGURE 1–13. A. Planes of section shown on the head. **B.** Coronal (frontal) slice of the brain. **C.** Horizontal slice of the brain. **D.** Midsagittal slice of the brain showing the medial surface of the left hemisphere.

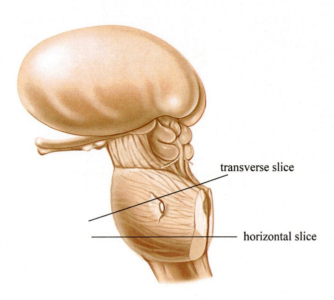

FIGURE 1–14. Horizontal and transverse slices of the brainstem.

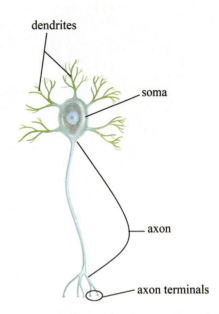

FIGURE 1–15. Components of a stereotypical neuron.

Neurons

Neurons have distinct regions with distinct functions (Figure 1–15). The cell body, or **soma**, contains the nucleus and the organelles. As with other cells in the body, the nucleus contains DNA. The various organelles do the work needed to keep the cells alive and to power their functions, such as synthesizing proteins, generating energy, and disposing of waste products.

Extending out from the soma are **dendrites**. Some types of neurons have a single dendrite that extends from the soma which then splits into multiple branches. Other types of neurons have many dendrites extending out from the soma. The dendrites are the "receivers" of the neuron and are designed with special receptor sites that receive chemical signals from other neurons or are specialized to respond to sensory inputs (e.g., taste, touch, temperature, sound, light). Some dendrites are spiny, covered with multiple enlarged regions that serve as receptor sites.

Neurons also have an **axon** extending out from the soma. The axon carries an electrical signal away from the soma to the distal axon terminal, where the signal is conveyed to a receiving neuron or structure (e.g., muscle, gland, organ). Each neuron has only a single axon extending out from the soma at a region called the **axon hillock**. Axons can have branches called axon collaterals. The axon is not simply an empty tube but, rather, contains a complex array of structures designed to provide a structural framework and to aid in the function of the neuron. These structures include microtubules, microfilaments, and neurofilaments. They facilitate movement of proteins and chemicals to and from the soma. Damage to the microtubules, primarily related to dysfunction of a tau protein, has been implicated in Alzheimer disease.

The distal end of an axon is called the **axon terminal** [also known as the synaptic knob or terminal bouton (French: *button*)]. Arborization, or extensive branches near the terminals, can occur, creating many terminal boutons and allowing a single neuron to synapse with up to 1,000 other neurons. The axon terminal is one component of a **synapse**, the point of communication between neurons. This is discussed in more detail later in this chapter.

The cell membrane of a neuron, like all other human cell membranes, is made up of a variety of cells, channels, proteins, and molecules (Figure 1–16). Just a few of them are described here:

- Ion channels allow ions (charged particles) to move in and out of the neuron. These channels can be opened, closed, and inactivated. Most channels are ion specific, such that sodium ions can only pass through sodium channels, and potassium ions can only pass through potassium channels. When ion channels are open, ions can freely move through the membrane. Ions will always passively move from areas of higher concentration to areas of lower concentration (along the concentration gradient) if not restricted by selective gating.

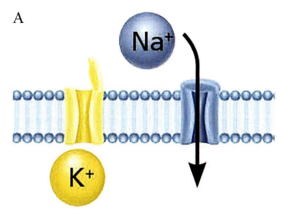
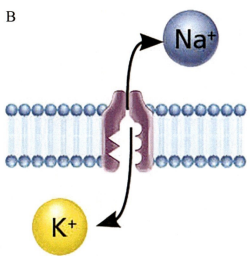

- Ion pumps are energy-using systems that will move ions across the cell membrane. Pumps are required to move ions from areas of lower concentration to areas of higher concentration (against the concentration gradient).
- Neurotransmitter receptors are places where neurotransmitters (brain chemicals) can bind, causing a change to nearby ion channels. Such receptors are most commonly found along the dendrites, but they are also found along the soma and the proximal and distal portions of the axon.

Within the CNS, the soma and dendrites create the gray matter, and axons create white matter. The color difference is based on the whitish, fatty substance called myelin that covers axons of larger neurons (Figure 1–17). Myelination speeds up the transmission of electrical signals down an axon. In unmyelinated axons, signals travel up to 10 m/sec, whereas myelination increases those speeds up to 120 m/sec. Myelination is not a solid covering of tissue around an axon but, rather, a series of internodes with tiny gaps in between in which the axon is exposed to the extracellular environment. These gaps, called **nodes of Ranvier**, are a critical architectural component for transmission of electrical signals in an axon (see Chapter 3).

Glial Cells

FIGURE 1–16. **A.** Neuron membrane with ion channels. **B.** Neuron membrane with ion pump.

Approximately 90% of the cells in the nervous system are glial cells (Latin: *glue*; plural: glia). These cells provide struc-

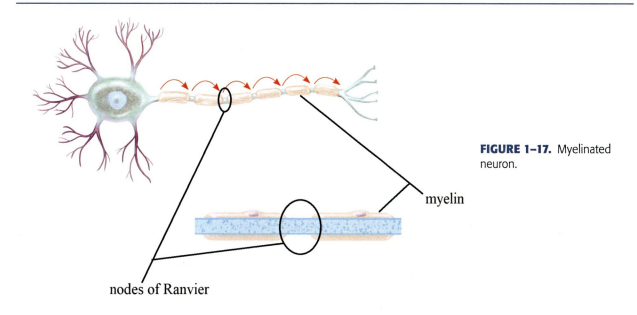

FIGURE 1–17. Myelinated neuron.

ture and protection for the nervous system. There are various types of glial cells with specific functions (Figure 1–18).

Microglia are tiny cells that act as immune cells within the CNS. They migrate to sites of damage and serve as macrophages that eat away, or clean up, dead and damaged tissues.

Ependymal cells are columnar (column-shaped) ciliated (with hairs) cells that form linings. They form the inside of the ventricles and the spinal canal, keeping the CSF from leaking into the tissue of the brain and spinal cord. The cilia assist in moving the CSF through the ventricular system.

Astrocytes make up the majority of glial cells. There are several types of astrocytes, each with different functions. Some, but not all, are star-shaped (hence the name astrocyte). Some serve as pathways during development

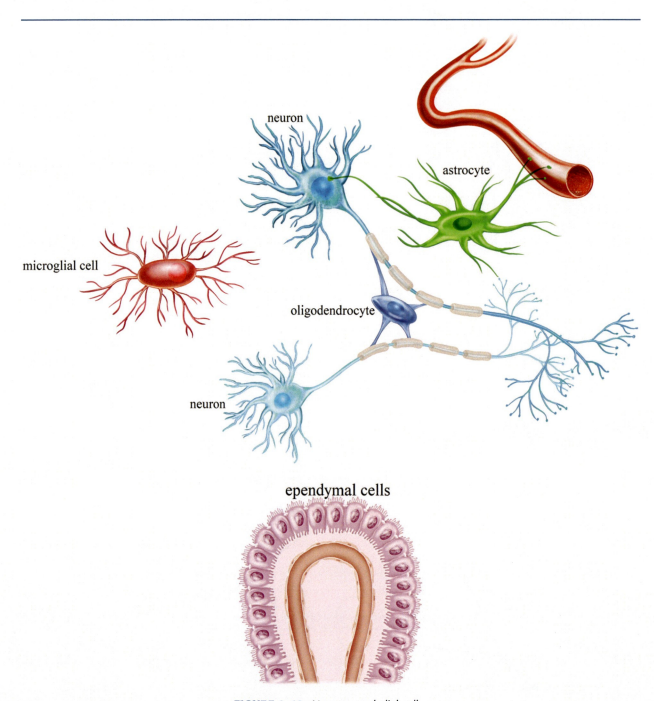

FIGURE 1–18. Neurons and glial cells.

to guide neuron migration. Others provide connections between blood vessels and neurons as part of the blood–brain barrier. In this role, they are the "bouncers" of the CNS, allowing some substances to pass from the bloodstream into the nervous system while blocking others. Astrocytes also control extracellular concentrations of potassium as well as certain neurotransmitters (glutamate and γ-aminobutyric acid).

Schwann cells (named after neurologist Theodor Schwann, who described them in the mid-1800s) produce myelin in the PNS (Figure 1–19). Each Schwann cell creates a single node of myelin. As it develops, it surrounds an axon segment and then spirals around the axon, creating multiple layers (Morell & Quarles, 1999).

Oligodendrocytes (Greek: *oligo–few*, *dendro–tree*, *cyte–cell*: *cell with few branches*) produce myelin within the CNS (Figure 1–20). Unlike the Schwann cells, each oligodendrocyte produces multiple nodes of myelin on multiple

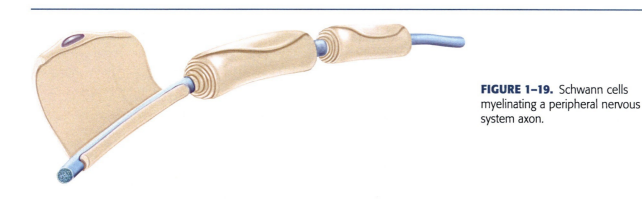

FIGURE 1–19. Schwann cells myelinating a peripheral nervous system axon.

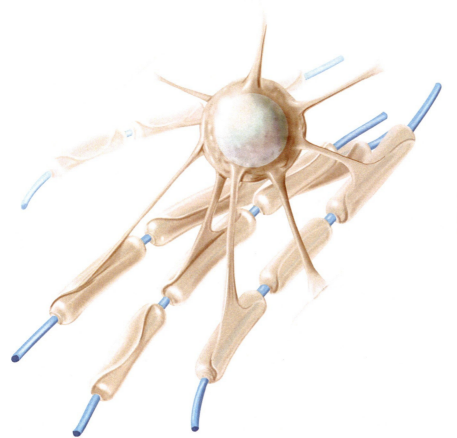

FIGURE 1–20. Oligodendrocyte myelinating central nervous system axons.

axons. The oligodendrocyte can be likened to an octopus with a single head (cell body) and multiple arms (cellular processes) that extend out to different axons and spiral around them to create nodes of myelin.

Structures and Landmarks

Each hemisphere is divided into four or five major lobes: frontal, parietal, occipital, temporal, and insula (insular lobe). All are paired structures with one in the right hemisphere and the other in the left. The lobes (all except the insula) share names with their adjacent cranial bones. Landmarks and general functions are discussed here. More details about specific regions will be covered in the relevant chapters based on their functions.

There are several distinct sulci and gyri that are consistent across all human brains that serve as landmarks or as borders between regions. From a superior view, the sagittal sulcus (also known as the longitudinal fissure) separates the right and left hemispheres (Figure 1–21). On the lateral surface (Figure 1–22) is the sylvian fissure (also known as the lateral sulcus), which divides the temporal lobe inferiorly from the frontal and parietal lobes superiorly. Deep in the sylvian fissure is the insula (Figure 1–23). The central sulcus (also known as the sulcus of Rolando) extends vertically from the sagittal sulcus down to the sylvian fissure. This sulcus is a clear, continuous groove on some brains, but on others it can be more difficult to identify. Pre- and postcentral gyri and sulci bookend the central gyrus.

On the medial surface, several important structures and landmarks are visible, including the cingulate gyrus,

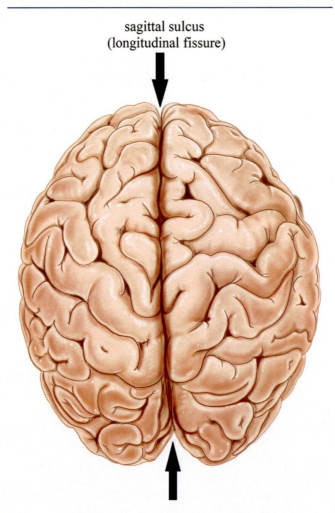

FIGURE 1–21. Superior view of the cerebra.

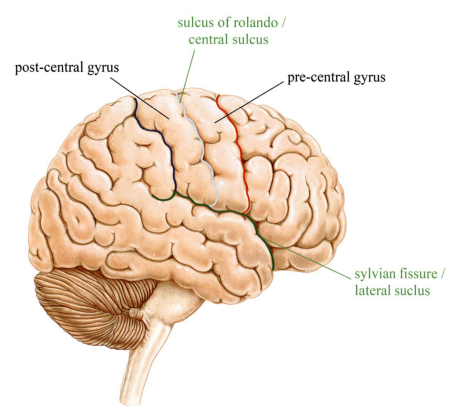

FIGURE 1–22. Landmarks on the lateral surface of the right hemisphere. Fissures/sulci are labeled in green; gyri are labeled in black.

corpus callosum, septum pellucidum, thalamus, and the calcarine sulcus in the occipital lobe (Figure 1–24). The cingulate gyrus, part of the limbic system, is important for emotions, motivation, and drive. Immediately inferior to that is the corpus callosum, a massive band of commissural axons that connect the right and left hemispheres. It appears light because of the myelination of the axons.

Inferior to that is a sickle-shaped piece of tissue called the septum pellucidum. This tissue separates two cavities in the brain: the left and right lateral ventricles. Inferior to that is the thalamus. As described later, the thalamus is a deep structure that has connections to most all other regions of the nervous system.

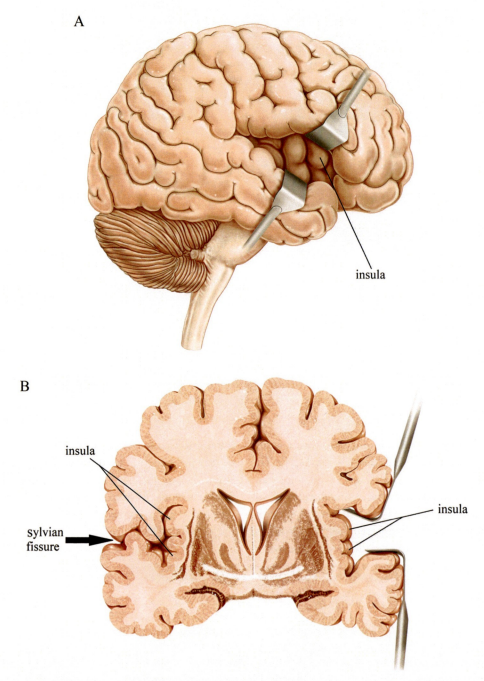

FIGURE 1–23. A. Lateral view of the insula deep to the sylvian fissure of the right hemisphere. **B.** Coronal slice showing insula deep to the sylvian fissure.

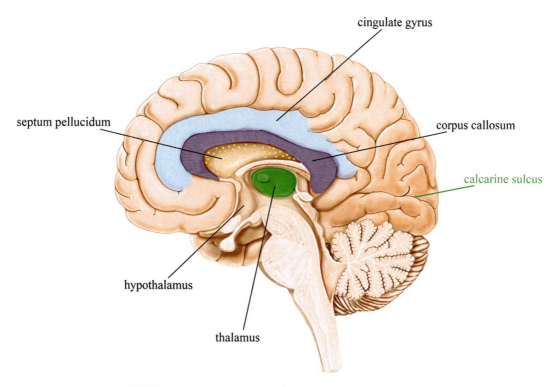

FIGURE 1–24. Landmarks on the medial surface of the brain.

Lobes

Frontal Lobes

The frontal lobes are the most anterior structures in the brain. They extend from the frontal pole posteriorly to the central sulcus. The frontal lobe is divided functionally into three regions. The anterior region is called the prefrontal area and is important for higher level cognition, including reasoning, planning, problem-solving, and working memory. These are often referred to as executive functions (see Chapter 14). The prefrontal cortex can be subdivided into dorsal and ventral sections on both lateral and medial surfaces: dorsolateral prefrontal, dorsomedial prefrontal, ventrolateral prefrontal, and ventromedial prefrontal cortices. The orbitofrontal region is the most inferior segment of the prefrontal region (Figure 1–25).

The posterior frontal region contains the motor cortices (Figure 1–26). From anterior to posterior, these include the supplementary motor areas, premotor area, and the primary motor area. The primary motor strip is housed within the precentral gyrus, the gyrus immediately anterior to the central sulcus. Finally, the posterior portion of the inferior frontal gyrus in the left hemisphere is critical for basic language expression. This region is called the frontal operculum and is further segmented into the pars orbitalis, pars triangularis, and pars opercularis.

Parietal Lobes

The parietal lobes are immediately posterior to the frontal lobes, divided by the central sulcus. The anterior-most portion is the postcentral gyrus, which houses the somatosensory map and is referred to as S1 (primary sensory area). The parietal lobes can roughly be divided into superior and inferior portions by the intraparietal sulcus (Figure 1–27). This sulcus is not always distinct.

The parietal lobes are important for sensory processing but also for your awareness of your own body (whether you are tall or short, thin or heavy, coordinated or clumsy) and movement of your body within space. They also are important for attentional processing.

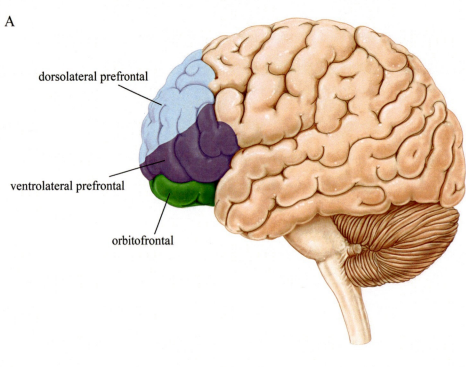

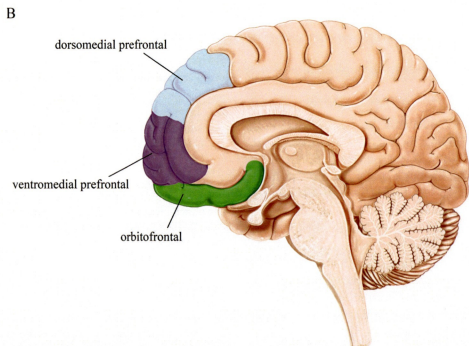

FIGURE 1–25. A. Lateral view of prefrontal lobe regions shown on the left hemisphere. **B.** Medial view of prefrontal lobe regions shown on the right hemisphere.

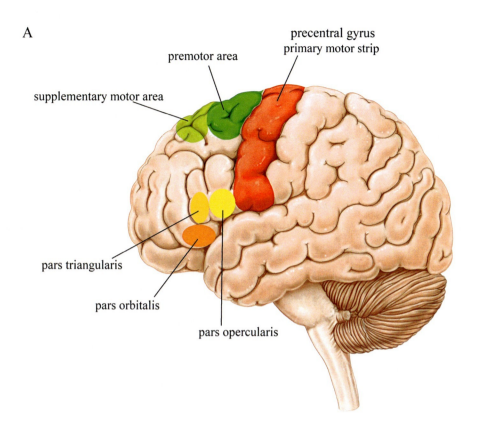

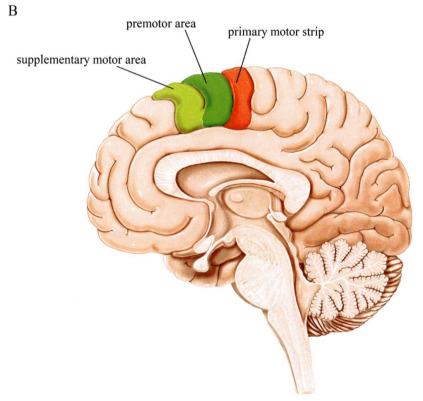

FIGURE 1–26. A. Lateral view of frontal lobe motor and language areas shown on the left hemisphere. **B.** Medial view of frontal lobe motor areas shown on the right hemisphere.

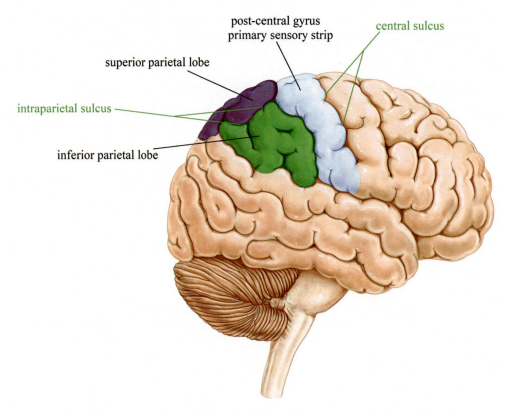

FIGURE 1–27. Regions of the parietal lobes shown on the right hemisphere.

Temporal Lobes

The temporal lobes lie inferior to the frontal and parietal lobes, separated by the distinctive lateral sulcus (sylvian fissure). The anterior-most point of the temporal lobes is called the temporal pole. The temporal lobes are roughly divided into three horizontal gyri: superior, middle, and inferior (Figure 1–28). The dorsal surface of the superior temporal gyrus lies in the sylvian fissure. The anterior portion is known as either the transverse temporal gyrus or Heschl gyrus, whereas the posterior segment is called the planum temporale. The transverse gyrus is the primary auditory processing area. The planum temporale tends to be larger in the left than the right hemisphere, suggesting that it is involved with basic language processes (see Chapter 14). The posterior superior temporal lobe on the lateral surface of the left hemisphere is known as Wernicke's area and is involved with language comprehension.

The inferior temporal gyrus can be seen on the lateral surface, but the bulk of it is on the inferior surface. Continuing medially on the inferior surface are the occipitotemporal gyrus (also called the fusiform gyrus), the parahippocampal gyrus, and the uncus. The fusiform gyrus is important for visual processing, particularly for faces.

Deep to the parahippocampal gyrus in the medial region of the temporal lobe is the hippocampus (Latin: *seahorse*), named for its squiggly appearance. This is the primary site of memory, where short-term memories are converted to long-term memory.

In the temporo-parieto-occipital area, where the three lobes come into contact posterior to the sylvian fissure, are two association areas: the angular gyrus and the supramarginal gyrus. In the left hemisphere, these regions integrate signals from the language areas of the temporal lobe with visual signals from the occipital lobe to aid in visual language, namely reading and writing.

Occipital Lobes

The occipital lobes form the posterior section of the cerebral hemispheres. There is no clear demarcation between the parietal/temporal and occipital lobes on the lateral surface.

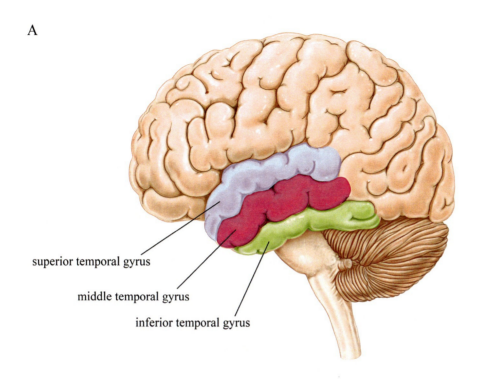
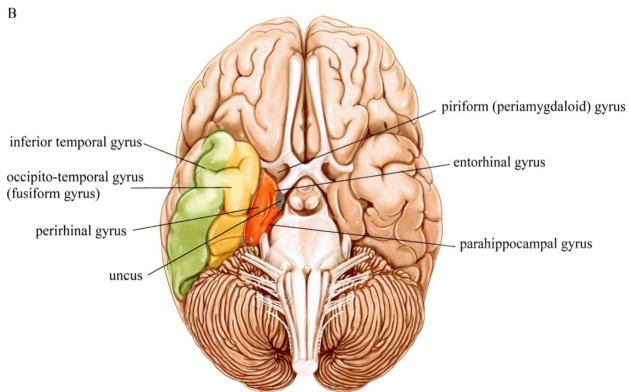

FIGURE 1–28. Temporal lobe structures on the lateral (**A**) and inferior (**B**) surfaces shown on the left hemisphere.

On the medial surface, the parieto-occipital sulcus divides those two lobes (Figure 1–29). Inferior to that is the roughly horizontal calcarine sulcus, which divides the occipital lobe into superior and inferior sections. Primary visual processing occurs in the occipital poles and around the calcarine sulcus.

Subcortical Structures

Basal Ganglia

The **basal ganglia** are a group of structures located deep within the cerebral hemispheres (Figures 1–30 and 1–31). Remember that the word ganglion (plural: ganglia) refers to a group of cell bodies. All of the structures within the basal ganglia thus are groups of cell bodies and will appear dark in comparison to the surrounding white matter in a brain slice. The major structures of the basal ganglia include the **caudate nucleus**, **putamen**, and **globus pallidus**. The **substantia nigra** and **subthalamic nuclei** are other structures commonly included in the definitions of the basal ganglia. All of these structures are bilateral, meaning that there is one each in the left and right hemispheres.

The caudate nucleus is a C-shaped structure that lies alongside the lateral ventricles. The head of the caudate lies deep in the frontal lobe, the body extends through the parietal lobe, and the tail extends into the temporal lobe. The putamen is egg-shaped and appears to lie within the curve of the caudate nucleus, inferior to the body of the caudate. Deep to the putamen is the globus pallidus. It is subdivided into the external and internal sections. On a frontal or coronal slice of the brain, the putamen and globus pallidus look a bit like a tipped-over candy corn, with a thin line of white matter between the putamen and globus pallidus external, and another thin line separating the external from the internal globus pallidus. The subthalamic nuclei and substantia nigra are in the superior-most extent of the brainstem.

The primary function of the basal ganglia is motor control. It has extensive connections to other motor regions of the brain (e.g., the precentral gyrus and other frontal lobe motor areas), the cerebellum, and brainstem. It also receives signals from the sensory regions of the CNS because motor and sensory functions are inextricably tied together. When you move, you sense where you are moving. In order to program goal-directed movements such as shooting a basketball, you have to know how far away and how high the basket is, the size and weight of the ball, how tall you are, and where your arms and hands are (are you holding the ball down low? Up high?) so your motor system can plan the direction of the movement.

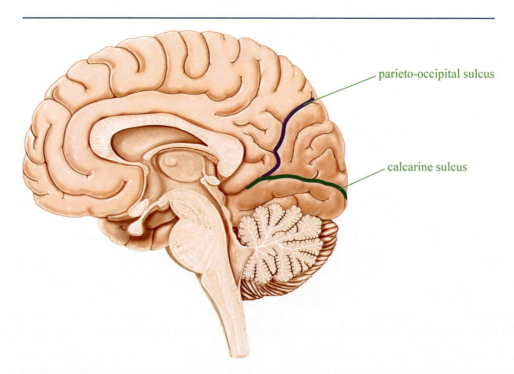

FIGURE 1–29. Occipital lobe landmarks on the medial surface shown on the right hemisphere.

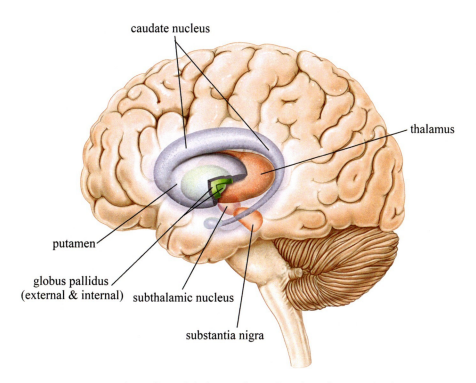

FIGURE 1–30. Basal ganglia and thalamus shown from lateral view of left hemisphere.

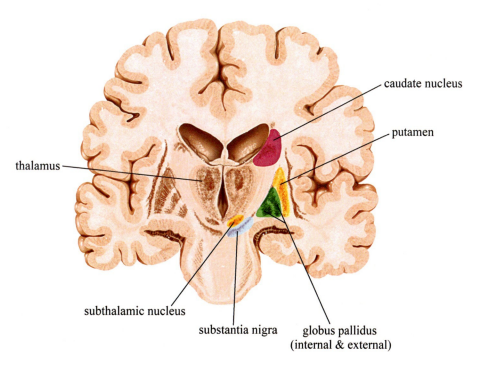

FIGURE 1–31. Subcortical structures in a coronal slice.

Thalamus

The **thalamus** is deep to the internal globus pallidus; the right and left thalami lie on either side of the midline (see Figures 1–30 and 1–31). The thalami are connected to nearly all other regions of the CNS: all lobes, the basal ganglia, cerebellum, brainstem, and spinal cord. All sensory signals with the exception of olfaction (smell) synapse in the thalamus before reaching the cortex. Thalamic connections with the basal ganglia and cerebellum influence the motor system. Areas of the brainstem responsible for cortical arousal are connected to the thalamus, along with other structures that control sleep–wake cycles, hunger/thirst responses, and hormonal systems.

Cerebellum

The **cerebellum** (Latin: *little cerebrum*) is located inferior to the occipital lobe and posterior to the brainstem. As the name suggests, it looks a bit like a little cerebrum, complete with sulci and gyri, although they are much thinner and more numerous than in the cerebrum and are called **folia** (Figure 1–32). The tightly packed shape is necessary to accommodate the large number of neurons. Indeed, the cerebellum makes up only 10% of the total brain volume yet contains approximately 50% of the neurons. The cerebellum has both right and left hemispheres with the vermis spanning the region between them. Each hemisphere can be divided into three lobes: anterior, posterior, and flocculonodular lobes. A slice of the cerebellum shows both gray and white matter, again like the cerebrum, with the gray matter located externally and the white matter situated deep within the structure. Three pairs of deep nuclei are embedded in the white matter (similar to the basal ganglia in the cerebrum). The cerebellum is attached to the brainstem by three **peduncles** (Latin: *foot*; common usage = *stalk*)—superior, middle, and inferior—made up of axon bundles carrying signals to and from the cerebellum.

Brainstem

The brainstem is aptly named because it really looks like the stem upon which the brain grew out of. It is subdivided into three segments (Figure 1–33). The most superior region is the **midbrain**. In an inferior view of the brain, it is situated right in the middle of the hemispheres, so again the name makes sense. The ventral (anterior) portion is called the tegmentum, and the dorsal (posterior) region is the tectum. Next is the **pons**, which bulges out anteriorly and is distinctive for its horizontal stripes. Posteriorly, the pons extends into the cerebellum through cerebellar peduncles, which are massive groups of axons sending signals to and from the cerebellum. Inferior to the pons is the **medulla oblongata** (or simply medulla). The medulla becomes the spinal cord when it exits the cranium through the foramen magnum (the large hole in the base of the occipital bone

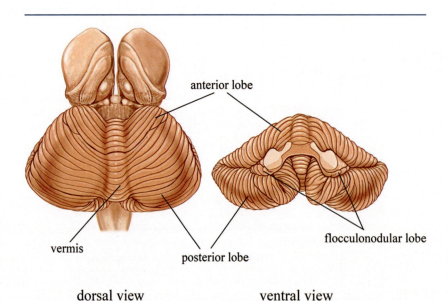

FIGURE 1–32. Posterior and anterior views of the cerebellum.

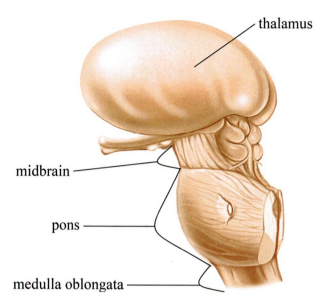

FIGURE 1–33. Lateral view of brainstem with cerebellum removed.

of the cranium). Thus, the brainstem is housed within the cranium, and the point at which it exits the cranium, the structure becomes known as the spinal cord.

Summary

The human nervous system has two main components, the CNS and the PNS. It is composed of neurons (communicating cells) and glial cells (supporting structures). The brain and spinal cord include gray and white matter (cell bodies and axons, respectively) that process and transmit information throughout the nervous system. The cerebrum can be divided into hemispheres (right and left) and lobes (frontal, parietal, temporal, and occipital). The lobes can be further divided into functional regions, often separated by sulci and gyri. Subcortical structures such as the basal ganglia and the thalamus as well as the cerebellum have crucial roles in sensory and motor systems, cognition, and communication. Finally, the brainstem carries out autonomic, life-sustaining functions, as well as housing cranial nerves crucial to speech and swallowing.

Key Concepts

- The nervous system has a systematic and function-oriented organization, which allows communication between structures to carry out complex motor and communication processes.
- The two sides of the brain are similar but not mirror images. Sensory and motor functions are represented in both hemispheres, but communication and cognition processes differ.
- Understanding the anatomy and functions of these structures and systems is foundational to understanding speech, language, swallowing, and cognitive functions for developmental, acquired neurological, and aging processes.

References

Blumenfeld, H. (2010). *Neuroanatomy through clinical cases* (2nd ed.). Sinauer.

Morell, P., & Quarles, R. H. (1999). The myelin sheath. In G. J. Siegel, B. W. Agranoff, R. W. Albers, et al. (Eds.), *Basic neurochemistry: Molecular, cellular and medical aspects* (6th ed.). Lippincott Williams & Wilkins.

Shipp, S. (2007). Structure and function of the cerebral cortex. *Current Biology, 17*(12), R443–R449.

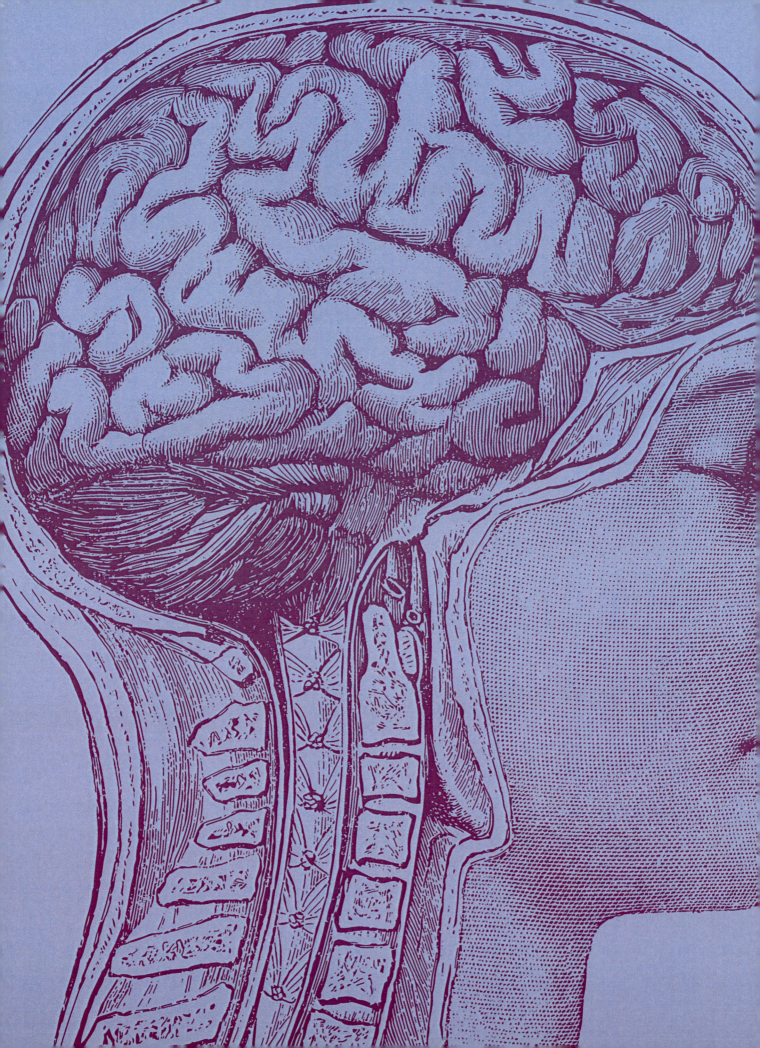

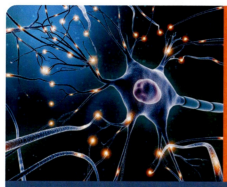

2
Ventricular System: Cranium, Ventricles, and Meninges

CHAPTER OUTLINE

Overview
Cranium, Cranial Vault, and Its Contents
Meningeal Layers
   Dura Mater
   Arachnoid Layer and Pia Mater
Ventricles
   Cerebrospinal Fluid Path and Functions
   Communication Through the
     Ventricular System

Disruptions to the Ventricular
   and Meningeal Systems
   Hydrocephalus
   Meningeal Damage
Summary
Additional Resources

Overview

The central nervous system (CNS) has multiple layers of protection. These include the boney casing of the cranium and vertebrae, a triple layer of tissues to restrict movement of the brain within the cranium, a fluid buffer that also restricts movement and transports nutrients and hormones, and a system of cavities and canals deep in the CNS where fluid is produced and circulated.

The connection between clinical practice and the inner environment of the cranium, ventricular system, meninges, and cerebral spinal fluid (CSF) may not be immediately apparent to speech–language pathologists, audiologists, and related professionals. Yet, these systems have relevance to clinical practice on several fronts, including protective functions, communication within the nervous system, and what happens when these systems are disrupted (e.g., hydrocephalus, meningitis, trauma). This chapter addresses the anatomy (including the practical purpose of anatomy in normal physiological conditions), physiology, and relevant clinical applications.

Cranium, Cranial Vault, and Its Contents

It is likely that you have learned previously about the external portions of the skull, particularly as they are relevant points of attachment for muscles of facial expression and mastication. You may have also discussed the relationship of inner cranium structures to speech and hearing mechanisms such as the petrous portion of the temporal bone or superior wings of the sphenoid bone. This chapter extends that knowledge to include the concept of the inner cranium as an environment for the cerebrum and surrounding ventricular–CSF systems.

On the inferior (ventral) surface of the cranium, you can clearly see foramen (larger holes) and foramina (smaller holes) where nerves or blood vessels enter and exit the skull (Figure 2–1). The largest of those foramina, the **foramen magnum** (Latin: *great hole*), houses the transition between the medullary brainstem and the cervical spinal cord. This is referred to as the **cervicomedullary junction** (Figure 2–2) and marks the transition from medullary brainstem to

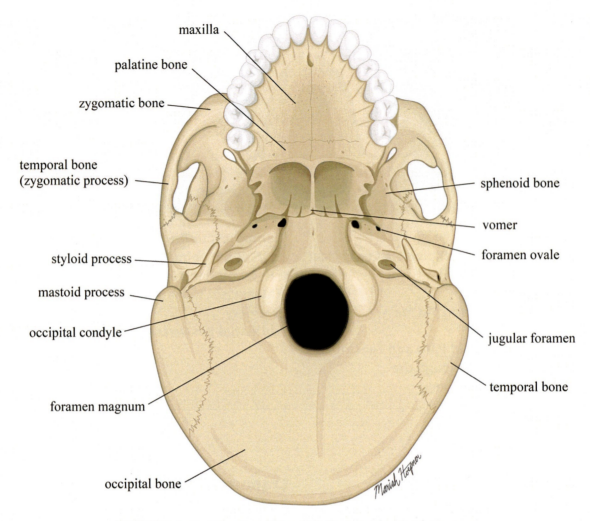

FIGURE 2–1. Ventral surface of the skull. Illustration by Mariah Hoepner.

cervical spine. This landmark has relevance to motor and sensory pathways, some of which **decussate** (cross over) near this landmark. In normal physiology, the caudal medulla should not pass below this level. However, sometimes swelling forces it to shift below the foramen magnum, called herniation, which represents a serious concern. Herniation typically occurs as a consequence of increased **intracranial pressure** but can occur due to low CSF volume/pressure as well. Other smaller foramen/foramina represent passages for smaller bundles of nerve fibers (e.g., cranial nerves) or blood vessels (e.g., carotid arteries).

The **cranial fossae** (Latin: *ditch*) divide the skull into three distinct regions. Figure 2–3 represents a mid-transverse slice through the cranium from a superior viewpoint denoting the cranial fossa. The anterior cranial fossa houses the frontal lobe, the middle cranial fossa houses the temporal lobes, and the posterior cranial fossa houses the parietal and occipital lobes as well as the cerebellum and brainstem structures. The foramen magnum is located in the posterior fossa. Figure 2–2 shows the correspondence between cranial fossa and the cerebral structures described here. In addition to serving as points of division, the cranial fossae are protective structures. Unfortunately, although these structures are protective in normal physiology/conditions, fossae and boney projections can damage brain tissue in traumatic head injuries, such as rapid acceleration and deceleration events, rotational forces, and through compression of surface structures against the boney protuberances with increased intracranial pressures and/or cerebral edema (see Chapter 14).

Key protuberances and projections in the anterior cranial fossa include the crista galli (Latin: *crest of the rooster*),

Chapter 2 – Ventricular System: Cranium, Ventricles, and Meninges 33

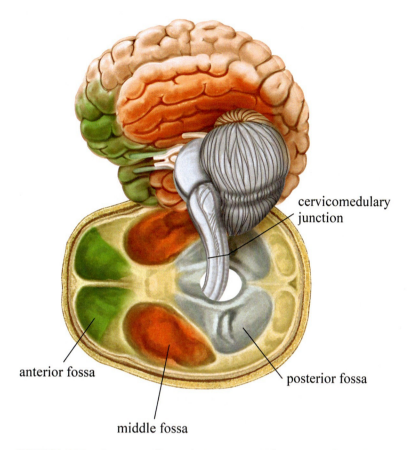

FIGURE 2–2. Correspondence between cranial fossa and cerebrum structures.

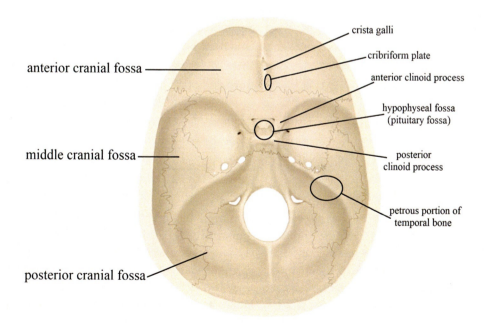

FIGURE 2–3. Cranial fossa. Illustration by Mariah Hoepner.

which is part of the ethmoid bone. This small projection lies between the left and right hemispheres of the ventromedial surface of the prefrontal cortices. It forms a perpendicular plate that extends out from the center of the cribriform plate, through which olfactory neurons extend from the nasal cavity into the CNS (see Chapter 9). Attached to the crista galli is a tissue (falx cerebri; see the section on dura mater) that separates the left and right hemispheres. In normal physiology, the falx cerebri helps stabilize the regions of the brain within the anterior cranial fossa. In trauma, in which rapid acceleration and deceleration forces and/or rotational forces are applied to the head, CSF can be displaced, causing the ventromedial surfaces of the cerebrum (which are crucial to executive functions and working memory; see Chapter 14) to come into contact with and be damaged by this projection. The anterior and posterior clinoid processes of the sphenoid bone project into the junction of the ventromedial prefrontal cortex, anterior–medial temporal lobes, and rostral brainstem. The depression present between the anterior and posterior clinoid processes, known variously as the pituitary fossa, the hypophyseal fossa, or the sella tursica, houses the pituitary gland. Again, morphologically this appears to serve a protective mechanism but may damage surrounding structures when rapid acceleration–deceleration and/or rotational forces are applied. The posterior border of the lesser sphenoid wing serves to separate the anterior and middle cranial fossa, lying in the region between the frontal and temporal lobes of the brain. If CSF is displaced by acceleration–deceleration and/or rotational forces, the anterior and medial surfaces of the temporal lobe may be susceptible to damage from this structure.

The petrous portion of the temporal bone marks the transition between the middle and posterior cranial fossa. You may recall that the petrous portion is a hill-like structure that houses the boney external auditory canal, the middle ear, and the cochlea (see Chapter 8). It is worth noting that the junction between the medial petrous portion, medial sphenoid wing, and the clinoid processes creates an X-like confluence. That X marks several crucial landmarks, as the optic chiasm crosses just superior to that landmark (see Chapter 7), the arterial circle of Willis centers just superior to this landmark (see Chapter 13), and the pituitary gland is positioned in the depression between the anterior and posterior clinoid processes. Within the cranium, most of the foramen, including the foramen magnum, are in the inferior portion of the skull, adjacent to the ventral surfaces of the cerebrum. The rest of the fully developed skull is a hard surface without openings. In cases in which intracranial pressure increases due to tumor, encephalitis, meningitis, stroke, trauma, hydrocephalus, or any other event that causes edema (swelling), brain tissues are compressed, potentially against or through (herniations) foramen. Because there are no openings along dorsal portions of the skull and the ventral surfaces have multiple foramen, the net force of swelling or increased intracranial pressure is on the ventral surfaces of the cerebrum, including the ventral prefrontal cortices, temporal lobes, cerebellum, and brainstem. Understanding this pathophysiology is crucial to making connections between the cranial environment and clinical applications.

Meningeal Layers

Three layers of tissue surround the external and medial surfaces of the cerebrum, cerebellum, brainstem, and spinal cord. These are, from superficial to deep, the dura mater, arachnoid membrane, and pia mater. Collectively, they are called the meninges (Figure 2–4).

Dura Mater

The **dura mater** (Latin: *tough mother*) is the outermost or most superficial layer of the meninges. If you ever have the opportunity to dissect a brain, you will see that you cannot tear the dura mater easily. Generally, you must use a scalpel to cut it. This is important because it protects the brain from the bony protuberances of the inner skull. As discussed previously, those sharp points include the sphenoid ridge, anterior and posterior clinoid processes, and the crista galli. The morphology of dura mater also prevents blood from passing through to the subdural space.

The dura mater consists of two layers: the periosteal layer, which adheres to the inner surface of the cranium and spinal column, and the meningeal layer, which adheres to the arachnoid layer. Under normal conditions, there should be no space between the periosteal dura mater and bones that protect the CNS; it adheres to the inner surface of those structures with the exception of spaces for meningeal blood vessels. Tears secondary to trauma or spontaneous hemorrhages in meningeal arteries can cause the potential space to become a real space, known as the **epidural space** and cause **epidural hematomas**. Hemorrhages between the dura mater and the arachnoid mater are known as **subdural hematomas**. Again, in normal physiology, there should not be a space between these layers, so the subdural space represents the second potential space.

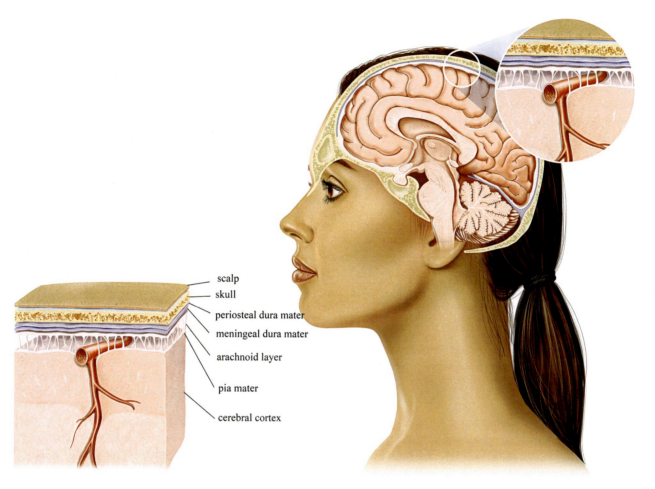

FIGURE 2–4. Meningeal layers.

Box 2–1. Hemorrhages and Hematomas

A hemorrhage is an escape of blood from arteries or veins. Damage to blood vessels due to trauma or bursting of an aneurysm (a weak spot in the wall of a blood vessel) will cause a hemorrhage. The blood that pools outside of the blood vessel is called a hematoma. Hematomas just under the skin are seen as bruises; the bluish-black coloring is caused by the blood that spilled out of damaged blood vessels. In the cranium, hemorrhages and hematomas are of significant concern because of the potential damage to the brain. As discussed in Chapter 14, large hemorrhages and hematomas can result in neuronal death due to loss of blood supply and behavioral symptoms related to increased intracranial pressure.

The dura mater has several enfoldings or extensions that provide separation between regions of the brain (Figure 2–5). These enfoldings attach to regions of the inner cranium to assist in minimizing movement of the brain. The **falx cerebri** (Latin: *falx = sickle or curved blade*) extends vertically from the dura covering the sagittal sulcus (longitudinal fissure) down into the gap between the left and right hemispheres, ending just superior to the corpus callosum. Anteriorly, the falx cerebri attaches to the crista galli of the ethmoid bone. The **falx cerebelli** is a second sickle-shaped structure, but it extends vertically between the right and left regions of the cerebellum. The third enfolding is the **tentorium cerebelli** (Latin: *tent of the cerebellum*), which extends horizontally in the space between the occipital lobe and the cerebellum. It is anchored to the inner cranium anteriorly at the clinoid processes of the sphenoid, laterally along the superior extent of the petrous temporal bone and inferior parietal bones, and posteriorly

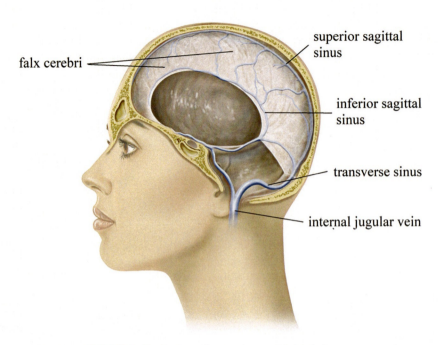

FIGURE 2–5. Meningeal extensions and dural sinuses.

to the occipital protuberance. Consistent with the role of meningeal layers throughout the cerebrum and spinal cord, these layers create spatial buffering between respective structures. Note that there is a double layer of meninges for each of these meningeal extensions (i.e., in the falx cerebri, the pia mater adheres to the medial surface of the left hemisphere followed by the arachnoid layer, followed by dura mater, which butts up to the dura mater associated with the right hemisphere, followed by the arachnoid layer, and then the pia mater, which is tightly adhered to the right hemisphere). Likewise, the falx cerebelli and tentorium cerebelli also are double-layered.

The **supratentorial space**, superior to the tentorium cerebelli, contains the cerebral hemispheres. The **infratentorial space** contains the cerebellum and brainstem in the posterior fossa. These terms can be used to describe the location of tumors or other pathologies (e.g., infratentorial mass).

At the origin of each enfolding, the periosteal and meningeal layers of the dura are separated to create dural venous sinuses that house meningeal veins (see Figure 2–5). Broadly, a sinus is a cavity or space; in this case, it serves as a drainage system. There are three primary dural venous sinuses, and their function is to drain venous blood from the brain and meninges. Deoxygenated blood runs through the meningeal veins in these sinuses and eventually flows into the jugular vein in the neck to return to the heart and lungs for reoxygenation. The **superior sagittal sinus** runs longitudinally (anterior to posterior) along the midline at the superior edge of the falx cerebri, within the longitudinal cerebral fissure. The **inferior sagittal sinus** lies within the sagittal sulcus at the base of the falx cerebri just superior to the corpus callosum. Laterally, there are bilateral **transverse sinuses** along the lateral portions of the tentorium cerebelli.

Arachnoid Layer and Pia Mater

Deep to the dura mater is the **arachnoid layer**, which includes the arachnoid trabeculae (Latin: *beam, timber*)—wispy, spiderweb-like extensions that create a physical space between the arachnoid and pia mater. This **subarachnoid space** is filled with CSF, which circulates around the brain and spinal cord. CSF protects the brain by creating spatial buffering and provides nutrients and hormone regulation. Hemorrhages in this space are known as **subarachnoid hemorrhages**. Along the superior sagittal and transverse sinuses are **arachnoid granulations** where the arachnoid membrane protrudes through the dura mater into the sinuses. These allow for CSF to be absorbed into the bloodstream after it has circulated around the CNS in the subarachnoid space.

Finally, the meningeal layer that adheres to the surface of the cerebrum (including extensions between lobes) is the pia mater. The **pia mater** (Latin: *gentle mother*) is very delicate and easily torn. It is also porous and adheres tightly to the surface of the brain and spinal cord. Because of this morphology, subarachnoid hemorrhages can come into contact with cortical brain tissue quite readily. Management of a subarachnoid hemorrhage is focused on minimizing the spread of the blood. This is done by reducing movement and external stimulation. Individuals with subarachnoid hemorrhages are placed in the reverse Trendelenburg position (supine position, head down, feet elevated), lights off and visual and auditory stimuli minimized (television off, radio/music off, limited interactions), in order to minimize spread of the hemorrhage and contact with brain/nervous tissue.

Box 2–2. Traumatic Brain Injury With Epidural Hematoma

A nurse, Penny, was walking briskly to work one morning, crossing the busy road from where she parked toward the hospital. Meanwhile, a 16-year-old boy who recently received his driver's license was on his way to school. He did not see my colleague and struck her with his car, which was traveling at approximately 25 miles per hour, before braking. Penny was propelled over the windshield, then over the roof of the car, and landed behind the car, a bit dazed. As the young man stepped out of the car, she apologized for walking in front of him and said she was fine. The young man pleaded with her to get into the car so he could take her to the emergency room, which was just around the corner. Moments later, they arrived and Penny was now unconscious.

She was admitted immediately and sent for a CAT scan, which revealed an epidural hematoma. Quickly, she was transferred to surgery for a burr hole procedure, which is a neurosurgical intervention whereby a small hole is made in the skull adjacent to a cerebral hematoma and a drain is placed to evacuate bleeding and reduce intracranial pressure. A couple of rough days passed, but the young man's quick thinking and honesty (despite knowing he would be charged with the accident by bringing her to the emergency department) ensured rapid care and a full recovery for this nurse. (See Case 16–1 in Chapter 16 for an extended version of this case.)

Ventricles

Ventricles are hollow cavities; in this case, cerebral ventricles are filled with CSF. There are four ventricles within the CNS: two lateral ventricles (one in each cerebral hemisphere), one third ventricle, and one fourth ventricle (Figure 2–6). As you might suspect because they are not paired structures, the third and fourth ventricles both lie along the midline. The third ventricle fills the space in between the right and left thalami. The fourth ventricle fills the space between the dorsal brainstem and the cerebellum. The ventricles are connected: The lateral ventricles are connected to the third ventricle by the **interventricular foramen**, also known as the **foramen of Monro**. The third ventricle is connected to the fourth ventricle by the **cerebral aqueduct** (**sylvian aqueduct**). There are four "exits" from the fourth ventricle: Laterally are the two **foramen of Luschka**, medially is the **foramen of Magendie**, and inferiorly the **spinal canal** extends down the center of the spinal cord.

The ventricles are filled with CSF. The CSF is produced by specialized ependymal cells called the **choroid plexus** (Figure 2–7). Given the opportunity to dissect a brain, you will find the choroid plexus in most of the ventricles but most prominently in the lateral ventricles. It is a pretty lavender color, so it is quite striking and beautiful. The choroid plexus serves as a pump, producing 600 to 700 ml of CSF each day. The ventricles account for 25 ml of the 140 to 270 ml of volume within the ventricular system at a given moment.

Cerebrospinal Fluid Path and Functions

The CSF travels from the lateral ventricles through the foramen of Monro to the third ventricle and through the sylvian (or cerebral) aqueduct to the fourth ventricle. From there, it flows through the foramina of Luschka and Magendie into the subarachnoid space surrounding the brain and spinal cord. It flows around the entire CNS and eventually is absorbed into the bloodstream through the arachnoid granulations.

Within the ventricular and meningeal system, CSF provides buoyancy, essentially keeping the brain afloat within the skull, and spatial buffering to prevent the brain and spinal cord structures from coming into direct contact with boney projections or foramen.

As described in detail later, CSF circulates neuroactive hormones, as well as transporting glucose and other nutrients to meninges. Note that it is faster and more efficient to distribute hormones through the CSF system than through

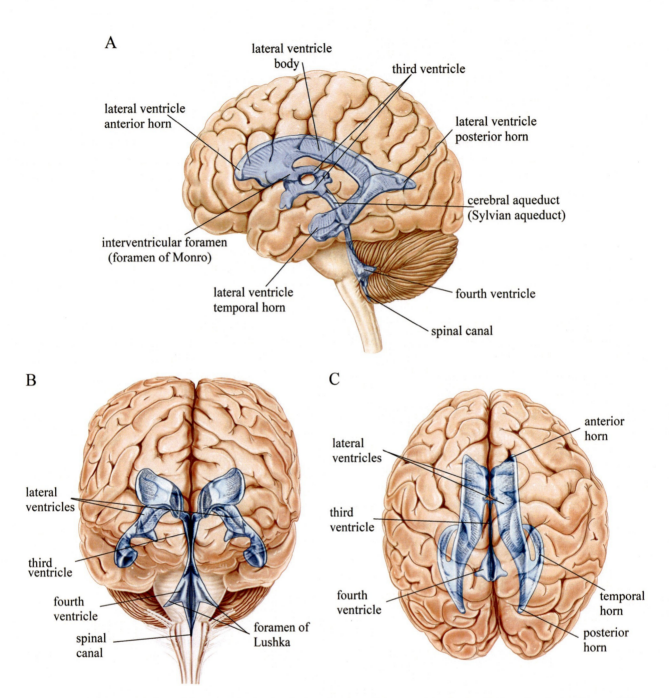

FIGURE 2–6. A. Lateral view of the ventricles in situ. **B.** Anterior view of the ventricles in situ. **C.** Superior view of the ventricles in situ.

the bloodstream. Furthermore, neuroactive hormones can alter brain behavior systemically, as opposed to hardwired signaling within neuronal pathways. Finally, CSF eliminates waste.

CSF composition can be an indicator of several pathologies. Typically, CSF is sampled by conducting a **lumbar puncture** (Figure 2–8). A needle is inserted between the third and fourth lumbar vertebrae, below the conus medullaris or end of the spinal cord, in order to reduce the likelihood of damage during the procedure. CSF is extracted and examined through visual and laboratory testing. The presence or absence of white blood cells can be an indicator of infection or dysfunction for acute bacterial meningitis or viral infections. Gross examination can determine

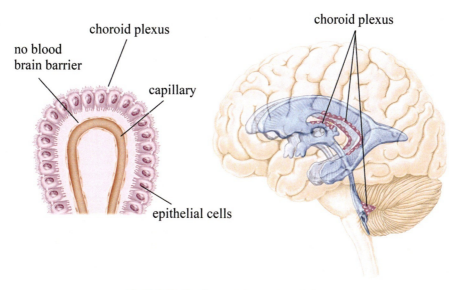

FIGURE 2–7. Choroid plexus morphology.

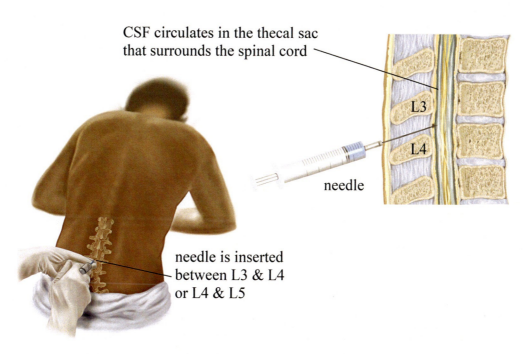

FIGURE 2–8. Lumbar puncture procedure.

the presence of cerebral hemorrhage as well. The presence of elevated proteins can indicate diseases such as multiple sclerosis or Guillain–Barré syndrome. The amount of pressure exerted by the CSF, called opening pressure, is an indirect measure of intracranial pressure and provides further information about potential neuropathologies such as hydrocephalus.

Communication Through the Ventricular System

The cerebrum is positioned within the cranium surrounded by a meningeal and ventricular system that has key roles in protection and communication within the nervous system. Although we typically think of communication in the nervous system as taking place through neuron-to-neuron signaling and perhaps even through the circulatory system by passing oxygen and nutrients to the brain cells, the cerebroventricular system communicates through the release of hormones. Interestingly, neurohormone release may affect structures at the local or systemic level. For instance, gonadotropin-releasing hormone is present in the third ventricle in an isolated manner. Note that the hypothalamus forms the inferior, lateral walls of the third ventricle. Recent investigations have shown that hormones released by the hypothalamus can be tracked in CSF. This includes hormones that stimulate hunger and thermoregulation. The connection also helps integrate the endocrine system with the autonomic nervous system. It may also have a role in emotional regulation. In summary, the cerebroventricular system regulates the extracellular fluid environment, which helps control behaviors and homeostatic regulation.

Circumventricular organs (those that lie in proximity to the perimeters of the ventricles) are found in the walls of the lateral, third, and fourth ventricles. Capillaries in the circumventricular organs lack a blood–brain barrier, the mechanism responsible for blocking larger molecules from crossing from the bloodstream to the brain (see Chapter 12). The lack of a blood–brain barrier in these regions allows monitoring of systemic circulation and the ability to detect and respond to noxious stimuli. Working as sensors, they have the ability to sense circulating concentrations of angiotensin II, a hormone that regulates renal function and, in turn, regulates blood pressure via vasoconstriction, controlling sodium, calcium, and ionic osmolality (i.e., the amount of ions such as sodium, potassium, chloride, urea, and glucose in blood helps regulate homeostasis), and autonomic outputs (i.e., direct regulation of hypothalamus and medulla). The absence of a blood–brain barrier also allows the circumventricular organs to secrete neurohormones directly into the CSF and circulatory systems.

Disruptions to the Ventricular and Meningeal Systems

Hydrocephalus

Trauma, blockages, and other disruptions to CSF flow and/or reabsorption can result in a buildup or shortage of CSF to carry out its roles. The resulting condition is called **hydrocephalus** (Greek: *water on the brain*). A failure of villi and arachnoid granulations to reabsorb results in **communicating hydrocephalus**. A blockage in flow of the CSF through the ventricular system creates **noncommunicating hydrocephalus**, which can create a buildup that compresses brain tissue medial or lateral to the ventricles (Figure 2–9). If not managed, that compression will eventually constrict blood flow, oxygen, and nutrients to that tissue and it will die.

Box 2–3. Exacerbation of Hydrocephalus

PJ was a 5-year old boy with severe developmental cognitive delay and progressive hydrocephalus due to Crouzon syndrome. PJ was nonverbal and communicated through vocalizations, some simple switches, and other cues such as joint attention and eye contact. In addition to dealing with feeding and nutrition issues, managing the boy's ventriculoperitoneal shunt [i.e., a surgically placed tube that runs from the ventricles to the gut (peritoneum) to remove excess or obstructed CSF] was a constant battle for his physicians, nurses, and parents. Medical staff and family dealt with shunt revisions and a regular regimen of antibiotics to deal with infections. As infections arose, the shunt did not function properly and thus did not remove excess CSF from his ventricles. The shunt malfunctions and infections led to increased communication difficulties. His interactions would become muted, and he became lethargic until the infection resolved. Hydrocephalus also damaged his hypothalamus (see Chapter 5), which compromised his ability to regulate body temperature. During infection, fevers would spike to high levels (e.g., above 105° Fahrenheit), and cooling him down with ice baths was necessary. When infections and malfunctions resolved, previous communicative interactions reemerged. Changes to cognition (alertness levels and communication) likely stemmed from several factors, including including compression of brain structures due to buildup of pressure within the ventricles and inflammation of the meninges, and homeostatic impairments due to the hypothalamic damage. (See Case 16–17 in Chapter 16 for an expanded version of this case.)

A. typical ventricle size

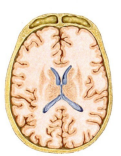
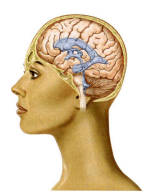

B. enlarged ventricles with hydrocephalus

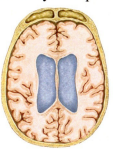
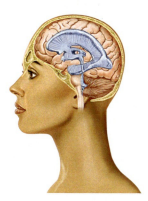

FIGURE 2–9. A comparison of typically sized ventricles (**A**) and those enlarged by hydrocephalus (**B**).

Box 2–4. Multiple Spinal Meningeal Diverticula and Low-Pressure CSF Syndrome

A speech–language pathologist (SLP) developed signs of postural headaches (these occur when standing but subside when laying down) and unrelenting nausea of unknown origin. Physicians could not identify a cause, although it contributed to an initial loss of 40 pounds and substantial restriction in activity level. As the problem progressed, weakness and fasciculations in the feet and calves began to accompany the other symptoms, along with hyperactive reflexes (see Chapter 10 for motor systems).

As quickly as it developed, the symptoms resolved and the SLP began to recover. Unfortunately, after a few months passed, the symptoms returned.

Eventually, a local neurologist had an epiphany, recalling a rare disease that affects the integrity of meningeal tissues, specifically the dura mater, leading to meningeal diverticula (outpouches). A key symptom is severe postural headaches that resolve upon lying flat. One cisternogram (a radiologic test that involves tracking a radioactive tracer within and outside of the ventricular system) later and the problem was finally identified, lighting up the nerve roots of the spinal cord like an inverted Christmas tree. The diverticula (upwards of 40) were at the junction of the spinal roots and the spinal cord. As they ballooned, the diverticula reached a point where they burst and CSF spilled out of the ventricular system. That led to compression of nerve roots (thus the fasciculations and lower motor neuron signs), and leaks caused the brain to sink down toward the foramen magnum (thus the hyperactive reflexes and upper motor neuron signs). (See Case 16–2 in Chapter 16 for an expanded version of this case.)

In some cases, a ventriculoperitoneal shunt will divert excess CSF from the ventricular space to the peritoneum (essentially the gut). This releases the pressure in the cranium and relieves the pressure on the brain tissue. The appearance of large, dilated ventricles is common among elderly individuals, particularly those with dementia. This is known as **normal pressure hydrocephaly** because the expanded ventricular size is due to the atrophy of cortical tissue and white matter rather than increased CSF pressure. Figure 2–10 shows drawings of magnetic resonance imaging and computed tomography scans of ventricles in normal versus hydrocephalic conditions.

Meningeal Damage

Holes in the meninges can cause low CSF pressure. Low pressure syndrome results in postural headaches that are worse when the individual is upright and improve when they are lying prone or supine. In this case, the CSF leaks out of the system and buoyancy cannot be maintained. Because of the lack of buoyancy, spatial buffering is disrupted and brain tissue is compressed along bony surfaces of the skull and vertebral column. Pressure of the brain on the dura causes the headache pain. When the person lies down, the pressure is relieved and thus the headache subsides. The problem occurs frequently after lumbar punctures and sometimes spontaneously. It is initially treated through rest and fluids. If that does not allow the puncture to heal spontaneously, sometimes an individual's own blood is injected into the epidural space of the spinal column in an attempt to clot off or seal the hole. This is known as an epidural blood patch.

If meninges are damaged through bacterial, viral, or mechanical trauma, they become swollen. That swelling can compress nearby brain or spinal tissue, restricting blood flow to those structures and altering function. Although we will not delve into specifics of bacterial versus viral infections, they can have substantive impacts on behavior and function throughout the brain or locally within structures affected directly. The same applies to mechanical meningitis, which can occur with surgeries, trauma, or spinal procedures.

Summary

The brain and spinal cord are surrounded and supported by a ventricular and meningeal system that protects, supports, and facilitates communication within the nervous system. The boney framework of the skull and vertebral columns serve as the first line of protection but can damage the same structures they protect in the presence of trauma and edema. Understanding normal anatomy and physiology of these environments of the brain and spinal cord allows us to better understand dysfunction and disruptions to these structures.

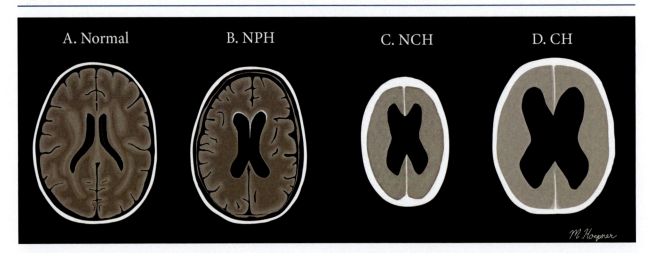

FIGURE 2–10. Comparison of ventricular morphology in normal versus impaired conditions. The black areas represent CSF. CH, communicating hydrocephalus; NCH, noncommunicating (obstructive) hydrocephalus; NPH, normal pressure hydrocephalus. Illustration by Mariah Hoepner.

Key Concepts

- There are four ventricles in the center of the CNS that convey CSF to the meningeal layer surrounding the CNS.
- The meninges are a set of three layers of tissue that provides buoyancy and tethers the brain within the cranium.
- The cranium and ventricular–meningeal-CSF systems protect CNS structures through encasing the CNS in CSF.
- The ventricular–meningeal-CSF system is a route for local and systemic hormonal control of the nervous system and body.
- Blockages in flow or leaks within ventricular–meningeal-CSF systems can have serious consequences on communication and cognition, and they can lead to death if not managed.
- Trauma and disease can disrupt the protective functions of the cranium as CNS structures are compressed against boney projections and foramen of the skeletal system.

Additional Resources

Blumenfeld, H. (2010). *Neuroanatomy through clinical cases* (2nd ed.). Sinauer.

Kandell, E., Schwartz, J., & Jessell, T. (2000). *Principles of neural science* (4th ed.). McGraw-Hill.

Noble, E. E., Hahn, J. D., Konanur, V. R., Hsu, T. M., Page, S. J., Cortella, A. M., . . . Kanoski, S. E. (2018). Control of feeding behavior by cerebral ventricular volume transmission of melanin-concentrating hormone. *Cell Metabolism, 28*(1), 55–68.

Nolte, J. (2002). *The human brain: An introduction to its functional neuroanatomy* (pp. 570–573). Mosby.

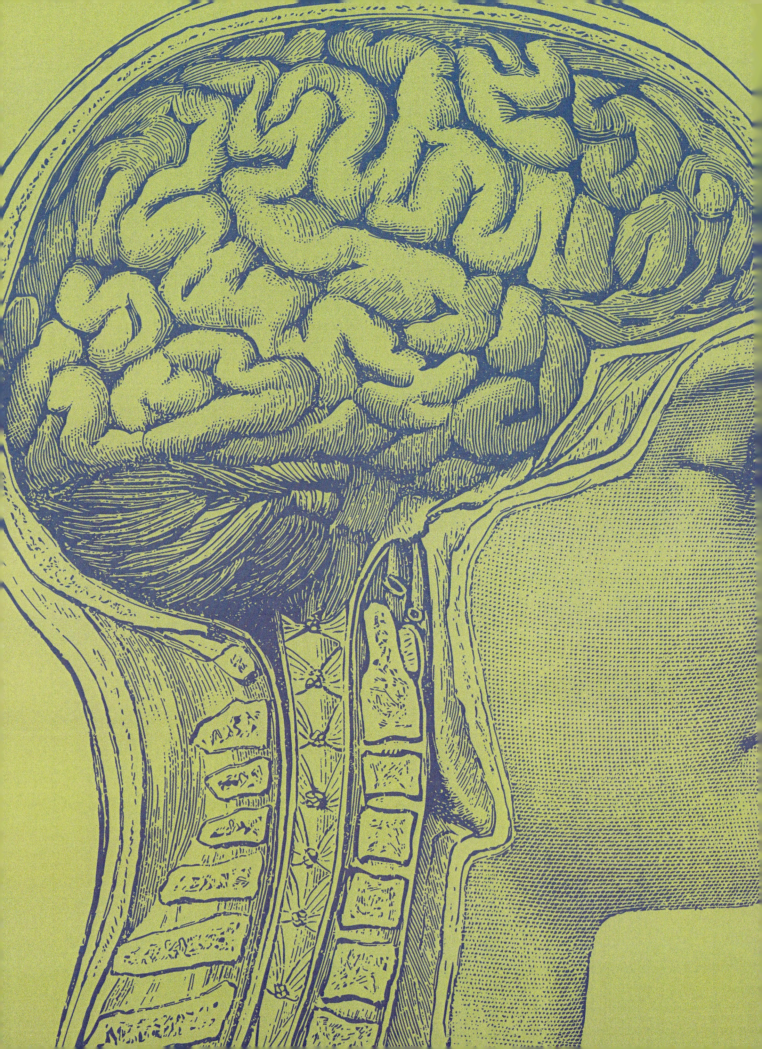

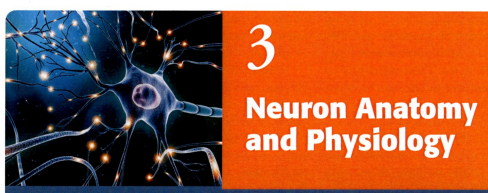

3
Neuron Anatomy and Physiology

CHAPTER OUTLINE

Overview
Classification of Neurons
Neuronal Communication
   Big Picture Overview
   Membrane Potentials
Synaptic Transmission
   Action Potentials
   Myelinated Versus Unmyelinated Axons
   Synaptic Transmission
     Types of Neurotransmitters
     Neurotransmitter Recovery and Degradation
Creating Meaning from Binary Signals
   Patterns of Signals
   Source of Signals
   Region or Location
Conditions That Alter Synaptic Transmission
Neurologic Disorders and Diseases That Affect Synaptic Transmission
   Parkinson Disease
   Multiple Sclerosis
   Myasthenia Gravis
Pharmacological Effects on Synaptic Transmission
   Blocking Effects
   Prolonging Effects
   Mimicking Effect
Summary
Reference and Additional Resources

Overview

Neurons are the specialized cells within the nervous system that convey the signals that combine to create movement, sensation, emotions, thinking, personality, and practically everything that you do. Although neurons can send only 2 different signals—excitatory (go) and inhibitory (no go)—humans have approximately 100 billion neurons, and each can receive up to 10,000 signals from other neurons. The vast number of neurons and extensive connections between them make it possible to think deep thoughts; feel and express a variety of emotions; communicate through speech, written word, gestures, body language, visual art, and music; feel the touch of a handshake; wiggle one's toes; and all other things that humans are capable of doing. In case it is not immediately evident, understanding neuron anatomy and physiology has great relevance to speech-language pathologists and audiologists. Communication between neurons is essential for processing sensory input, sending motor signals to the body (including muscles of the speech and hearing mechanism), and processing thoughts and language. A better understanding of the underlying mechanisms of these functions leads to a better understanding of what occurs when they are disrupted or fail to develop normally.

Classification of Neurons

The basic structure of neurons was covered in Chapter 1. Remember that neurons generally consist of a soma or cell body, dendrites (receive signals), and an axon (sends signals). There are more than 100 different types of neurons; just a few are mentioned here. Neurons can be classified in various ways: by shape, size, or function.

Shape: There are three major types of neuronal shapes, named for the number of structures extending from the soma (Figure 3–1). **Multipolar neurons** have multiple extensions from the soma. These neurons have a single axon and many dendrites extending from the soma. The majority of neurons within the human nervous system are multipolar, including motor neurons within the corticospinal tracts and Purkinje cells found in the cerebellum. **Bipolar neurons** have two extensions: one dendrite and one axon. Although there is only one dendrite extending from the soma, it can have extensive branching. **Unipolar neurons** have a single extension from the soma. The main section of this extension is the axon, with branches off of the axon that serve as dendrites. Unipolar neurons in vertebrates are found primarily within the autonomic nervous system. A **pseudounipolar neuron** has a single extension from the cell body, the majority of which functions as an axon, with the peripheral portion serving as dendrites. First-order neurons in the somatosensory system, which carry pain, touch, and temperature information from the body to the spinal cord, are pseudounipolar neurons.

Size: Large neurons, called **Golgi type I**, have axons that are long (can be 3 feet or more) and relatively large in diameter. Primary neurons within the motor and somatosensory systems typically are Golgi type I cells. Smaller neurons, called **Golgi type II**, are considerably shorter in length and diameter. The smallest of these can be called **microneurons**. Some are called **anaxonic** because their axons are roughly the same length as the dendrites and can be difficult to identify.

Function: Neurons also can be classified by their function within the nervous system. **Motor** or **efferent** neurons conduct signals from the brain out to the body to innervate muscles. **Sensory** or **afferent** neurons conduct signals from the body to the brain for conscious awareness and processing of sensation. **Interneurons** provide connections between neurons, establishing local circuits. They can provide connections between sensory and motor systems, for example, in a typical reflex arc in which a sensory signal is sent into the spinal cord, where it is conveyed to the motor system either directly or through an interneuron.

Millions of neurons do not fit nicely into these classification schemes. The cerebral neurons that connect regions of the cerebral hemispheres, for example, are predominantly multipolar neurons but do not easily fit into function or size classifications.

Neuronal Communication

Communication between neurons requires a combination of electrical and chemical signals. Electrical signals occur within a neuron, whereas chemicals called **neurotransmitters** convey signals between neurons or between a neuron

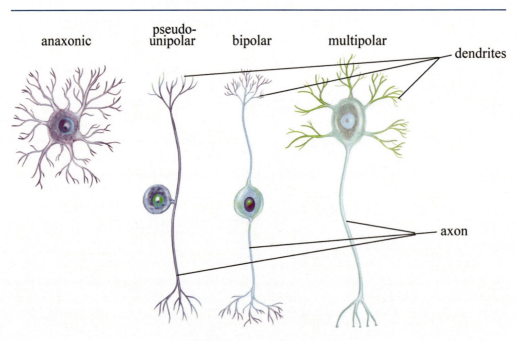

FIGURE 3–1. Types of neurons.

and a peripheral structure such as a muscle, organ, or gland. For purposes of this book, the focus is on communication between neurons in the central nervous system (CNS) and between neurons and muscles via the neuromuscular junction in the peripheral nervous system (PNS).

Big Picture Overview

Neurons communicate with one another in a region called a **synapse**. **Presynaptic neurons** are "senders," and **postsynaptic neurons** are "receivers." Neurons do not physically touch at the synapse but, rather, are separated by a small space called a synaptic gap or synaptic cleft. An electrical signal created by the movement of ions (charged particles) is generated within the soma of a neuron and is sent down the axon (from proximal to distal) until it reaches the presynaptic neuron's axon terminal. This electrical signal is called an **action potential**. At this point, the action potential triggers the release of a chemical known as a neurotransmitter. This chemical moves through the synaptic cleft and binds to a receptor on the postsynaptic neuron. The presence of the neurotransmitter causes ion channels to open, allowing movement of charged particles across the membrane of the postsynaptic neuron. This then creates an electrical change in the soma, and the process repeats.

Membrane Potentials

Within the nervous system there is a difference in electrical charge inside versus outside of neurons. This is called **polarization**. The inside of a neuron at rest has a negative charge in relation to the extracellular matrix outside of the neuron. The cell membrane is the barrier between the inter- and extracellular spaces. Although the exact level of intercellular negativity differs across types of neurons, −65 millivolts (mV) is typically used as a standard. Thus, the outside of the neuron is considered to be neutral, at 0 mV, compared to the −65 mV **resting membrane potential** within the neuron. Changes to this membrane potential affect the likelihood that an electrical signal will be generated and sent through the neuron. When the membrane potential becomes more negative (e.g., −80 or −90 mV), the neuron is **hyperpolarized** and is less likely to generate and send a signal. In contrast, when the membrane potential becomes more positive (or less negative, such as −60 or −50 mV), the neuron is said to be **depolarized** and is more likely to generate and send a signal. In order for an electrical signal to be sent down an axon, the neuron has to be depolarized to a critical threshold. Once this threshold is reached, a cascade of events occurs to open, close, and inactivate ion channels and allow depolarization and repolarization along the length of the axon. Negative 50 mV is commonly used as a standard threshold, although the actual threshold can differ across neurons, just as the exact resting membrane potential differs.

> **Box 3-1.** Key Terms Related to Membrane Status
>
> **Hyperpolarization:** The difference in electrical charge between the inside and outside of the cell becomes greater as the inside of the cell becomes more negative, thus increasing the polarization.
>
> **Depolarization:** The difference in electrical charge between the inside and outside of the cell becomes smaller (and may disappear altogether or reverse) as the inside of the cell becomes more positive, thus decreasing the polarization.
>
> **Repolarization:** The process by which the resting (baseline) electrical polarization of a neuron is reestablished.
>
> **Resting membrane potential:** A net negative, intracellular charge (i.e., net positive extracellular to net negative intracellular) that is maintained through the sodium–potassium ion pump at rest in order to create a gradient and energy potential when membrane permeability is altered.

The membrane potential is created by two different gradients, or different levels of concentration across the cell membrane. The first is an electrical gradient. There are more negatively charged ions inside the neuron and more positively charged ions outside the neuron. If ions could move freely through the membrane, positive ions would move into the cell—down their concentration gradient—to equalize the positive charge and create neutral or equilibrium status. Likewise, negative ions would move from higher to lower concentrations; in this case, however, they would move out of the cell to equalize the negative charge. The second gradient is the ion concentration gradient. There is an unequal distribution of the number (concentration) of different types of ions inside and outside of the neuron. When ion channels are open, the ions move down their concentration gradient from an area of high concentration to an area of lower concentration.

There are three key ions for understanding neuronal communication: sodium (Na^+), potassium (K^+), and calcium (Ca^{2+}). In the CNS, there is more sodium (Na^+) and calcium (Ca^{2+}) outside the cell and more potassium (K^+) inside the cell. As described previously, nature likes to be in balance, so if there was a way for ions to cross the membrane, then sodium and calcium ions would move in—down their concentration gradient—until the number (concentration) of those types of ions was equivalent inside and outside of the cell membrane. Likewise, potassium would move out of the cell to balance out its ion concentration differential.

There are ion channels within the cell membrane (Figure 3–2). When they are open, ions can move freely, and they will always passively move down their gradients from areas of higher concentration to areas of lower concentration. This free movement, along the concentration gradient, is known as passive transport because no energy is expended. There are several types of ion channels that differ in how and when they open. Ionotropic (also called ligand-gated) ion channels open in response to the presence of a neurotransmitter. Mechanically gated ion channels open in response to a mechanical displacement of the cell membrane. Finally, voltage-gated channels open when the electrical charge (voltage) of a neuron reaches a specified threshold.

Box 3–2. Types of Ion Channels

Ligand-gated: Also called ionotropic, these channels open when a neurotransmitter binds to a receptor. These are found in synapses throughout the CNS and PNS. (Ligand = substances that bind to others; in neuroscience, it is used to refer to substances that bind to receptors.)

Mechanically gated: These channels open in response to mechanical displacement. They are found in somatosensory systems, responding to touch or vibration, and in the auditory system, responding to the movement of cilia on cochlear hair cells (see Chapter 8).

Voltage-gated: These channels open when the electrical charge or the voltage of a neuron reaches a specific level. Sodium channels along the axon and calcium channels in the axon terminal are voltage gated and will open when depolarization occurs.

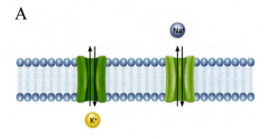

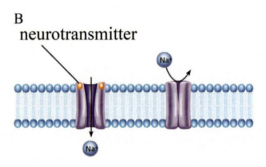

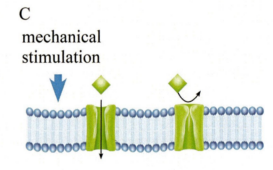

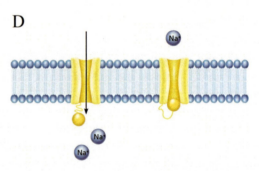

FIGURES 3–2. Cell membranes and ion channels. **A.** Basic ion channels, always open, allow free movement of ions. **B.** Ligand-gated (ionotropic) channels open in response to the presence of a neurotransmitter (ligand) binding to the channel. **C.** Mechanically gated channels open in response to mechanical stimulation to the cell membrane. **D.** Voltage-gated channels open in response to changes in the voltage (electrical charge) within the neuron.

Box 3–3. Ion Charges and Abbreviations

Sodium (Na; Latin: *Natrium*) has a single positive charge and thus is represented as Na^+.

Potassium (K; derived from Potash, neo-Latin: *Kalium*) has a single positive charge and thus is represented as K^+.

Calcium (Ca) has a double positive charge and thus is represented as Ca^{++} or Ca^{2+}.

Chloride (Cl) has a single negative charge and thus is represented as Cl^-.

Synaptic Transmission

Neuronal communication involves several stages. The process is circular and cyclical, and thus it is difficult to determine exactly where to start with the explanation. There are several important concepts to know before diving into the details.

Box 3–4. Important Concepts in Neuron Communication

- Neurons can send (and receive) only two signals: excitatory and inhibitory. Excitatory signals assist in triggering the next neuron in the chain to "fire" or send a signal. Inhibitory signals assist in preventing the next neuron from "firing" or sending a signal. Essentially, neurons convey either "go" (excitatory) or "no go" (inhibitory). All thoughts, actions, sensations, emotions, opinions, knowledge, etc. are created by patterns of excitatory and inhibitory signals; this is somewhat akin to the binary (0, 1) code that computers use.
- Neurons can send electrical signals only in one direction: from the soma to the axon terminal.
- Electrical signals exist within a neuron, and chemical signals exist between neurons. For one neuron to communicate with another, an electrical signal travels through the first neuron to the axon terminal, which results in a chemical signal that affects the second neuron, causing an electrical change in the second neuron.

As described previously, a neuron at rest is polarized, meaning that the inside of the cell is negatively charged (–65 mV) compared to the outside of the cell (0 mV). Each neuron receives signals from hundreds of other neurons. Each of those hundreds of signals is either excitatory or inhibitory. Excitatory signals cause depolarization, which will push the neuron toward sending a signal to the next neuron in the chain; inhibitory signals cause hyperpolarization, which decreases the chance that the neuron will send a signal. These are called excitatory postsynaptic potentials (EPSPs) and inhibitory postsynaptic potentials (IPSPs), respectively. They are called "potentials" because each signal has the potential to either excite or inhibit the postsynaptic (receiving) neuron, but no one signal is strong enough to cause an action potential.

Initially, signals alter the permeability of neuron membranes, allowing for movement of ions into or out of the neuron. EPSPs create depolarization by opening sodium (Na^+) channels. Remember that there is a higher concentration of sodium outside the cell, so when the sodium channels open, Na^+ will flow into the cell through diffusion (passive transport). The influx of many positively charged ions will result in an increase in positive charge within the cell, or depolarization. IPSPs will result in hyperpolarization by opening either potassium (K^+) or chloride (Cl^-) channels. Remember that there is a higher concentration of potassium inside the cell, so when the potassium channels open, K^+ will move out of the cell, also through diffusion (passive transport). The exodus of positively charged ions will leave the inside of the neuron even more negative than it was before, thus creating hyperpolarization. Cl^- has a higher concentration outside of the neuron; when Cl^- channels open, the ions will flow into the cell, taking in negative charges.

Box 3–5. Summary of Excitatory and Inhibitory Signaling

An **excitatory postsynaptic potential (EPSP)** is the result of a neurotransmitter that opens Na^+ channels, causing Na^+ to move into the neuron and begin to depolarize the cell by increasing positivity. "Excitatory" refers to the fact that it is moving the neuron closer to the depolarization threshold, which will result in an action potential. "Postsynaptic" refers to

continues

> **Box 3–5.** *continued*
>
> the fact that it occurs in the receiving or postsynapticneuron. It is a "potential" because a single signal will not be strong enough to reach the depolarization threshold, but it adds to the potential for depolarization and the creation of an action potential.
>
> An **inhibitory postsynaptic potential (IPSP)** is the result of a neurotransmitter that opens K^+ channels, causing K^+ to move out of the neuron and begin to hyperpolarize the cell by increasing negativity. It also can trigger opening of chloride channels (Cl^-) that allow chloride to move into the neuron, again beginning hyperpolarization by increasing intercellular negativity. "Inhibitory" refers to the fact that it is moving the neuron further from the depolarization threshold, which will prevent the generation of an action potential. "Postsynaptic" refers to the fact that it occurs in the receiving or postsynaptic neuron. It is a "potential" because a single signal will not be strong enough to counteract the EPSPs, but it adds to the potential for hyperpolarization and the prevention of an action potential.

Whether or not the depolarization threshold is met depends on the **summation** of EPSPs and IPSPs. If there are enough excitatory signals that result in enough Na^+ ions moving in so that the electrical charge moves from –65 mV (resting) to –50 mV (threshold), then an action potential will be created, causing a signal to be sent down the axon to the axon terminal. In contrast, if there are not enough excitatory signals, or if there are IPSPs that keep the intracellular charge below (more negative than) the threshold, then the neuron will do nothing; it will not create an action potential and thus will not transmit a signal. Following a subthreshold signal, the sodium–potassium ion pump uses active transport [i.e., energy in the form of adenosine triphosphate (ATP)] to restore the cell to resting membrane potential.

There are two primary types of summation that occur: temporal and spatial. In temporal summation, a large number of either excitatory or inhibitory signals occur close in time. The influx or efflux of ions from multiple signals that arrive all within a small time frame can cause a rapid change in polarization. Although each of those smaller signals is inadequate to meet threshold individually, adding multiple subthreshold signals together meets the threshold (whether it be a typical, resting membrane potential or a more elevated threshold that follows recent EPSP or IPSP). Spatial summation occurs when there are multiple EPSPs or IPSPs that occur close together spatially, or within the same small region of a neuron. In the case of excitatory signals, the influx or efflux of ions within that small region of space can quickly add up and create depolarization that will trigger an action potential. Similarly, a large number of IPSPs that occur within a small region of the soma can hyperpolarize the neuron and prevent an action potential from being generated. Like temporal summation, multiple subthreshold signals in close physical proximity to each other are added together (summed) in order to produce an EPSP or IPSP. See Figure 3–3 for a visual of summation.

Synapses can be named according to their location: axodendritic, axosomatic, and axo-axonic. Synapses that result in EPSPs generally are **axodendritic**, found on the dendrites or dendritic spines, but also can be **axosomatic**, on the soma. Those that tend to result in IPSPs are found typically on the soma and often near the axon hillock. Inhibitory synapses also can be **axo-axonic**, found at the proximal and distal ends of the axon. Due to this pattern of distribution, summation of many EPSPs is necessary to reach the depolarization threshold at the axon hillock as the accumulation of positive ions must diffuse from the dendrites into the soma in order to trigger an action potential, but a small number of IPSPs can spatially summate near the axon hillock and prevent the action potential from being created.

In the soma, the EPSPs and IPSPs "add up" in terms of the amount of negativity or positivity within the soma. If there is enough of an increase in positivity near the axon hillock that the depolarization reaches the threshold, then an action potential is created. This action potential sets off a series of changes to the ion channels and ion pumps along the axon, creating a "wave" of depolarization that runs down the entire length of the axon. When the action potential reaches the axon terminal, it signals the release of chemicals (neurotransmitters) that are housed within the axon terminals. This release from the presynaptic neuron is referred to as exocytosis (you can think of it as exporting from a neuron). The neurotransmitters spill into the synaptic cleft and bind to receptors on a receiving (postsynaptic) neuron. When the neurotransmitters bind, they will create either (1) an inhibitory signal and aid in hyperpolarization or (2) an excitatory signal and aid in depolarization. The process then begins again in the receiving neuron, in which case it then becomes a sending (presynaptic) neuron.

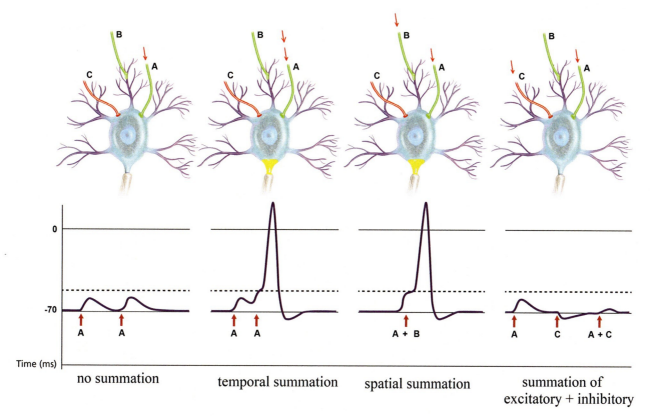

FIGURE 3-3. Summation in postsynaptic neurons.

Action Potentials

Once summation of EPSPs occurs and the threshold is reached at the axon hillock, an action potential is generated (Figure 3-4). Action potentials are often referred to as nerve impulses or the "firing" of a neuron. The cell membrane surrounding the axon includes voltage-gated Na$^+$ and K$^+$ ion channels. As described in Box 3-2, voltage-gated channels open or close in response to changes in electrical charge. When there is sufficient summation of EPSPs near the axon hillock, the depolarization (reduced negative voltage) in the cell triggers the opening of many Na$^+$ channels in the proximal axon. When the channels are open, Na$^+$ rapidly flows into the neuron, creating a depolarizing spike that can reverse the polarization, making the inside of the neuron positive (up to +40 mV) compared to the extracellular matrix.

The sodium ions that entered the neuron diffuse down the axon, creating depolarization in the adjacent segment and triggering the opening of voltage-gated sodium channels in that region; more sodium flows in, and the depolarization once again spreads. This staged influx of Na$^+$ down the length of the axon essentially renews the action potential at each point along the axon, thus maintaining the strength of the action potential throughout the entire length.

Soon after the Na$^+$ flows in, the K$^+$ channels open. K$^+$ ions then move out of the axon, down the potassium concentration gradient. The efflux of positive ions restores the polarization of the neuron. K$^+$ channels open and close relatively slowly, which allows too much K$^+$ to leave the neuron, resulting in a hyperpolarized state in which the intercellular voltage is more negative (e.g., -75 mV) than the resting membrane potential. This period of hyperpolarization can be referred to as an "undershoot," in which the polarization exceeds that of the resting state.

As Na$^+$ channels open on each adjacent region of the axon, those more proximally will close. In addition, they are inactivated or "locked" for a brief amount of time. While they are inactivated, they cannot be opened, even if the neuron remains depolarized. This inactivation forces the action potential to move in only one direction—proximal

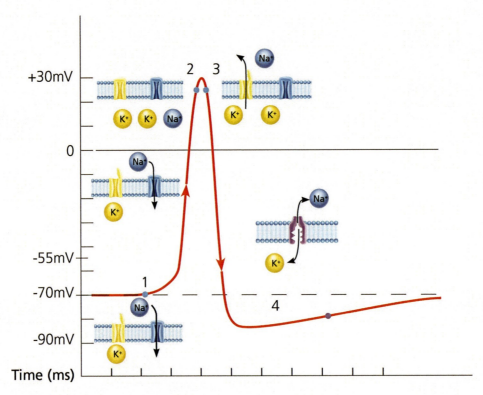

FIGURE 3–4. Graph of an action potential. **1.** EPSP opens Na+ channels; Na+ moves into the cell, creating depolarization. **2.** Na+ channels close and inactivate. **3.** K+ channels open; K+ moves out of the cell, creating repolarization. **4.** Na+/K+ pumps move K+ in and Na+ out to restore the resting membrane potential.

to distal—and prevents it from spreading back toward the soma. It also prevents a new action potential from being generated until the Na+ channels are activated (unlocked). This period of Na+ channel activation is called the **absolute refractory period**, in which no new action potential can be generated (because there is no way for Na+ channels to be opened, even in the presence of depolarization). This allows the neuron to "reset." The channels are reactivated (unlocked) once the neuron returns to its resting membrane potential.

A second phase of the refractory period, called the **relative refractory period**, then occurs. During this time frame, a new action potential is possible but requires a greater stimulus (more EPSPs or greater depolarization). This occurs after the efflux of K+ ions when the inside of the neuron is hyperpolarized. Imagine enough K+ leaves the neuron to change the voltage to –80 mV. To reach the depolarization threshold of –50 mV, a 30 mV change is necessary; this is greater than the 15 mV change required (moving –65 to –50 mV) for the prior action potential to be generated. The original resting membrane potential is reestablished through the closure of K+ channels and the working of the Na+/K+ pump.

The movement of sodium and potassium ions across the axonal membrane changes the ion concentrations: Na+ is no longer as imbalanced with greater concentration outside the neuron, and K+ is no longer as imbalanced with greater concentration inside the neuron. Although the alteration of the ion concentrations is relatively small after a single action potential, the additivity of multiple rapid action potentials could lead to rather large alterations. Thus, to restore the resting ion concentration gradients and prevent long-term changes, K+ must be pushed back into the cell and Na+ must be pushed back out of the cell. This restoration is achieved by the work of sodium–potassium pumps. These pumps require energy in the form of ATP because they are pushing ions against their gradients. Each cycle of a sodium–potassium pump moves three Na+ ions out and two K+ ions in. Once the ionic concentrations are restored, the neuron is again "at rest." Figure 3–5 illustrates

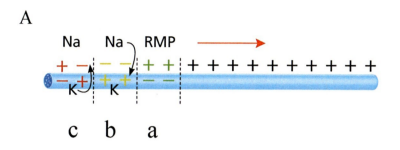

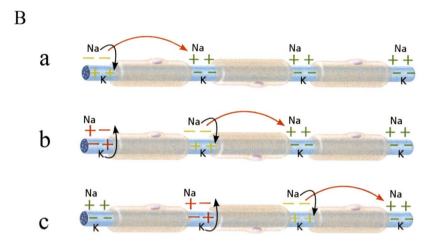

FIGURE 3–5. A. Action potential propagation in an unmyelinated neuron. **a.** Neuron resting potential, more negative inside the cell than outside. **b.** Na⁺ moves into the neuron, creating depolarization. **c.** K⁺ moves out of the neuron, repolarizing the neuron to return it to the resting membrane potential. **B.** Action potential propagation in a myelinated neuron. **a.** Depolarization begins as Na⁺ moves into the neuron. Na⁺ ions diffuse down the axon surrounded by myelin to the next node of Ranvier. **b.** Voltage-gated Na⁺ channels at the second node of Ranvier open and allow Na⁺ in to create depolarization at the second node. At the first node, K⁺ channels are opening, allowing K⁺ to move out to repolarize the neuron. **c.** The progression moves down the axon, proximal to distal at each node of Ranvier.

propagation of action potentials down unmyelinated and myelinated axons.

The sequence of events of the action potential can be summarized as follows:

- Depolarization beyond the threshold occurs near the axon hillock, stimulating an action potential.
- The depolarization opens voltage-gated Na⁺ channels in the proximal axon, allowing lots of Na⁺ to move rapidly into the axon.
- The Na⁺ ions diffuse down the axon, triggering the opening of new Na⁺ channels in an adjacent region.
- As Na⁺ flows into the ion, too much Na⁺ enters the neuron, causing an "overshoot" at the peak of the action potential.
- The original Na⁺ channels close and become briefly inactivated or "locked." This creates an absolute refractory period in which no new action potential can be generated.
- Voltage-gated K⁺ channels open in response to the depolarization, allowing K⁺ to move out of the axon, resulting in repolarization. Some refer to this as the "rectifying" response.
- The slowed closure of the K⁺ channels results in hyperpolarization or "undershoot" in the return of polarization.
- K⁺ channels close, preventing the efflux of further potassium ions.
- The Na⁺ channels "unlock," or are reactivated, resetting the neuron for a new action potential.

- The hyperpolarization creates a relative refractory period in which a new action potential can be generated but a stronger stimulus (more EPSPs) is required to achieve the threshold.
- The Na^+/K^+ pump pushes Na^+ ions back outside of the neuron and pushes K^+ neurons back into the neuron to reestablish the ion concentration gradients.

Action potentials are an "all-or-none" phenomenon. Once an action potential is begun, it will continue unless stopped by an external input such as an inhibitory axo-axonic synapse. The movement of an action potential down an axon is called **propagation** of the action potential. All action potentials are the same strength; there are no weaker or stronger electrical signals. In addition, because of the physiology of the action potential, with ion channels opening in sequence all the way down an axon, the electrical signal maintains the same strength throughout the entire axon; it does not weaken the farther it extends distally. In neurons with axon collaterals, or branches, the action potential continues down each branch at the same rate and strength. For example, imagine an axon with a single collateral. When the action potential reaches the branch, voltage-gated sodium channels in each of the branches will open when the depolarization reaches the split point, thus allowing the action potential to be conducted separately in each of the collaterals.

Box 3–6. Toxins and Sodium Ion Channels

Several toxins affect the function of voltage-gated sodium channels. Tetrodotoxin, produced by puffer fish, blocks Na^+ channels, preventing the influx of sodium. Action potentials cannot be created without the sodium influx, and thus neuronal signals cannot be sent. Other toxins, such as those from buttercups, lilies, scorpions, and sea anemones, result in Na^+ channels opening at a lower threshold; thus, instead of opening only when the –50 mV threshold is achieved, the channels may open at –60 mV; this would lead to too many action potentials.

Once the action potential reaches the axon terminal, the depolarization signals the opening of voltage-gated calcium (Ca^{2+}) channels. Remember that calcium has a higher concentration outside the cell and thus will flow into the cell, down its gradient. The presence of calcium in the axon terminal signals the release of neurotransmitters, thus beginning the chemical phase of synaptic transmission. This process is described in detail in the section titled Synaptic Transmission.

Myelinated Versus Unmyelinated Axons

In unmyelinated axons, the sequence of events described previously occurs along the extent of the entire axon from proximal (soma) to distal (axon terminal). You can think of this as gate-by-gate or channel-by-channel transmission, which is slower and results in more signal loss. In myelinated axons, the myelin covers much of the surface of the axon membrane. There are exposed sections, however, in the nodes of Ranvier, which have a high density of ion channels. It is within these nodes that the ion channels and pumps are located, and where the ion exchanges take place. Once the Na^+ ions enter the axon at one node, they diffuse down the axon to the next node, where a new set of sodium channels open in response to the depolarization. Thus, the action potential appears to "jump" down the axon from node to node. This action is called **saltatory conduction** (Latin: *soltare* = *to hop or dance*). The presence of myelin, as noted previously, speeds up the transmission of the electrical signal down the axon. Figure 3–6 illustrates the differences.

Synaptic Transmission

There are two types of synapses: electrical and chemical. Electrical synapses occur in regions in which neurons are in extremely close proximity to each other, separated by spaces called gap junctions. Ions can move from one neuron to another, creating a direct exchange of electrical signals. Electrical synapses are important for very fast signal transmission. They exist not only between neurons but also between neurons and glia, epithelial cells, and some muscle tissues (smooth and cardiac muscles). Electrical synapses are important for regions in which close synchrony of neural signals is necessary.

Although electrical synapses are spread throughout the CNS and PNS, they are relatively rare in comparison to chemical synapses. In chemical synapses, neurotransmitters act as between-neuron messengers of the electrical signals that exist within neurons. As described previously, once the action potential reaches the axon terminal, the depo-

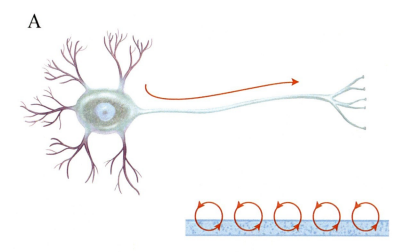

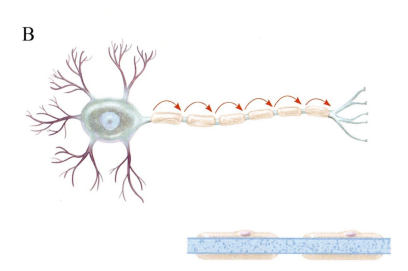

FIGURE 3–6. Action potentials in unmyelinated versus myelinated axons. **A.** In an unmyelinated axon, the exchange of ions in the action potential must occur along the entire length of the axon. **B.** In a myelinated axon, the exchange of ions occurs only at the nodes of Ranvier.

larization causes Ca^{2+} channels to open, allowing Ca^{2+} to enter the terminal. The presence of Ca^{2+} signals actions of several proteins that cause synaptic vesicles to move toward the **active zones** of the cell membrane. The vesicles then fuse with the cell membrane, allowing the neurotransmitter to be released into the synaptic gap (i.e., exocytosis; Figure 3–7). The vesicle membrane then detaches and moves back into the axon terminal for recycling. The amount of neurotransmitter released depends on two factors. First, is the size of the synaptic vesicle. Small vesicles have smaller quantities of neurotransmitter than larger synaptic vesicles. Second, is the amount of calcium that enters the axon terminal: more calcium will result in the release of more vesicles and thus more neurotransmitters.

Once released into the synaptic cleft, the neurotransmitters diffuse through the cleft to the postsynaptic neuron, where they bind to specific receptors. The neurotransmitters and receptors work as "lock and key" mechanisms. When a neurotransmitter binds to a receptor, it causes a change to ion channels. For ionotropic channels (see Box 3–2), neurotransmitter binding will directly open ion channels. Other receptors, called G protein-coupled receptors

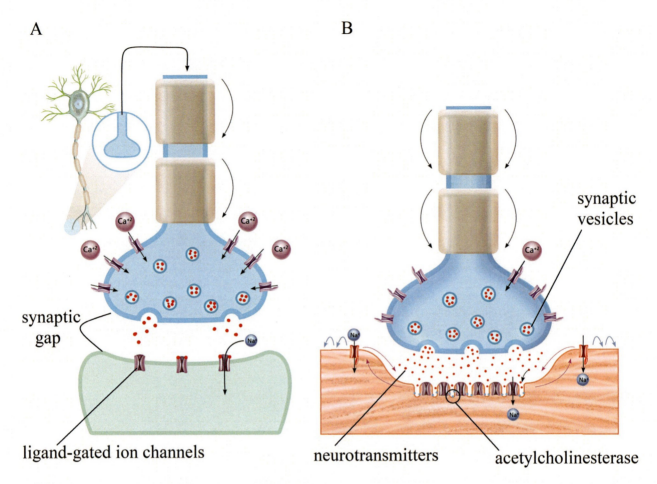

FIGURE 3–7. Actions at the synapse. When the action potential (*noted by arrows*) reaches the axon terminal, the depolarization triggers the opening of voltage-gated calcium (Ca^{2+}) ion channels. Calcium flows into the cell, triggering the release of neurotransmitters. **A.** In a neuron–neuron synapse, the neurotransmitters bind to ligand-gated ion channels, which opens those channels and allows the flow of ions. **B.** In a neuron–muscle synapse, the neurotransmitter binds to receptors that trigger the opening of sodium channels.

(GPCRs), have a more complicated response. When the neurotransmitter binds to a GPCR, it triggers a change to the structure of a G protein within the postsynaptic neuron, which in turn will either open ion channels or trigger additional proteins or enzymes (second messengers) that impact the ion channels. Second messengers serve to relay signals received at receptors but also substantially amplify signal strength. As you might guess, synaptic transmission is much faster via ionotropic receptors given the direct connection to the ion channels and occurs within milliseconds. In contrast, the effects of G protein and second-messenger systems can take hundreds of milliseconds or longer. In either case, after binding to the receptor, the neurotransmitter is then released and moves back into the synaptic cleft. It is removed from the synaptic cleft—either recycled through endocytosis or destroyed—so that the synaptic cleft is left clear of chemicals and in essence is reset for the next transmission.

The ion channels that are opened determine the resulting effect on the postsynaptic neuron. If sodium or calcium channels are opened, Na^+ or Ca^{2+} will move into the postsynaptic neuron, creating an EPSP. If potassium or chloride channels are opened, the movement of K^+ out or Cl^- in results in an IPSP. The creation of EPSPs and IPSPs takes us back to the beginning of the explanation of neuronal communication; these potentials can summate and either depolarize or hyperpolarize the cell. This neuron now becomes the presynaptic neuron.

Types of Neurotransmitters

There are a variety of different neurotransmitters that can be categorized into three groups: amino acids, amines, and peptides. The three amino acids include the 3 G's: glutamate (Glu), gamma-aminobutyric acid (GABA), and glycine (Gly). The amines include acetylcholine (ACh), dopamine (DA), norepinephrine (NE), and serotonin (5-HT). Enkephalins, endorphins, and substance P are examples of peptides. There are several important differences between peptides and the small molecule neurotransmitters. First, peptides are stored in secretory granules instead of synaptic vesicles, and these granules are not in close proximity to the active zones or the Ca^{2+} channels. Second, because of their placement, a greater influx of Ca^{2+} is required to trigger their release. Third, the release time is much slower: 50 mV compared to 0.2 mV for the amines and amino acids. Finally, they are not removed from the synapse as quickly as other neurotransmitters (see the following section), allowing them to have a longer lasting effect.

Specific neurotransmitters are associated with different systems and functions within the CNS and PNS. Although most neurotransmitters tend to have either excitatory or inhibitory effects, the determination is made by the receptors. As described later in relation to DA, a single neurotransmitter can have either excitatory or inhibitory effects depending on the receptor to which it binds.

Table 3-1 lists these neurotransmitters, regions of concentration, and effects of disruption to the neurons or neurotransmitter levels. Those that have direct relevance to cognition, communication, and swallowing processes are described in more detail.

Neurons that release or respond to GABA are widely spread throughout the cortex as well as the hippocampus and cerebellum. GABA's function is primarily inhibitory. Loss of GABAergic neurons (those that release and/or respond to GABA) in the caudate nucleus results in Huntington disease, which is characterized by slow, writhing, unwanted movements and cognitive deficits. This movement disorder can interrupt speech production and nonverbal communication modes such as facial expression and gestures. The unwanted movements are a result of the loss of inhibition within the motor system so that excitatory signals are not in balance with inhibitory signals, thus causing too many signals to be sent to the muscles.

As described later, GABA agonist drugs can be used to treat disorders of anxiety, insomnia, and epilepsy, for which there is too much excitability within regions of the nervous system. The drugs facilitate the effects of GABA, thus increasing the number of inhibitory signals to balance out the excess excitability.

Glutamate is the primary excitatory neurotransmitter in the CNS. Most neurons and some glial cells have glutamate receptors, and the vast majority can release glutamate. When glutamate binds to its receptors, sodium and/or calcium channels are opened, resulting in influx of these ions and depolarization and EPSPs in the postsynaptic neuron. The glutaminergic system is incredibly complex, with multiple receptor types with different functions and a precise mechanism for glutamate reuptake. The reuptake systems are critical because excess glutamate can result in excitotoxicity, in which too much Ca^{2+} enters the cell, disrupting the cells' energy production and limiting the effectiveness of the ion pumps. The continued influx of Ca^{2+} causes continued release of glutamate, which results in repeated EPSPs. The result is too much excitation in the region, hence excitotoxicity. Excitotoxicity results in damage and/or death to neurons.

Acetylcholine is the primary neurotransmitter in the PNS as it is released at the neuromuscular junction and causes muscle contractions. As such, it is involved in most voluntary movements of the body as well as some involuntary movements. ACh is also found in some cortical networks, including those that connect the frontal lobes and the hippocampi. ACh has been implicated in Alzheimer disease.

Dopamine is an important part of the motor system and is found in many regions of the basal ganglia. Dopaminergic neurons (those that release and/or respond to DA) are found within the reward systems of the brain as well as circuits for cognitive processing and motivation. Parkinson disease is associated with disruption to DA production and results in motor system deficits as well as cognitive impairment. Dopaminergic neuron systems have also been implicated in schizophrenia.

As noted previously, DA can have either excitatory or inhibitory effects depending on the receptor to which it binds. In the motor system, there are two types of DA receptors: D1 and D2. When DA binds to D1 receptors, the result is excitatory; when it binds to D2 receptors, the result is inhibitory. This dual function of DA is one of the reasons that Parkinson disease, which is caused by destruction of DA-generating neurons in the brainstem, results in seemingly contradictory symptoms: both too much movement (tremors) and not enough movement (facial masking, reduced range of motion, slowed movement).

Table 3-1. Common Neurotransmitters

Neurotransmitter	Location	Function	Effects of Disruption
Amino acids: small organic molecules released at synapses from synaptic vesicles			
Gamma-aminobutyric acid (GABA)	Cortex, hippocampus, cerebellum	Inhibitory effects and regulation	Huntington disease
Glutamate (Glu)	Various areas within the CNS	Fast synaptic transmission	Schizophrenia
Amines: small organic molecules released at synapses from synaptic vesicles			
Acetylcholine (ACh)	Neuromuscular junction	Voluntary movement; some involuntary movement	Myasthenia gravis, weakness, paralysis
	Frontal lobes, hippocampi	Cognitive networks, memory processes	Alzheimer disease
Dopamine (DA)	Basal ganglia	Motor system	Parkinson disease
	Frontal lobes, limbic system, reward centers	Reward behaviors, motivation	Gambling/sex addictions; cognitive deficits
Epinephrine	Sympathetic nervous system, through bloodstream	Increases heart rate, muscle activation, blood pressure, and sugar metabolism	Anxiety, depression, blood pressure changes (low levels) Tachycardia, hypertension, anxiety, weight loss, excessive sweating (elevated levels)
Norepinephrine (NE)	Brainstem (locus coeruleus), thalamus, cortex, limbic system	Attention and vigilance	Anxiety, depression, lethargy, inattention (low levels) Hypertension, sweating, irregular heartbeat, headaches (elevated levels)
	Sympathetic nervous system	Fight-or-flight response	
Serotonin (5-HT)	Various areas within the CNS	Sleep cycles, mood, modulation of pain input	Depression
Peptides: large molecules released from axon terminal from secretory granules			
Enkephalin	Opioid receptors	Regulate nociception and reduce substance P release in dorsal horn of spinal cord to inhibit pain	Parkinson disease (low levels) Diabetes and Alzheimer disease (high levels)
Substance P	Sensory nerve endings and inflammatory cells (macrophages, eosinophils, lymphocytes)	Transmits pain information from PNS to CNS	Inflammation, arthritis, fibromyalgia (elevated levels)

Although each synaptic vesicle contains only one type of neurotransmitter, within any one axon terminal there may be different sets of vesicles containing different neurotransmitters. For example, peptides and either amines or amino acids often reside in the same axon terminal. Whether or not one or both are released depends in part on how much Ca^{2+} enters the axon terminal.

Neurotransmitter Recovery and Degradation

There are two methods of removing neurotransmitters from the synaptic cleft after they bind to receptors on the postsynaptic membrane. One method is reuptake (endocytosis). Reuptake essentially allows for the neurotransmitter molecules to be recycled. They diffuse back toward the presynaptic axon terminal and are taken back into the axon terminal. From there, they can be repackaged into a new synaptic vesicle for future release.

The second method is degradation. Some neurotransmitters are destroyed by enzymes in the synaptic cleft. A prime example is ACh. Acetylcholine esterase (AChE) is an enzyme that destroys ACh. Once ACh binds to its receptors and then releases, AChE enters the synaptic cleft and "eats up" the ACh, thus leaving the cleft clear for the next synaptic transmission.

Creating Meaning from Binary Signals

As described previously, neurons can only send two signals: excitatory (go) and inhibitory (no go). From this binary system, all human activity, including reflexes and patterned responses as well as complex emotions, thoughts, and reasoning, is created. The complex responses arise from patterns of excitatory and inhibitory signals, the source of the signals, and the region or location within the brain that receives the signals.

Patterns of Signals

Remember that each neuron receives signals from, and sends signals to, hundreds or thousands of other neurons. It is not a simple 1:1 relay system. Patterns also can be created by the timing and concentration of signals. Remember that action potentials are all the same strength; there are no stronger versus weaker action potentials. In addition, although the speed of action potentials differs across neurons based on the diameter of the axon and the presence of myelin, each individual axon transmits action potentials at the same speed, so there is no way for a neuron to send faster or slower action potentials. One factor that can be manipulated is the number of action potentials sent within a span of time. Throughout the sensory systems, intensity of sensations generally is coded by the number of action potentials created within a time frame. For example, in the somatosensory system, a touch with light pressure will result in fewer action potentials per millisecond compared to deeper pressure. In the somatosensory strip in the brain, a greater number of action potentials results in more releases of neurotransmitters, which are interpreted by cortical neurons as greater pressure. Similarly, louder sounds result in more action potentials in inner ear neurons than do softer sounds.

Signals of different strength can be sent at the synapse. The amount of neurotransmitter released can vary, thus creating EPSPs and IPSPs that vary in strength. A few large EPSPs can summate faster than multiple small EPSPs, resulting in faster generation of an action potential in the postsynaptic neuron.

Patterns of neuron connections and circuits also aid in conveying meaning (Figure 3–8). Neurons can be arranged in divergent circuits in which a small number of neurons connect to increasingly larger pools to convey signals more broadly throughout the system. Alternately, there are convergent circuits in which axons from many neurons converge onto just a few neurons, resulting in multiple signals concentrated onto a small region of cells. In addition, some systems include reverberating circuits in which one axon collateral extends back to its own soma. In this arrangement, each time the neuron fires an action potential, it receives an EPSP from that collateral. This aids in keeping the neuron continuously firing until it is inhibited by a different neuron. In a sequential system, signals are processed in serial, one at a time. In a parallel circuit, signals are processed synchronously along multiple neuron chains.

An illustration of patterns of connections can be found in **lateral inhibition**. Lateral inhibition occurs in the sensory system to aid in precise perception of sensory stimuli. The ability to identify the borders of objects visually, the ability to identify the specific location of a touch on one's hand, and the ability to perceive a specific pitch are all aided by lateral inhibition.

When a touch is applied to the hand, the mechanoreceptors directly at the site are stimulated, sending excitatory signals up to the brain (Figure 3–9). Axon collaterals branching off from these target neurons synapse onto interneurons that send an inhibitory signal to neighboring mechanoreceptive neurons, thus decreasing the probability that they will generate action potentials and send signals to

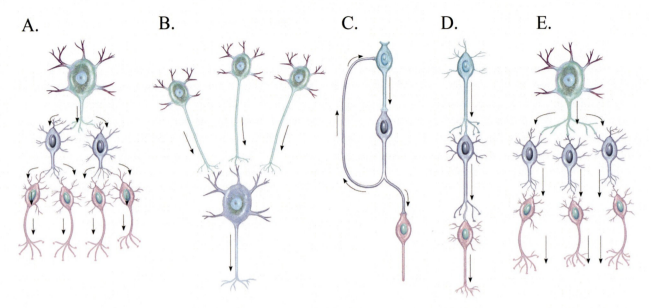

FIGURE 3–8. Neuron circuits. **A.** Divergent circuit. **B.** Convergent circuit. **C.** Reverberating circuit. **D.** Serial circuit. **E.** Parallel circuit.

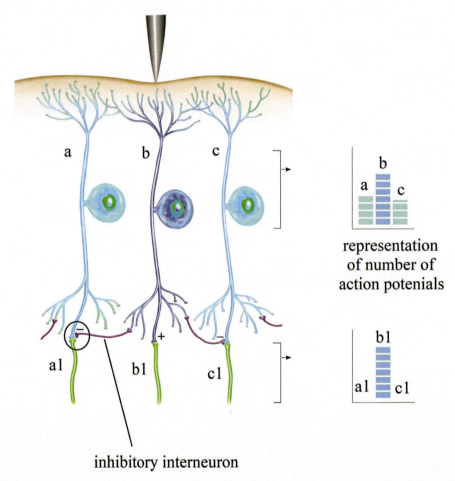

FIGURE 3–9. Lateral inhibition. Mechanical stimulation creates a large number of action potentials at the exact site of the simulation and fewer action potentials in nearby neurons. Inhibitory interneurons synapse with the nearby neuron pathways, reducing the number of action potentials so that the signals that reach the brain are nearly all from the path leading from the exact site of the stimulation.

the brain. This aids in localization of touch because excitatory signals will be conveyed to the cortical neurons representing the exact location of the touch on the hand while the neurons representing nearby locations will receive fewer signals because the stimulus was inhibited at a lower level of the pathway. Without lateral inhibition, more action potentials would be sent from the target mechanoreceptive neurons than from those in the adjacent regions because of the difference in pressure. This still would aid in localization, but the precision would not be as good as when the adjacent regions receive few, if any, signals, as opposed to simply fewer signals.

Source of Signals

Interpretation of signals also is related to the source. The contribution of the source also can be illustrated by the sensory systems. As described in Chapter 6, there are different somatosensory neurons specialized to respond to different types of sensation. Mechanoreceptors respond to touch, nociceptors respond to pain, and thermoreceptors respond to temperature. Stepping onto sand on the beach, the feel of the coarseness of the sand will result in action potentials sent via the somatosensory touch pathways, whereas signals for the temperature will be sent via the thermoreceptor pathways. If the sand is hot enough to burn the skin, then signals also will be sent along nociceptive (pain) pathways. The combination of these signals reaching the cortex will be interpreted as coarse or fine sand that is hot or cool and whether it is hot enough to be painful.

Region or Location

Intraoperative monitoring provides examples of the contribution of location. During brain surgery, it is possible to apply electrical stimulation to regions of the cortex. Experiments by William Calvin and George Ojemann (1994) during surgery for epilepsy contributed to our knowledge of localization of function in the brain. An electrical pulse is, by itself, uninformative. It carries no meaning. Application of an electrical stimulus will create an EPSP in the targeted neurons. If those neurons are in the motor strip, the stimulus will cause movement, such as twitching of the thumb. If that same neutral, nonmeaningful stimulus is applied to neurons in the sensory strip, the person will report feeling a sensation. If the stimulus is applied in the primary auditory area, sound will be reported. Thus, the location of the neurons stimulated influences the interpretation of what is, in isolation, a meaningless signal.

Box 3–7. That Neuron Rings a Bell: Location Determines Function

The interpretation of neural signals based on source or location is analogous to interpreting the meaning of a "ding" of a bell. If you are in an elevator and hear a ding, you know that it means you have reached a new floor. If you are in a kitchen and you hear a ding, you know it is a timer (perhaps the microwave?) signaling that something is done cooking. If you are in a busy diner, a ding may mean an order is ready. If you are in a car, a ding can signal that someone is not wearing a seat belt. If it arises from your smartphone, it indicates you have a new message. In each case, the signal is the same—a simple ding—yet in each location/context it means something completely different. In the nervous system, each excitatory signal can be thought of as the ding of a bell. If it occurs in the auditory cortex, it signals a sound; in the visual cortex, it signals an image. If that ding was created by a somatosensory mechanoreceptive neuron, it signals touch or pressure, whereas if it was transmitted by a somatosensory thermoreceptive neuron, it signals temperature.

Conditions That Alter Synaptic Transmission

Neurologic Disorders and Diseases That Affect Synaptic Transmission

There are many diseases and disorders that affect neuronal function with consequences for swallowing and communication. Some, such as strokes, amyotrophic lateral sclerosis, Alzheimer disease, or traumatic brain injury, result in neuronal death. These are discussed in later chapters because the consequences depend on the location of the damage within the nervous system. Others, such as Parkinson disease (PD), multiple sclerosis, and myasthenia gravis (MG), affect the functions of neurons. These are discussed briefly here to illustrate the effects of disruptions to different stages of synaptic transmission.

Parkinson Disease

Parkinson disease is caused by degeneration of neurons within the substantia nigra (black substance) located in the midbrain. These are dopaminergic neurons that synapse within regions of the basal ganglia. As a result, there is not enough dopamine at dopaminergic synapses, particularly within the basal ganglia. Remember that there are two forms of dopamine receptors: D1 receptors, which are excitatory, and D2 receptors, which are inhibitory. As described in more detail in Chapter 10, a delicate balance of excitatory and inhibitory signals throughout the structures of the basal ganglia is required for just the right amount of movement. Loss of dopamine alters this balance and results in both too much movement and not enough movement.

Too much movement is apparent in the resting tremors characteristic of PD. Such tremors are a result of either too much excitation or not enough inhibition within the motor system, resulting in action potentials traveling down the motor tracts to the muscles and creating unwanted movement. Not enough movement is apparent in the masked face; individuals with PD often have limited facial expression and, in severe cases, can appear to be wearing a mask because there is little or no movement of facial muscles. Voice and speech production are also affected by too much inhibition. In this case, the range of motion of the articulators is reduced. The result is that articulation is less precise but also faster: When the tongue and lips do not move as far as they should, they can move faster than typical to create speech sounds, albeit with reduced articulatory precision. In addition, the voice can be weak and breathy because of reduced adduction of the vocal folds.

The characteristic shuffling gait is also a result of not enough excitation or too much inhibition. As with speech production, there is a reduced range of motion of the legs when walking so that the person takes short shuffling steps. In PD, the movements become increasingly smaller over time. This is called festination. Although the steps are fast, amplitude of movement is low, resulting in bradykinesia (slow movement). The net effect is hypokinesia (less movement).

Multiple Sclerosis

Multiple sclerosis is an autoimmune disease in which the body's immune system attacks the oligodendrocytes that create myelin in the CNS. When the myelin is destroyed, action potentials move more slowly down the axon. This will alter the timing of neural signals. Once the myelin is destroyed, the axons also can degenerate, which will in turn lead to neuronal death.

Multiple sclerosis is a progressive disorder, meaning that it gets worse over time. However, there are different courses of progression. The most common is a relapsing–remitting progression in which symptoms get worse for a period of time (relapse), and then the immune system slows or stops its attack and the myelin regenerates. This is accompanied by a reduction in symptoms (remission). An individual may or may not return to their original level of function during the remission. This depends in part on whether or not axonal damage and neuronal death occur or if only the myelin is damaged. A second pattern is slowly progressive, in which the symptoms just slowly worsen over time without periods of remission or recovery.

Symptoms of multiple sclerosis vary depending on which neurons are affected. Slowed thinking (bradyphrenia) and other cognitive symptoms occur if neurons in the frontal lobe are affected or if there is widespread damage. Motor deficits including poor coordination, weakness, or muscle spasticity can occur if the neurons in the motor system are affected, and double vision and loss of vision are a result of attacks to the visual pathways.

Swallowing and speech production can be affected if motor systems are compromised. Communication can be affected by changes in cognition, including slowed processing, memory deficits, or attentional deficits.

Myasthenia Gravis

Myasthenia gravis is an autoimmune disease that affects ACh receptors in the neuromuscular junction. In MG, antibodies block and destroy ACh receptors on skeletal muscles. In early stages of the disease, the antibodies block the ACh receptors. When ACh is released at the neuromuscular junction, there are not many open receptors to which the neurotransmitter can bind. This results in weakened muscle contraction. Muscle weakness increases over time with continued use of a muscle. Essentially, the ACh that was not absorbed through reuptake is broken down by AChE and not available for immediate use. This depletes the store of ACh available for subsequent calls for muscle contractions. When a person rests, muscle strength can return because ACh components (broken down by AChE) can be recycled into useable ACh in nearby neurons.

One of the tests for diagnosing MG is the injection of an anticholinesterase drug such as neostigmine, prostigmine, tensilon, or Mestinon. (Note that tensilon was formerly used for testing but has been discontinued in the United States.) These drugs block the cholinesterase enzymes that break down ACh in the synaptic cleft, leaving the ACh in the synaptic cleft for longer periods of time. The ACh will then be able to bind, release, and bind again to the ACh receptors on the muscle and create stronger muscle contractions.

Weakness of the articulators can be observed if the individual is asked to talk for a long period of time (e.g., count for several minutes). Decreased precision of articulation will be noticed along with increased hypernasality as weakness affects the soft palate. In relation to swallowing, individuals with MG may have to plan their meals carefully. They may select softer foods that do not require excessive chewing because that will cause increased weakness. They also may eat several small meals a day so that they do not become too weak to finish a meal or to safely swallow. Furthermore, coordinating timing of medications, such as Mestinon, with mealtimes is often crucial in order to benefit optimally from the effects of the medication.

Pharmacological Effects on Synaptic Transmission

Pharmacological agents, both legal and illegal drugs, can affect the transmission of signals at the synaptic cleft. Drugs that have neurological effects can block, prolong, or mimic the actions of natural neurotransmitters. Brief explanations of these help illustrate the different stages of synaptic transmission.

Blocking Effects

Drugs that have blocking effects can prevent the release of neurotransmitters from the synaptic vesicles or prevent the binding of the neurotransmitters to the receptors. Several poisons and toxins have a blocking effect.

Botulinum toxin (Botox) prevents synaptic vesicles from releasing neurotransmitters into the synaptic cleft, thus blocking synaptic transmission. Botox works primarily at the neuromuscular junction, causing weakness or paralysis of muscles.

The poison curare also causes paralysis, but in a slightly different way. Curare blocks ACh receptors on the postsynaptic membrane at the neuromuscular junction. Thus, when ACh is released, it is unable to bind to the blocked receptors, and no muscle contraction is created. Early South American hunters would dip their arrow tips in curare, which would cause paralysis of the animals hit by the arrows. In the mid-1900s, it was used as a component of anesthesia to paralyze patients undergoing surgery. Curare cannot pass through the blood–brain barrier, and thus it does not affect cholinergic synapses in the CNS.

Atropine and tropicamide are anticholinergic drugs used by optometrists and ophthalmologists to dilate the pupil. They work via the same mechanism as curare, preventing ACh from binding to postsynaptic receptors. The muscles that constrict the pupil are temporarily paralyzed, resulting in dilation of the pupil.

Prolonging Effects

Drugs that have prolonging effects increase the amount of time neurotransmitters stay within the synaptic cleft. As described previously, after neurotransmitters bind to postsynaptic receptors and then are released back into the cleft, they are either recycled in the axon terminal through reuptake or cleaned out via enzymatic destruction. Prolonging effects are created by limiting these actions. One example is the class of drugs called selective serotonin reuptake inhibitors (SSRIs). As the name suggests, these drugs inhibit or slow down the reuptake process specifically for serotonin. After serotonin binds and then is released from the postsynaptic receptors, it should be absorbed back into the axon terminal. The presence of SSRIs prevents or slows this reuptake process, leaving the serotonin in the synaptic cleft, where it can then bind again to the receptors.

Box 3–8. Botox

In the United States, the first US Food and Drug Administration-approved use of Botox was for spasmodic dysphonia (SD), a speech disorder in which the laryngeal adductor muscles (those that adduct, or close the vocal folds) spasm and create tight closure of the vocal folds, making voicing exceedingly difficult. Botox can be injected into the thyrovocalis muscle so that the vocal folds cannot adduct too tightly. In the first few days after an injection, the client's voice is weak and breathy, and they must be cautious about swallowing to prevent aspiration (food/liquid passing through the vocal folds and entering the bronchi and lungs). The toxin wears off after several months, so individuals with SD have to return for repeat injections. It was several years later that Botox was approved for use in facial muscles, such as the frontalis muscle, to "erase" wrinkles on the forehead related to aging.

In this way, the postsynaptic neuron responds as if there was more serotonin released initially. Serotonin generally results in EPSPs and thus repeated binding of serotonin will increase the number of EPSPs and increase the probability of generating an action potential in the postsynaptic neuron. Serotonin stabilizes mood and is associated with happiness and sense of well-being; thus, keeping it in the cleft increases these outcomes. SSRIs such as fluoxetine (Prozac) and citalopramare (Celexa) are commonly used to treat depression.

Acetylcholinesterase inhibitors are another class of drugs that have a prolonging effect. These reduce the enzymatic destruction of ACh by interfering with the action of AChE. Slowing of ACh destruction allows the neurotransmitter to stay in the synaptic cleft longer and re-bind to the postsynaptic receptor. Examples of AChE inhibitors include donezepil (Aricept), used to treat Alzheimer disease, and pyridostigmine (Mestinon), used for MG. Neostigmine (Prostigmine) is a short-acting AChE inhibitor that can be used to diagnose MG.

Mimicking Effect

Some pharmaceuticals are designed to be similar enough in shape and chemical makeup that the nervous system "mistakes" them for natural neurotransmitters and they bind to the neurotransmitter-specific postsynaptic receptors. Benzodiazepines can mimic natural GABA, which has an inhibitory effect. When GABA binds to its receptors, chloride channels open, allowing chloride into the cell, which causes hyperpolarization through IPSPs. Benzodiazepines can bind to GABA receptors and thus cause IPSPs. The increased inhibition leads to the "downer" effect of benzodiazepine drugs, which can be useful for anxiety disorders in which there is too much excitation in neural circuits.

Summary

Neurons are specialized cells that are designed to send and receive signals. Signals within a neuron are electrical, whereas signals sent between neurons or between neurons and muscles are almost always chemical. Electrical signals are created by the movement of ions across the cell membrane. Chemical signals are created by neurotransmitters released from one neuron that bind to and create electrical change in another neuron. Synaptic transmission results in either excitatory or inhibitory signals. The patterns and locations of these signals are interpreted by the nervous system as meaningful messages. Dysfunction of neurons or synaptic transmission can result in specific disorders that affect movement, sensation, language, or cognition, depending on the location.

Key Concepts

- Neurons can send two types of signals—excitatory (go) and inhibitory (no go).
- Neurons maintain an intentional ionic differential (imbalance) in order to create membrane potentials that allow for energy creation (action potential) to propagate signals along axons.
- At resting membrane potential, there is a net positive charge in extracellular space and a net negative charge within intracellular space, with more Na^+ and Ca^{+2} outside and more K^+ inside.
- During passive transport, ions move freely or diffuse from areas of greater concentration to lesser concentration, seeking equilibrium.
- Depolarization occurs with EPSPs, as sodium diffuses into neurons via passive transport.
- Hyperpolarization occurs with IPSPs, as either potassium diffuses out or chloride diffuses in via passive transport.
- The sodium–potassium ion pump uses active transport, fueled by ATP, to move ions against their concentration gradients to restore ion differentials to resting membrane potential.
- Summation is the process of adding up subthreshold signals that are in close physical proximity to each other (spatial summation) or that occurred in close time proximity to each other (temporal summation).
- When a presynaptic axon terminal is depolarized, calcium diffuses into the end terminal, which signals synaptic vesicles to migrate to the surface of the terminal and release neurotransmitters into the synapse. This process is called exocytosis.
- Neurotransmitters selectively bind to receptors on the postsynaptic neuron, activating that neuron and returning to the action potential process.
- The neuromuscular junction is a synapse involving neuron-to-muscle communication, rather than

neuron-to-neuron communication. ACh is the only neurotransmitter present at this synapse.
- There are three neurotransmitter categories: amino acids, amines, and peptides.
- Neurological disorders can disrupt the functions of neurons. Symptoms reflect the regions of the CNS or PNS affected.
- Drugs with neurological effects have three basic actions: blocking, prolonging, or mimicking the actions of natural neurotransmitters.

Reference and Additional Resources

Calvin, W. H., & Ojemann, G. A. (1994). *Conversations with Neil's brain: The neural nature of thought and language.* Addison-Wesley.

Web links for myasthenia gravis testing
- Prostigmine demonstration for MG (1935): https://www.youtube.com/watch?v=uRoRsmvkhTI
- Positive tensilon test in a dog: https://www.youtube.com/watch?v=k7YX9kuWrxA

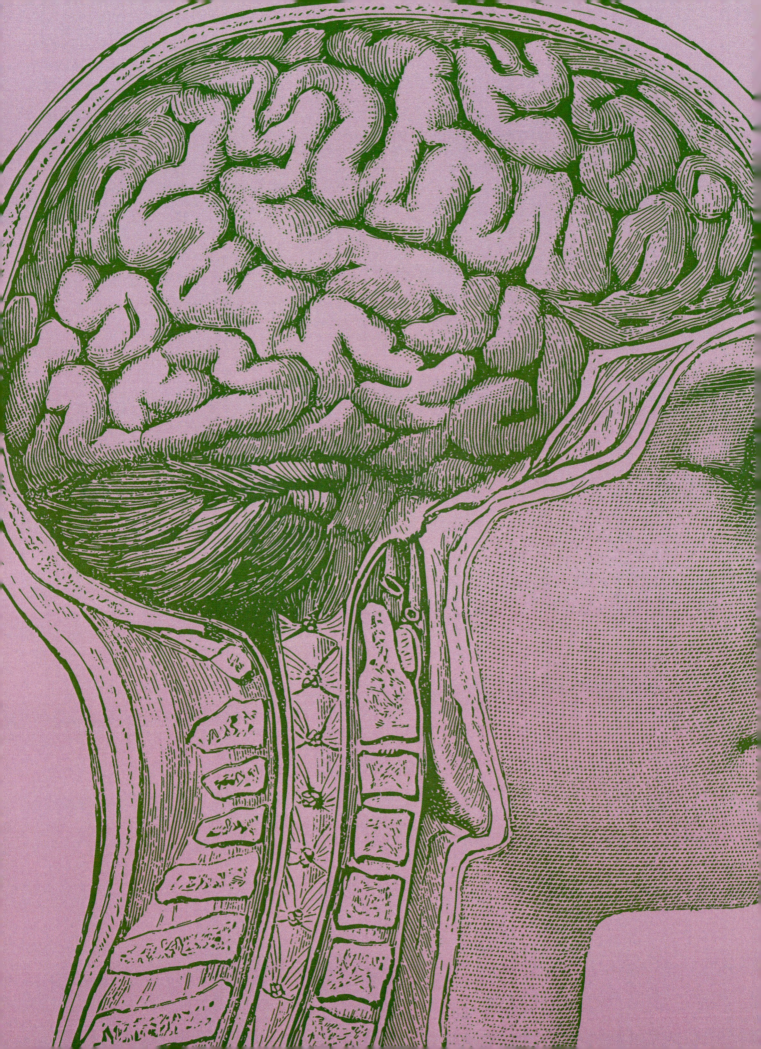

4

Neuroembryology

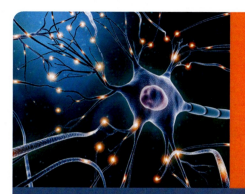

CHAPTER OUTLINE

Overview
The Neural Tube
   Developmental (Embryologic) Precursors
   Sulcus Limitans
   Lamina Terminalis (Precursor to the Corpus Callosum)
   Vesicles of the Neural Tube (CNS Precursors)
Landmark Timelines
Telencephalon and C-Shaped Development
Disruptions to Development and Consequences
Summary
References and Additional Resources

Overview

Neuroembryology can sound complex or intimidating, but this concept simply relates to development of the nervous system. This development is certainly crucial to communication, cognition, and swallowing functions. It provides an explicit connection between biological functions and speech, language, hearing, and swallowing functions. Thus, neuroembryology is pertinent to professionals working in birth-to-three contexts, school-based settings, and medical contexts. Knowledge of typical development helps one better understand disruptions to development or aging that can result in disorders of communication, cognition, or swallowing exhibited by clients in those clinical contexts. Any **teratogens** (i.e., viruses or toxins) or events that disrupt development at any given point in gestation have the potential to lead to a variety of impairments that result in developmental communication disorders. Furthermore, neurodevelopment provides insights into typical aging processes.

To begin, it is helpful to recall what you already know about basic organization of the nervous system. These basic principles will help you make sense of the more complex elements of neurodevelopment. The first foundational concept is the **dichotomy of motor and sensory systems** within the central nervous system (CNS; Figure 4–1). Anterior structures, whether in the cerebrum, brainstem, or spinal cord, primarily house motor functions (*anterior = motor*). Motor functions include gross motor signals, motor planning, and executive functions (prefrontal functions involved in initiating or inhibiting motor actions or thoughts). Posterior structures, throughout the CNS, primarily house sensory functions (*posterior = sensory*). Note that there are a few key exceptions to this, particularly locations of subcortical structures such as the basal ganglia and cerebellum. The neuroembryological precursor to this anterior-to-posterior dichotomy is the **sulcus limitans**, which is discussed later in this chapter.

The second concept relates to communication within the nervous system. As described in previous chapters, **gray matter** processes information, whereas **white matter** transmits it. In the context of development, white matter includes all axons connecting one part of the brain with another or brain-to-body/body-to-brain connections. These connections are formed during development. Initially, those connections are incomplete and often there is more than one pathway to carry out specific functions. Pruning is a selective process of keeping the most efficient

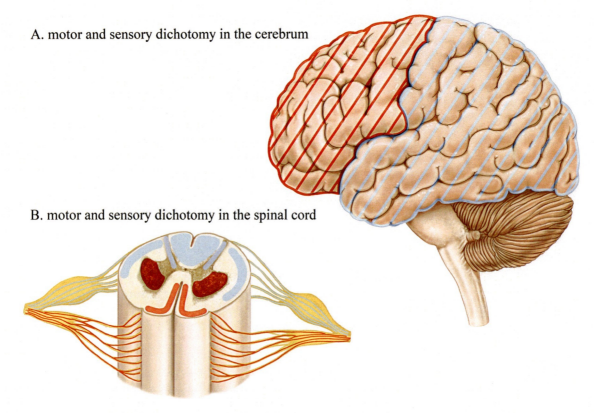

FIGURE 4–1. Motor (*red*) and sensory (*blue*) dichotomy in the central nervous system.

pathways and eliminating (pruning) less efficient pathways. Remember that myelin insulates and protects axons and increases the speed of signal transmission. All infants are born with some myelin, but the cerebral neurons are not fully myelinated until young adulthood. The sensorimotor cortices are fully myelinated by 4 to 6 years, the parietal and temporal association cortices by 10 years, and the prefrontal cortices by 15 to 20 years (Casey et al., 2005). The processes of myelination and pruning occur throughout development. Understanding that these processes are not completed until the adolescent and early adulthood years provides a biological explanation for why cognitive processing is less efficient and less consistent among children and teenagers compared to adults.

The **corpus callosum** is a crucial bundle of pathways that connects the two hemispheres of the brain (Figure 4–2). Development of this complex network of pathways connecting left and right sides, initially known as the **lamina terminalis**, is a key developmental milestone. Gestational week 6 is a crucial week for development of the lamina terminalis, which is the precursor to the corpus callosum. Failure of development of either of these structures is called agenesis of the corpus callosum (ACC; Box 4–1). ACC most typically occurs given a disruption in weeks 12 to 22 of gestation.

The final foundational concept is called **C-shaped** development. Several structures within the cerebrum follow this pattern of development. In short, the brain develops in a C-shaped manner. Posterior structures (near the curve of the C) develop earlier and are preserved later in the aging process. In contrast, anterior structures (toward the upper/lower extent of the C) develop later and decline earlier in typical aging. Details of this concept are explained later in this chapter, but it may help you understand developmental behavior basics. Because the front of the C develops late, knowing what structures are at the front is pertinent. The prefrontal cortex and anterior medial temporal lobe are the two anterior-most portions of the C-shaped development of the cerebrum. The prefrontal cortex has a key role in executive functions (see Chapter 14), and the anterior medial temporal lobe has an important role in new learning and memory formation (see Chapter 12).

As a precursor to discussion of embryologic development, it is helpful to consider the relevance of this knowledge to speech–language pathologists and audiologists. Often, clinicians fail to recognize the relevance of such

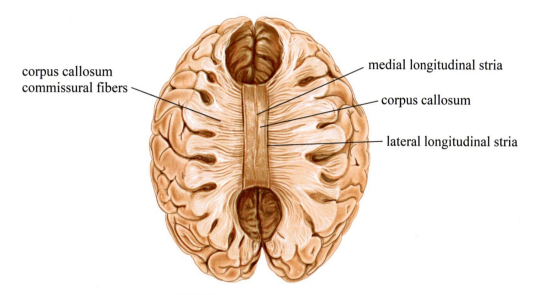

FIGURE 4–2. The corpus callosum.

Box 4–1. Agenesis of the Corpus Callosum

Selika was a 30-year-old female with agenesis of the corpus callosum. There was a lack of development of the corpus callosum in the medial portion of the brain; however, there was a compensatory commissure anteriorly between the two hemispheres of the prefrontal cortex and posteriorly within the parieto-occipital regions between the two hemispheres. Evidence of more substantial than usual connections was indicated on a magnetic resonance imaging (MRI) scan (although prominence may not correlate with efficiency or effectiveness in interhemispheric communication). Etiology of Selika's agenesis is unknown; however, disruptions to development of the corpus callosum can include teratogens (medications or environmental toxins) that chemically block the development process, or trauma. Note that although *agenesis* literally means "lack of development," the term is used to refer to a continuum of disrupted development spanning from a complete lack of commissural fibers between the hemispheres to a reduction in the number of connecting fibers. Selika had moderate impairments in social communication and pragmatics. She displayed limited empathy for others and a lack of theory of mind. She struggled with social conventions in general. One day during a session, she shared "I have a gun in my car." She did not seem to have any malintent by making that statement; she was simply reporting the facts. That being said, it resulted in an obligatory report to security. (See Case 16–19 in Chapter 16 for an extended version of this case.)

developmental steps until there is an impairment due to a lack of complete development. Understanding typical development can help one better understand key timelines for development of neuronal structures and what happens when that development is disrupted.

1. When reviewing a medical record, clinicians should take note of anything that may have disrupted preterm, embryologic development, such as a mother's exposure to medications or toxins, trauma, or inadequate nutrition. Key timelines are discussed in the following section regarding the neural tube and its vesicles.
2. Likewise, one can work backwards by identifying the impairment or lesion to determine likely timelines for disruptions to development.
3. Understanding typical development has relevance for the emergence of abilities such as language and cognition. This is particularly relevant for postnatal development, such as myelination and pruning. In addition, this helps one understand the process of declining functions in typical aging as well as disorders of aging.

The Neural Tube

Developmental (Embryologic) Precursors

The embryo begins as a sheet of cells that divides into three layers (Figure 4–3). The **ectoderm** is a precursor to skin, eyes, and nervous tissue. The **mesoderm** is a precursor to bones, muscles, and blood. Finally, the **endoderm** is a precursor to organs, such as the lungs and liver, and linings of the gut.

The notochord, a component of the mesoderm, provides a structure for the developing embryo and also secretes signals that guide developmental changes. It is a precursor to the vertebral column. A chemical signal from the mesoderm causes thickening of a longitudinal section of the ectoderm. That thickened region becomes the **neural plate** at approximately week 3. Soon after, this neural plate folds inward, creating a neural groove at midline with a neural fold on each side (Figure 4–4). **Dorsal induction** is the process of forming and closing the neural tube. In

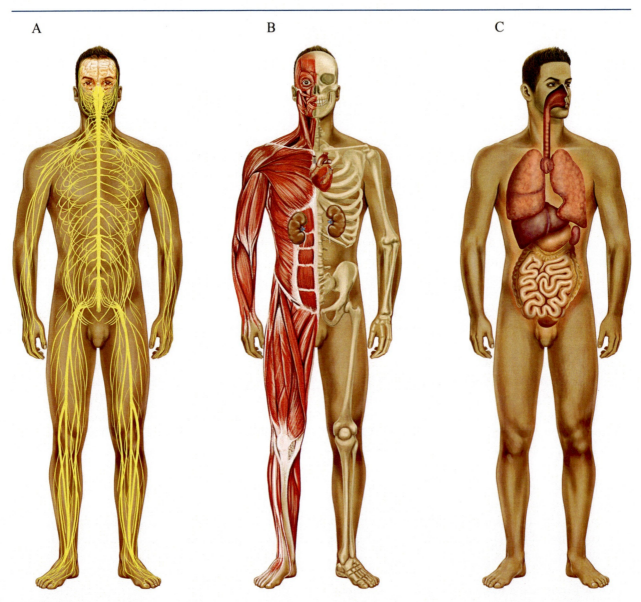

FIGURE 4–3. Embryologic precursors and their roles at maturity. **A.** Ectoderm is a precursor to skin, eyes, and nervous tissue. **B.** Mesoderm is a precursor to bones, muscles, and blood. **C.** Endoderm is a precursor to organs, such as the lungs and liver, and linings of the gut.

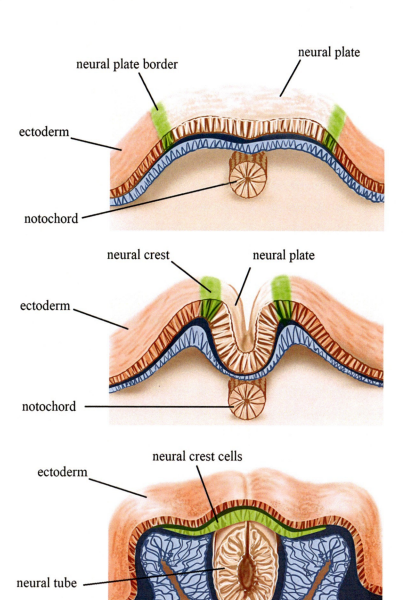
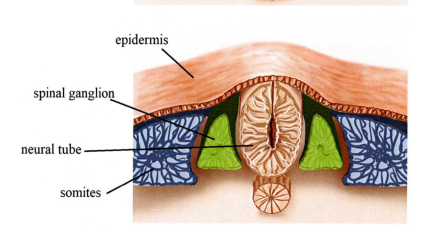

FIGURE 4-4. Development of the neural tube.

this process, also known as primary neurulation, the neural plate bends upwards. See Box 4–2 for anomalies of dorsal induction. By the end of the third week of gestation, the two folds begin to fuse, initiating the formation of the **neural tube**. Closure is complete by the end of the fourth week. As it closes, it leaves cells known as the **neural crest cells**, which are precursors to dorsal root (sensory) ganglia for spinal and sensory cranial nerves, Schwann cells (myelin), and the autonomic nervous system. The neural crest is on the dorsal surface, whereas the notochord is on the anterior surface. The neural tube eventually develops into the entire CNS. The inner cavity becomes the ventricular system. Secondary neurulation includes formation of the distal spinal cord, including sacral and coccygeal segments.

Sulcus Limitans

During the fourth week of gestation, a longitudinal groove begins to separate the dorsal and ventral halves of the neural tube. This is known as the **sulcus limitans**, separating the anterior and posterior halves of what will become the spinal cord and brainstem. The dorsal gray matter becomes the **alar (sensory) plate**, whereas the ventral half forms the **basal (motor) plate**. These are the precursors to the posterior horn and anterior horns of gray matter in the adult spinal cord (Figure 4–5). As described in Chapter 1, the posterior horn houses sensory neurons, whereas the anterior horn houses the somatic and autonomic motor neurons. This sensory/motor dichotomy extends through the entire brainstem and can be partially seen in the cerebrum, although the distribution of functions is less discrete in the cerebrum.

Lamina Terminalis (Precursor to the Corpus Callosum)

The lamina terminalis, a precursor to the corpus callosum, is a thin membrane that connects the two initial swellings of the telencephalon (precursor to the cerebral hemispheres). This takes place at gestational week 6. The corpus callosum is nearly fully developed by gestational weeks 12 to 16. Ultimately, the corpus callosum is a collection of pathways made up of more than 200 million axons that connect the two hemispheres (Luders et al., 2010).

Vesicles of the Neural Tube (CNS Precursors)

Vesicles of the neural tube are developmental precursors to CNS structures, including the brainstem, thalamus, hypothalamus, and cerebral hemispheres (Figure 4–6). Three primary vesicles comprise the neural tube: the **rhombencephalon**, **mesencephalon**, and **prosencephalon**. The face and brain develop from those three vesicles in a process called **ventral induction**. Essentially, this is closure of the cerebral and facial midline. This takes place between gestational weeks 5 and 18. See Box 4–3 for anomalies of ventral induction. The three primary vesicles then divide into secondary vesicles. The rhombencephalon divides into the **myelencephalon**, which is a precursor to the medulla (and spinal cord), and the **metencephalon**, which becomes the pons and cerebellum. The mesencephalon has no secondary vesicles but becomes the midbrain. The tectum arises from the dorsal mesencephalon, eventually becoming the dorsal midbrain. It has two main elements—the

---

Box 4–2. Anomalies of Dorsal Induction

The first two anomalies, anencephaly and exencephaly, are rare and generally result in death preterm or soon after birth.

- Anencephaly: Lack of development of the cerebral hemispheres; absent frontal, parietal, and occipital bones; accompanied by anomalies to the cerebellum, brainstem, and spinal cord.
- Exencephaly: Brain tissue that protrudes outside of the cranial vault and is not encompassed by skin due to partial or complete lack of skull development. Exposure of brain tissue to amniotic fluid and trauma (due to lack of protection of the brain) leads to severe brain damage.
- Cephaloceles: Protrusion of brain, spinal, or meningeal tissues through skin and bony structures.
- Chiari malformation: Herniation of the cerebellum through the foramen magnum.
- Spinal dysraphism and spina bifida: failure of the bony posterior spine to develop and/or failure of neuronal tissues to fuse. Can lead to herniation of the meninges and spinal cord through the posterior spine, known as a myelomeningocele.

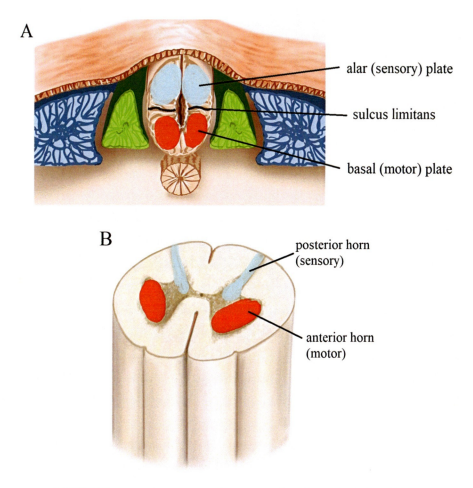

FIGURE 4–5. Cross sections of the neural tube (**A**) and spinal cord (**B**).

superior colliculus, which controls eye movement, and the inferior colliculus, which is part of the auditory pathway. Finally, the prosencephalon expands to form the **diencephalon** and **telencephalon**. The diencephalon gives rise to the thalamus, hypothalamus, retina, and parts of the basal ganglia. It is notable that the basal ganglia sometimes appear to be a part of the telencephalon vesicle; however, it is an embryonic derivative of the diencephalon. Finally, the telencephalon is a precursor to the cerebral hemispheres.

Initial development of cerebral structures begins as the vesicles of the neural tube begin to differentiate (Figure 4–7). Specifically, the prosencephalon becomes the cerebrum, including the cerebral hemispheres, thalamus, hypothalamus, and basal ganglia. Each cerebral hemisphere begins with a smooth surface and becomes increasingly convoluted with sulci and gyri. Those increased convolutions (gyrification) create more surface area for gray matter processing (Zilles et al., 2013). Massive neuronal proliferation and migration of neurons and glial cells account for these morphological changes to the surfaces of the cerebrum. Neuron precursors proliferate along the central zone of the neural tube, which becomes the ventricles. At the peak of proliferation, 250,000 new neurons form every minute. Neuronal migration is the process of neurons migrating from their embryological origin to their final position in the brain/CNS. Much of the neuronal development and migration takes place during months 3 to 5 of gestation. There are two main types of migration—radial and tangential. It may help to think of this process as covering development of all of the necessary angles and spaces of the brain. Radial migration is when neurons are displaced laterally and perpendicularly by new neurons. Tangential migration is when neurons are displaced by new neurons, parallel and orthogonally (imagine a honeycomb, where the neuron moves from one octagon to the next). This process is essential to development of proper neuronal circuits,

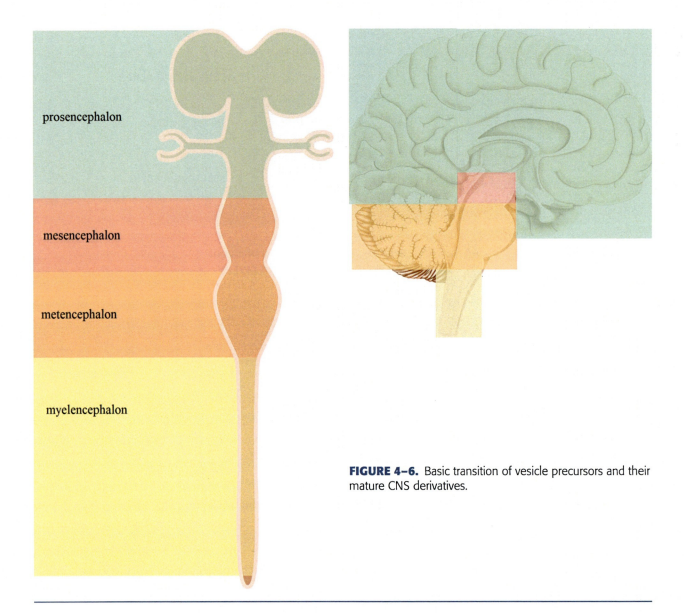

FIGURE 4–6. Basic transition of vesicle precursors and their mature CNS derivatives.

putting neurons in the correct places within the mature nervous system. Neuronal migration disorders result in missing or underdeveloped structures within the cerebral hemispheres, cerebellum, brainstem, or hippocampus. This includes a variety of disorders, including ACC and agenesis of cranial nerves. Consequences include decreased muscle tone and motor function, seizures, developmental delays, developmental cognitive impairments, failure to thrive, difficulties with feeding, and small head circumference. When neuronal proliferation and migration go as planned, the maturing circuits continue to develop. Development of neuronal pathways and myelination occur primarily after birth. The adult brain has approximately 100 billion neurons, 20 billion of which are located within the cerebral cortex (Herculano-Houzel, 2009).

Landmark Timelines

Development is most relevant to clinical practice when considering relatable timelines during gestation (pregnancy/preterm) and postnatal development (Figure 4–8). Just as the neural tube achieves closure, three bulges or vesicles become evident. They are delineated by a cephalic/mesencephalic flexure between the forebrain and midbrain and a cervical flexure between the rhombencephalon and spinal cord. The sulcus limitans separates the basal and alar plates

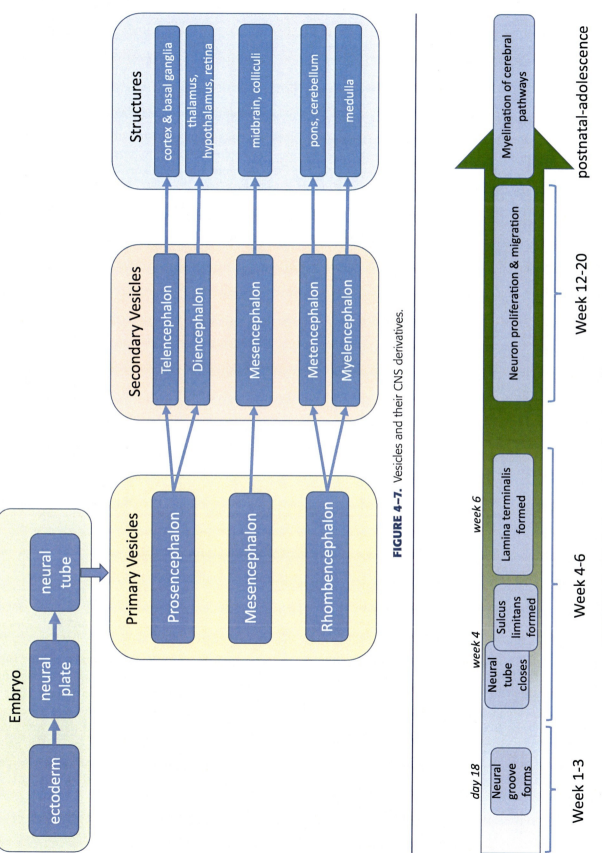

FIGURE 4–7. Vesicles and their CNS derivatives.

FIGURE 4–8. Key developmental timelines during prenatal and postnatal periods.

> **Box 4–3.** Anomalies of Ventral Induction
>
> Ventral induction leads to closure of the cerebral and facial midline. It may help to think of the hemispheres and sides of the head/face like a compact mirror (half on one side, half on the other, and hinged in the back). Ventral induction is the process of bringing those sides together. Thus, disruptions of this process result in craniofacial anomalies and cerebral anomalies due to problems with anterior closure.
>
> Craniofacial anomalies
>
> - Cleft lip and palate: Median cleft, orbital hypotelorism (eyes too closely spaced), flat nose
> - Ethmocephaly: Severe hypotelorism, arrhinia (absence of nose) with prosboscis (elongated, nose-like facial appendage)
> - Cebocephly: Orbital hypotelorism, prosboscis-like nose, no cleft
> - Cyclopia: Single eye or single orbit, arrhinia with prosboscis
> - Agnathia-astomia: Mandibular hypoplasia or absent mandible (small or underdeveloped jaw), small or absent mouth, abnormal position of ears
>
> Cerebral (proencephalon) anomalies
>
> Lack of prosencephalon development
>
> - Aprosencephaly: More rostral elements of the telencephalon and diencephalon fail to develop while more caudal structures are normal or only mildly affected.
> - Atelencephaly: A rudimentary telencephalon forms; microencephaly.
>
> Disorders of prosencephalon cleavage
>
> - Holoprosencephaly: The diencephalon and telencephalon do not develop into right and left hemispheres.
> - Holotelencephaly: The telencephalon does not develop into right and left hemispheres.
>
> Disorders of prosencephalon midline development
>
> - ACC, a continuum of severity
> - Agenesis of septum pellucidum, often includes hydrocephalus
> - Septo-optic dysplasia: Characterized by underdevelopment of the optic nerves, abnormal development of midline brain structures, and underdevelopment of the pituitary gland.

at this time, creating the anterior/posterior, motor/sensory dichotomy. By the fifth week of gestation, transition of primary vesicles to secondary vesicles becomes evident. During this process, particularly as the telencephalon develops, the lamina terminalis (or precursor to the corpus callosum) is formed. Note that a period of intensive neuronal development and proliferation follows for several weeks, leading to an eventual migration to mature morphology of cerebral structures. Ongoing development, including myelination, continues and takes place primarily during the postnatal periods through adolescence.

By the second year of life, the human brain reaches nearly 80% of adult weight (Kretschmann et al., 1986). By age 5 years, there are no additional major changes in cerebral volume as measured by MRI-based anatomical studies (Giedd et al., 1996a, 1996b). This does not mean that neural development is complete. As described later, brain development continues through adolescence.

Telencephalon and C-Shaped Development

Understanding the concept of C-shaped development provides a basis for understanding the timing of development, particularly within the cerebrum (telencephalon), and typical aging processes. Returning to the basic concept, several structures within the brain (i.e., the cerebrum/telencephalon, basal ganglia, fornix, ventricles, cingulate gyrus, and corpus callosum) develop in a C-shaped pattern (Figure 4–9). Posterior portions of those structures develop early and tend to be preserved late in life, amid declines in function that occur in typical aging. In contrast, anterior portions of those structures develop later and tend to decline earlier with aging. For instance, the prefrontal cortex and anterior medial temporal lobes of the cerebrum (telencephalon) begin to demyelinate in typical aging beginning as early as one's late 60s.

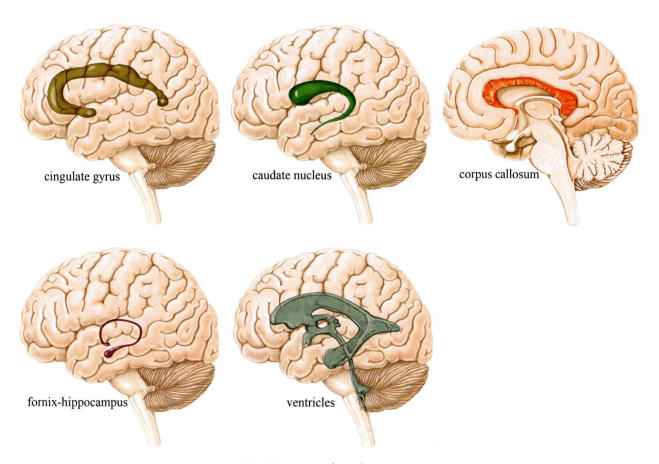

FIGURE 4–9. C-shaped structures.

To better orient to this concept, imagine your hand as the C shape for the cerebrum (Figure 4–10). In this case, the tips of your fingers represent the prefrontal cortices, whereas the tip of your thumb represents the anterior–medial temporal lobe. Broadly speaking, these two structures house the highest level cognitive function: executive functions and memory systems/emotional regulation functions, respectively. In typical development, these "develop" last in terms of gray matter development, myelination, and pruning.

Gray matter develops last in the dorsolateral prefrontal cortex and superior temporal gyri (Gogtay et al., 2004; Sowell et al., 2003). In terms of myelination, the frontal lobes and anteromedial temporal lobes are not fully myelinated until approximately age 12 to 16 years in females and 18 to 20 years in males. In particular, axons that connect subcortical structures to cortical structures myelinate during adolescence to early adulthood (Barnea-Gorlay et al., 2005). With regard to aging, there is approximately a 10% decrease in myelin volume per decade, accounting

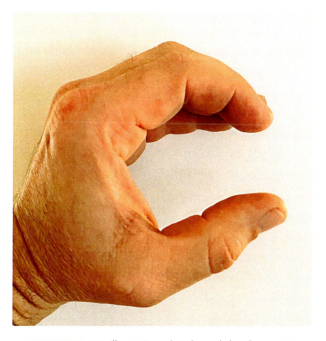

FIGURE 4–10. Illustration of C-shaped development.

for a total decrease of 45% from age 20 years to 80 years (Marner et al., 2003). There is no significant difference in rate of loss by sex (Marner et al., 2003).

Pruning of synaptic connections and pathways also continues throughout the entire life span, removing unnecessary and less efficient connections (Craik & Bialystok, 2006). The occipital lobe undergoes substantial pruning from ages 2 to 4 years, whereas pruning in the prefrontal cortices peaks near age 20 years (Goswami, 2004). Furthermore, functional MRI studies on language development, verbal fluency, and reading in children show that functional activity increases in the prefrontal and temporal areas with age, despite pruning and decreases in synaptic density (Szaflarski et al., 2006; Vannest et al., 2009; Price, 2012). Synaptic pruning and myelination occur last in the frontal lobes and prefrontal cortices (Rivkin, 2000). Altogether, myelination, pruning, cortical development, and cortical activation coincide with cognitive development (Amso & Casey, 2006).

Putting all of this into context, it makes sense why children have less self-regulation, emotional regulation, and less efficient declarative learning than adults. It makes sense why they may throw a tantrum or watch the same cartoon movie 30 times. In typical aging, those same cerebral structures experience demyelination in typical aging, accounting for changes to problem-solving capacity in complex contexts, mild changes to working memory, and perhaps other subtle changes with aging. See Box 4–4 for an everyday application of typical changes with aging.

Disruptions to Development and Consequences

Many adverse events, teratogens, deficiencies, or excesses can disrupt normal development processes and timelines. Adverse events can include in utero cerebral vascular accidents, direct or indirect trauma, and exposure to infectious agents or toxins. Teratogens often include medications given to the mother for other medical purposes (e.g., thalidomide, a drug formerly used to treat morning sickness but caused birth defects), illicit drugs, alcohol, or exposure to environmental toxins (e.g., lead). Developmental deficiencies may be linked to dietary factors (e.g., folic acid), absorption of nutrients, or impaired secretion of hormones. Excesses that interrupt development can include elevated blood serotonin or hormone levels. In any of these

Box 4–4. Cognition and Communication Changes With Typical Aging

Mildred is in her late 70s and is aging normally. She does things, however, that she would not have done in years past. For instance, she will begin a conversation by saying, "Do you know what Phyllis did?" Her conversational partner might be thinking, "I don't even know who Phyllis is, so no, I don't know what she did." This is a problem with presupposition, a higher order executive function that involves being able to take the perspective of your audience and adjust the level of background information you provide, depending on your knowledge of that person's degree of joint knowledge of your experiences. In the past, she would have contextualized the question or at least checked the listener's level of knowledge about Phyllis. "Do you know Phyllis?" or perhaps "Phyllis is a lady that comes to Women's club." This and other small interactional missteps are a part of typical aging but nonetheless highlight changes to anterior portions of the "C" eloquently.

Box 4–5. Etiologies of Cerebral Palsy

In speech–language pathology and audiology, individuals with cerebral palsy (CP) are commonly encountered across a range of settings (i.e., neonatal intensive care units, birth-to-three programs, schools, outpatient, hospitals, and long-term care contexts) and throughout the life span. Despite the widespread potential for clinical interactions, practitioners may be less aware that there are three basic etiologies of CP: teratogenic, static–prenatal, and at/during birth. In the case of teratogenic CP, the disruption occurs early in development, in which brain structures never develop appropriately. In static, prenatal cases, there is trauma or stroke that alters development. Finally, trauma or stroke during the birthing process can also lead to CP. There is evidence from the medical (pharmacological) and surgical disciplines that the outcomes of these diverse etiologies are different, and individuals with CP may respond differently to interventions or perhaps benefit from different interventions. In this case, understanding such developmental principles is thus central to identifying the best interventions for those individuals.

cases, timing and degree of the disrupting factors or perhaps a combination of multiple factors can halt or alter the normal development timelines and processes. Because of the timing of structural development, any disruptive factors will differentially affect the later developing structures and functions, many of which are predominantly related to communication and cognition. See Box 4–5 for an everyday clinical application of such disruptions to development.

Summary

In basic terms, the process of neurodevelopment includes the transformation of single cells to ectoderm and the subsequent proliferation of cells that results in the formation of a human being. Although the process is complex and includes a host of terminology associated with structures and stages, the relevance to clinical practice is found in the timing of structure development and understanding the potential impact of anything that disrupts that process (see several examples of disruptions to the developmental process in Chapter 15). Teratogens, nutritional deficiencies, and trauma can all potentially disrupt development. Normal aging and neurodegenerative diseases first impact the later developing structures. Awareness of key points along the timeline can help one understand the nature of impairments and prevention at both ends of the life span. Perhaps most important, late-developing structures are differentially susceptible, and many of those structures are crucial for communication and cognition functions.

References and Additional Resources

Amso, D., & Casey, B. J. (2006). Beyond what develops when: Neuroimaging may inform how cognition changes with development. *Current Directions in Psychological Science, 15*(1), 24–29.

Barnea-Goraly, N., Menon, V., Eckert, M., Tamm, L., Bammer, R., Karchemskiy, A., . . . Reiss, A. L. (2005). White matter development during childhood and adolescence: A cross-sectional diffusion tensor imaging study. *Cerebral Cortex, 15*(12), 1848–1854.

Casey, B. J., Tottenham, N., Liston, C., & Durston, S. (2005). Imaging the developing brain: What have we learned about cognitive development? *Trends in Cognitive Sciences, 9*(3), 104–110.

Craik, F. I., & Bialystok, E. (2006). Cognition through the lifespan: Mechanisms of change. *Trends in Cognitive Sciences, 10*(3), 131–138.

Giedd, J. N., Vaituzis, A. C., Hamburger, S. D., Lange, N., Rajapakse, J. C., Kaysen, D., . . . Rapoport, J. L. (1996a). Quantitative MRI of the temporal lobe, amygdala, and hippocampus in normal human development: Ages 4–18 years. *Journal of Comparative Neurology, 366*(2), 223–230.

Giedd, J. N., Snell, J. W., Lange, N., Rajapakse, J. C., Casey, B. J., Kozuch, P. L., . . . Rapoport, J. L. (1996b). Quantitative magnetic resonance imaging of human brain development: Ages 4–18. *Cerebral Cortex, 6*(4), 551–559.

Gogtay, N., Giedd, J. N., Lusk, L., Hayashi, K. M., Greenstein, D., Vaituzis, A. C., . . . Thompson, P. M. (2004). Dynamic mapping of human cortical development during childhood through early adulthood. *Proceedings of the National Academy of Sciences of the USA, 101*(21), 8174–8179.

Goswami, U. (2004). Neuroscience, education, and special education. *British Journal of Special Education, 31*(4), 175–183.

Herculano-Houzel, S. (2009). The human brain in numbers: A linearly scaled-up primate brain. *Frontiers in Human Neuroscience, 3*, 31.

Key Concepts

- Vesicles of the neural tube are precursors to mature nervous system structures.
- Neuronal proliferation and migration is the process of generating neurons and sending them to their final position within the "mature" nervous system.
- Dorsal induction is the process of closing the neural tube, whereas ventral induction is the process of forming the brain and face, along with bringing the hemispheres and sides of the face together at midline. Disruptions to these processes result in several developmental neurological disorders.
- The sulcus limitans creates a division between motor and sensory portions of the nervous system, particularly the brainstem and spinal cord.
- The lamina terminalis divides the left and right portions of the telencephalon and is a precursor to the corpus callosum, which is crucial for interhemispheric communication.
- The concept of C-shaped development is relevant to understanding the timing of development within the cerebrum. The anterior-most portions of the C develop late and typically decline earlier, even within typical aging. Those late-developing portions include cognitive and communication functions that represent our highest order thinking.

Luders, E., Thompson, P. M., & Toga, A. W. (2010). The development of the corpus callosum in the healthy human brain. *Journal of Neuroscience, 30*(33), 10985–10990.

Marner, L., Nyengaard, J. R., Tang, Y., & Pakkenberg, B. (2003). Marked loss of myelinated nerve fibers in the human brain with age. *Journal of Comparative Neurology, 462*(2), 144–152.

Price, C. J. (2012). A review and synthesis of the first 20 years of PET and fMRI studies of heard speech, spoken language and reading. *Neuroimage, 62*(2), 816–847.

Rivkin, M. J. (2000). Developmental neuroimaging of children using magnetic resonance techniques. *Mental Retardation and Developmental Disabilities Research Reviews, 6*(1), 68–80.

Sowell, E. R., Peterson, B. S., Thompson, P. M., Welcome, S. E., Henkenius, A. L., & Toga, A. W. (2003). Mapping cortical change across the human life span. *Nature Neuroscience, 6*(3), 309–315.

Szaflarski, J. P., Holland, S. K., Schmithorst, V. J., & Byars, A. W. (2006). fMRI study of language lateralization in children and adults. *Human Brain Mapping, 27*(3), 202–212.

Takahashi, E., Folkerth, R. D., Galaburda, A. M., & Grant, P. E. (2012). Emerging cerebral connectivity in the human fetal brain: An MR tractography study. *Cerebral Cortex, 22*(2), 455–464.

Vannest, J., Karunanayaka, P. R., Schmithorst, V. J., Szaflarski, J. P., & Holland, S. K. (2009). Language networks in children: Evidence from functional MRI studies. *American Journal of Roentgenology, 192*(5), 1190–1196.

Zilles, K., Palomero-Gallagher, N., & Amunts, K. (2013). Development of cortical folding during evolution and ontogeny. *Trends in Neurosciences, 36*(5), 275–284.

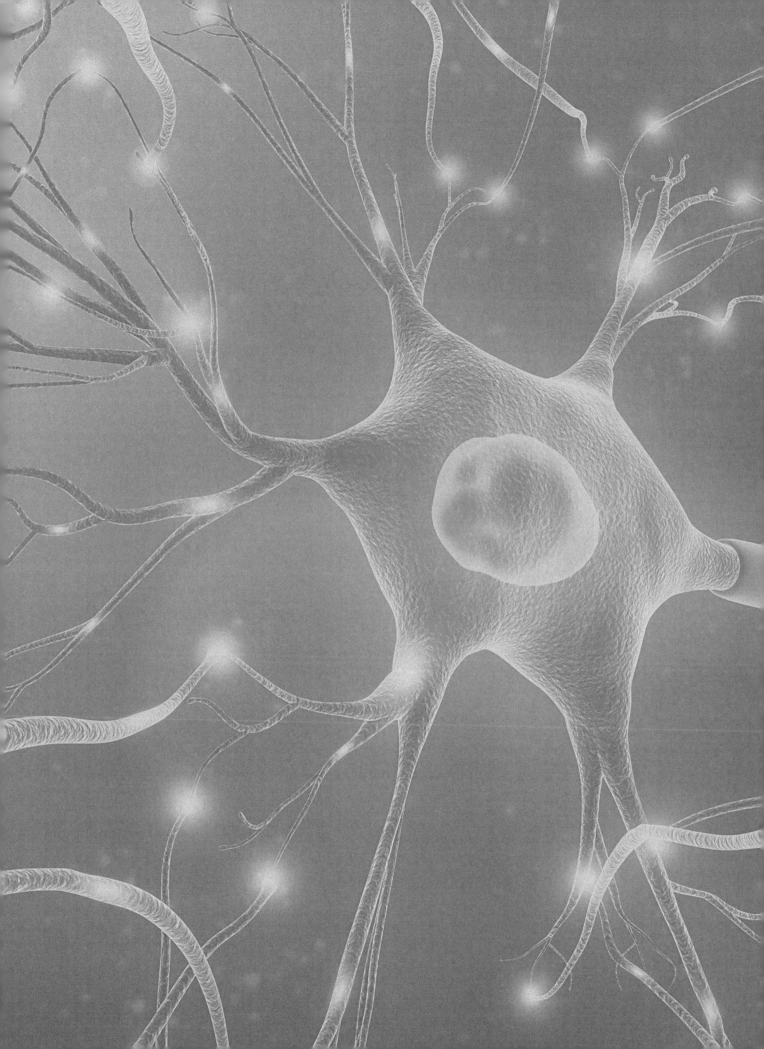

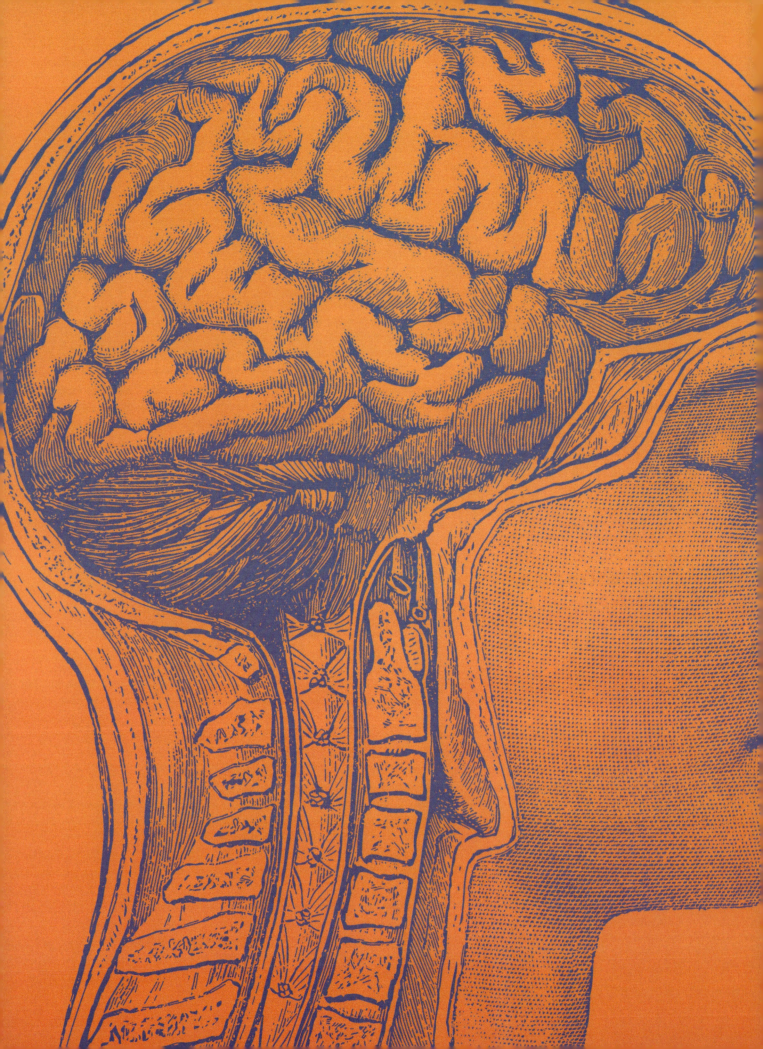

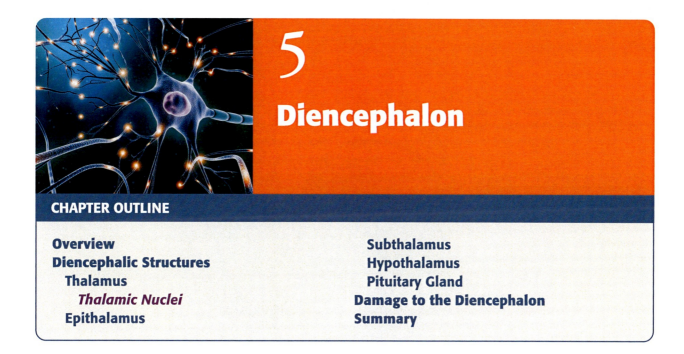

5
Diencephalon

CHAPTER OUTLINE

Overview
Diencephalic Structures
  Thalamus
    Thalamic Nuclei
  Epithalamus

Subthalamus
Hypothalamus
Pituitary Gland
Damage to the Diencephalon
Summary

Overview

The diencephalon's role in communication is related to its extensive interconnections between regions of the central nervous system (CNS) and between the body and the brain. These connections facilitate cognition, language, sensory functions (including audition), motor control (important for speech and swallowing), and homeostatic regulation. The thalamus, the largest of the diencephalic structures, mediates messages between the reticular formation and cognitive systems that are needed to carry out these higher order functions effectively (emotion, mood, personality, judgment, reasoning, memory, and language). The thalamus has reciprocal (back and forth) connections to most structures in the cortex, serving a key role in intracerebral communication.

The diencephalon consists of the **thalamus** and **hypothalamus** along with the **epithalamus**, **subthalamus**, and the **optic tract** (Figure 5–1). All are paired structures and thus technically should be referred to as the thalami, hypothalami, etc. By convention, they are described in the singular, but remember that there are two of each structure. As described in Chapter 4, the diencephalon, along with the telencephalon, develops from the prosencephalon. It lies at the superior extent of the midbrain, deep within the right and left hemispheres. Structures in the diencephalon are extensively connected with a variety of cognitive, language, motor, and sensory areas of the cortex as well as brainstem nuclei. For their relatively small size, they have a large effect on the CNS.

Diencephalic Structures

Thalamus

The thalami are separated by the third ventricle, although they are connected by the thalamic adhesion or massa intermedia in approximately 75% of people. It is unclear why this adhesion does not appear in all people, nor is it clear what the function of the structure is because there are no obvious differences between people who do and do not have one. The thalamus is made up primarily of gray matter as it houses more than 120 definable nuclei. Not to worry, only a few are described here. Amid the nuclei is a Y-shaped region of white matter called the **internal medullary lamina**. Some nuclei, collectively referred to as **intralaminar nuclei**, are embedded within this white matter region.

The thalamus is primarily known as a gatekeeper for somatosensory and special sensory signals because, with the exception of olfaction, all sensory pathways synapse in the thalamus prior to reaching the appropriate cortical regions. In addition to relaying sensory signals, the thalamus also integrates motor information through extensive

84 Clinical Neuroscience for Communication Disorders: Neuroanatomy and Neurophysiology

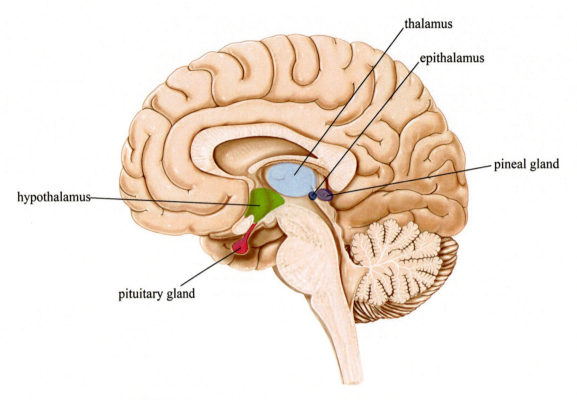

FIGURE 5–1. Diencephalic structures seen in a midsagittal slice.

connections with the basal ganglia, cerebellum, and limbic system and the primary and premotor cortices. Finally, the thalamus regulates cortically mediated cognitive functions through reciprocal connections with the reticular formation and speech and language processing areas. One of these connections is the thalamo-cortico-thalamic loop, a reverberating circuit. As described in Chapter 3, reverberating circuits are self-sustaining: Axon collaterals synapse onto their own cell bodies so that each action potential stimulates another one.

Thalamic Nuclei

Thalamic nuclei can generally be classified as either specific, with bidirectional connections to specific cortical areas, or nonspecific, with connections to brainstem arousal systems but no direct connection to the cortex. Thalamic nuclei are classified into six major complexes based on their location and function. Although the thalamus has multiple functions and connections and can be confusing because the location-based names of the nuclei all sound similar, the functions of the nuclei are logical given the inputs and outputs. For example, the ventroposterolateral (VPL) nucleus receives inputs from the spinal cord and sends outputs to the primary sensory strip. Given only this information, you can guess that the VPL is part of the somatosensory system. Table 5–1 summarizes the connections and functions of these six nuclear complexes, and Figure 5–2 illustrates those connections; descriptions of these complexes and their functions follow in the text.

The medial or **mediodorsal (MD) nuclear complex**, as might be predicted, is located in the medial and superior (dorsal) region. It is densely interconnected with prefrontal and orbitofrontal cortical regions, hippocampus, and the limbic system including the amygdala and hypothalamus. Thinking about the functions of these cortical areas, it should not be surprising that the medial thalamic nuclei are important for regulating mood, emotion, cognition (judgment and reasoning), personality, memory, and language. Due to connections with the hypothalamus and limbic system, this region aids in integration of visceral information with affect, emotion, thought processes, and personality.

The **anterior nuclear complex** has a role in memory due to its extensive connections to the hippocampus. It also connects to the frontal lobes and cingulate gyrus, which influence emotion and executive functioning processes.

Table 5–1. Connections and Functions of Thalamic Nuclear Groups

Thalamic Nuclear Complex	Primary Functions	Connections (Inputs and Outputs)
Mediodorsal (MD)	Mood, emotion, cognition, personality	Hippocampus, cortical association areas, prefrontal, orbitofrontal, limbic, hippocampus, hypothalamus
Anterior (Ant)	Memory, emotion, executive function	Hippocampus, frontal lobes, cingulate gyrus
Lateral dorsal (LD) and lateral posterior (LP)	Complex sensory integration	Cortical association areas
Ventral lateral (VL) and ventral anterior (VA)	Motor integration	Primary motor, basal ganglia, cerebellum
Ventroposterolateral (VPL) and ventroposteromedial (VPM)	Sensory relay	Afferent spinal somatosensory neurons
Pulvinar (P)	Language, vision	Superior colliculus, angular, marginal gyri
Medial geniculate nucleus (MGN)	Auditory	Inferior colliculus, brainstem nuclei along auditory pathway
Lateral geniculate nucleus (LGN)	Vision	Optic nerve (cranial nerve II)

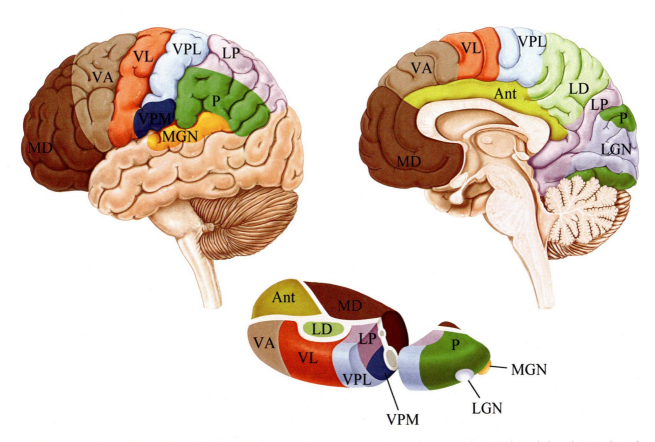

FIGURE 5–2. Thalamic nuclei and their cortical connections. Ant, anterior nuclear complex; LD, lateral dorsal; LGN, lateral geniculate nucleus; LP, lateral posterior; MD, mediodorsal; MGN, medial geniculate nucleus; P, pulvinar; VA, ventral anterior; VL, ventral lateral; VPL, ventroposterolateral; VPM, ventroposteromedial.

The **lateral nuclear complex**, consisting of the **lateral dorsal (LD)** and **lateral posterior (LP)** nuclei in the superior lateral region, is important for sensory integration. This includes integrating visceral and sensory information and integrating multiple sensory modalities. Connections include the superior and medial regions of the parietal lobes.

The **ventral nuclear complex** includes four smaller nuclei, two linked to the motor system and two to the sensory system. The **ventrolateral (VL)** and **ventroanterior (VA)** nuclei are located inferior (ventral) to the lateral posterior nuclei and aid in motor integration and coordination. This is clear given the connections to the globus pallidus, substantia nigra, primary motor cortex, and the cerebellum. Body position, muscle tone, and coordination of movement all are influenced by signals through the VL and VA nuclei.

The **ventral posterolateral (VPL)** and **ventral posteromedial (VPM)** nuclei lie inferior (ventral) to the lateral posterior nucleus and are "relay stations" for the somatosensory system. Inputs from spinal nerves providing somatosensory signals from the body below the neck synapse in the VPL. Afferent signals from cranial nerves carrying somatosensory information from the head and neck synapse in the VPM. Outputs from the VPL/VPM synapse in the primary sensory strip (S1) in the postcentral gyrus of the parietal lobe. Pain signals are sent not only to the sensory strip but also to the insula. The neurons within these nuclei are somatotopically organized, with separate columns of nuclei representing different areas of the body. Neurons carrying different sensory modalities also may be organized separately, with proprioceptive signals synapsing in a separate region from touch signals.

The **pulvinar** is a large nucleus in the posterior region of the thalamus. Inputs come from the visual cortex, superior colliculus, visual reflex center of the midbrain, and inferior parietal lobes. Outputs extend to the inferior parietal, angular, and supramarginal gyri. Functions include mediating visual reflexes and language processing, including reading and writing.

The last two regions covered here are the **medial and lateral geniculate nuclei (MGN and LGN)**. Both appear to grow out of the inferior pulvinar. The MGN (sometimes called the medial geniculate body) is a stop along the auditory pathway, receiving signals passed from the VIIIth cranial nerve through brainstem nuclei and the inferior colliculus and in turn sending signals to the temporal lobe (for details of the auditory pathway, see Chapter 8). The LGN (or lateral geniculate body) is part of the visual pathway, receiving signals from axons of the optic nerve (cranial nerve II) and sending signals to the occipital lobe (discussed in Chapter 7).

As described previously, the traditional characterization of the thalamus is as a sensory relay station. But only a few nuclei are dedicated specifically to sensory systems, and even in those, signals can be amplified or muted before being sent to the cortex. Thus, the notion of a simple relay station vastly underrepresents the function of the thalamus. In addition, the thalamus also plays a role in cognition, speech, and language. The nonspecific connections to the brainstem also provide a role for the thalamus in consciousness and the flow of information to the cortex.

Intralaminar nuclei are connected to a variety of areas and play a role in visual processing, motor systems, attention, cognition, and pain perception. Some receive pain signals conveyed through the spinothalamic tract (see Chapter 6) as well as inputs from the reticular formation in the brainstem and influence pain perception. Others are connected to the motor system, and still others have connections to prefrontal cortical areas and impact cognitive processing.

Blood supply to the thalamus is carried through branches of the posterior cerebral arteries and posterior communicating arteries (see Chapter 13). As described later, strokes in these branches result in deficits associated with the region of the thalamus affected.

Epithalamus

The epithalamus consists of three structures: the **pineal gland, habenulus,** and **stria medullaris**. The pineal gland (Figure 5–3), made up entirely of glial cells, is a small structure located between the superior extent of the midbrain and the ventral–posterior extent of the thalamus. The pineal gland is part of the endocrine system and secretes melatonin. It plays an important role in the sleep–wake cycle and influences the gonadal (sex) systems.

The habenulae (or habenular nuclei) are small, paired nuclei located superior to the pineal gland. They are connected to both the limbic system and the globus pallidus of the basal ganglia as well as brainstem nuclei involved in both dopaminergic and serotonergic networks. The **stria medullaris** is a white matter tract connecting the anterior limbic system to the habenula. Given these connections, the habenula plays a role in motivation, responses to rewards, goal-directed behavior, and motor behaviors. Damage or dysfunction has been linked to addiction and psychiatric disorders including schizophrenia and depression.

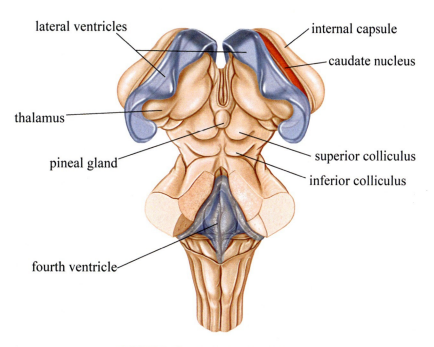

FIGURE 5–3. Pineal gland and thalamus.

Subthalamus

The **subthalamus**, as the name suggests, is located inferior to the thalamus and contains both the subthalamic nucleus and the substantia nigra. Although physically and developmentally part of the diencephalon and thus related to the thalamus, these two structures are functionally part of the motor system and often considered to be part of the basal ganglia. The subthalamus is discussed in Chapter 10.

Hypothalamus

The **hypothalamus** is located at the ventral and rostral extent of the thalamus (Figure 5–1). Like the thalamus, it is made up of many distinct nuclei. Despite being a relatively small structure, it has wide-ranging influences on the brain and body because of its influence on the autonomic nervous system; the endocrine (hormonal) system; and regulatory functions such as body temperature, blood volume, eating/drinking, and circadian rhythms. It is discussed further in Chapter 12 in the context of the limbic system.

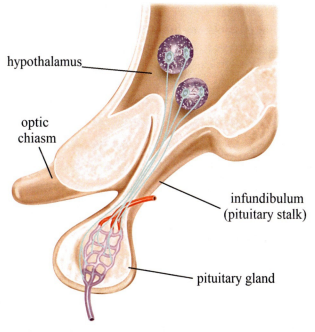

FIGURE 5–4. Hypothalamus and pituitary gland.

Pituitary Gland

Extending inferiorly from the hypothalamus is the **pituitary stalk** or **infundibulum**, which ends in the **pituitary gland** (Figure 5–4). This gland has a primary role in synthesis and excretion of hormones, including growth hormone, testosterone, estrogen, oxytocin, endorphins, and thyroid hormones. The pituitary gland is surrounded by blood vessels into which hormones are excreted.

Damage to the Diencephalon

Lesions in the thalamus, caused, for example, by thalamic strokes, can have a variety of effects depending on the size and location of the damage. Thinking about the major nuclei described previously, it is clear how a thalamic stroke could affect movement, sensation, language, memory, or auditory and visual processing. Thalamic strokes also can result in aphasia or dysarthria or can have an impact on cognition. Commonly, patients will acutely experience disorders of consciousness, even coma. Cognitive deficits can include disorientation, amnesia, problems creating new memories, apathy, and abulia (reduced initiation of responses).

Motor deficits include hemiparesis, abnormal movements, and vertical eye gaze palsy. Thalamic syndrome, first described in 1906, comprises a variety of abnormal movements, including hemi-ataxia (incoordination affecting half of the body), hemidystonia (unwanted movements on half of the body), and jerking movements. Thalamic pain syndrome is characterized by intractable, severe pain that can include burning, tingling, or needle sensations. It often is not responsive to traditional pain medications. Additional somatosensory disorders associated with damage to the thalamus are discussed in Chapter 6.

Left thalamic lesions are more likely to result in language deficits (thalamic aphasia) and difficulties with verbal memory, whereas right thalamic lesions can cause unilateral neglect (an attentional deficit in which the patient appears not to process visual, auditory, or somatosensory signals from the opposite side) or visual memory deficits. In addition, pain syndromes are more likely after right thalamic lesions.

Hypothalamic lesions can interrupt normal regulatory functions, resulting in fluctuations in body temperature and changes in fluid retention, appetite, and eating patterns. Pituitary tumors are not uncommon, comprising 10% to 15% of all intracranial tumors, with approximately 10,000 detected annually. Fortunately, they are rarely cancerous, and in many people they are asymptomatic, meaning that you may never know that you have one. Pituitary tumors can cause over- or underproduction of hormones. Although overproduction may seem odd, some of the tumors themselves produce hormones, such as adrenocorticotropic hormone-secreting tumors that stimulate production of cortisol from the adrenal glands or tumors that produce growth hormones that affect hand/foot size and cause sweating, joint pain, increased body hair, and other symptoms.

Box 6–1. Thalamic Aphasia

Mario was a 69-year-old Hispanic male with a history of hypertension and diabetes. He presented to the emergency department with difficulty producing speech and mild right-sided hemiparesis. A computed tomography scan revealed an ischemic lesion in the left thalamus in the region of the ventral anterior and ventrolateral nuclei. Evaluation by a speech–language pathologist indicated the presence of aphasia characterized by difficulty naming and phonemic paraphasias (e.g., sound errors involving substituting one sound for another, as in "pog" for "dog"). His word and sentence repetition was intact. Over the course of several days, both the hemiparesis and the aphasia resolved, and by the time Mario was released from the hospital, his language was essentially back to pre-stroke levels.

Summary

Although the thalamus makes up only a small portion of the cerebrum, it is connected to multiple areas of the cortex and influences most cerebral functions, including cognitive, emotional, motor, sensory, and regulatory functions, as well as cortical arousal. Lesions can affect any of these areas, including language and speech.

Key Concepts

- The thalamus is made up of many functionally defined nuclei that influence nearly all cortical functions.
- The thalamus is a sensory gateway. All sensory information with the exception of olfaction is relayed through the thalamus prior to reaching the cortex.
- The thalamus is interconnected with brainstem regions to control consciousness and cortical arousal.
- Extensive connections with the basal ganglia create an essential role for the thalamus in motor function.
- The hypothalamus and epithalamus influence regulatory body systems.
- The epithalamus influences the endocrine system and a variety of cognitive functions, including goal-directed behaviors and responses to rewards, through its connections to serotonergic and dopaminergic systems.
- The hypothalamus and pituitary glands regulate the release of hormones.

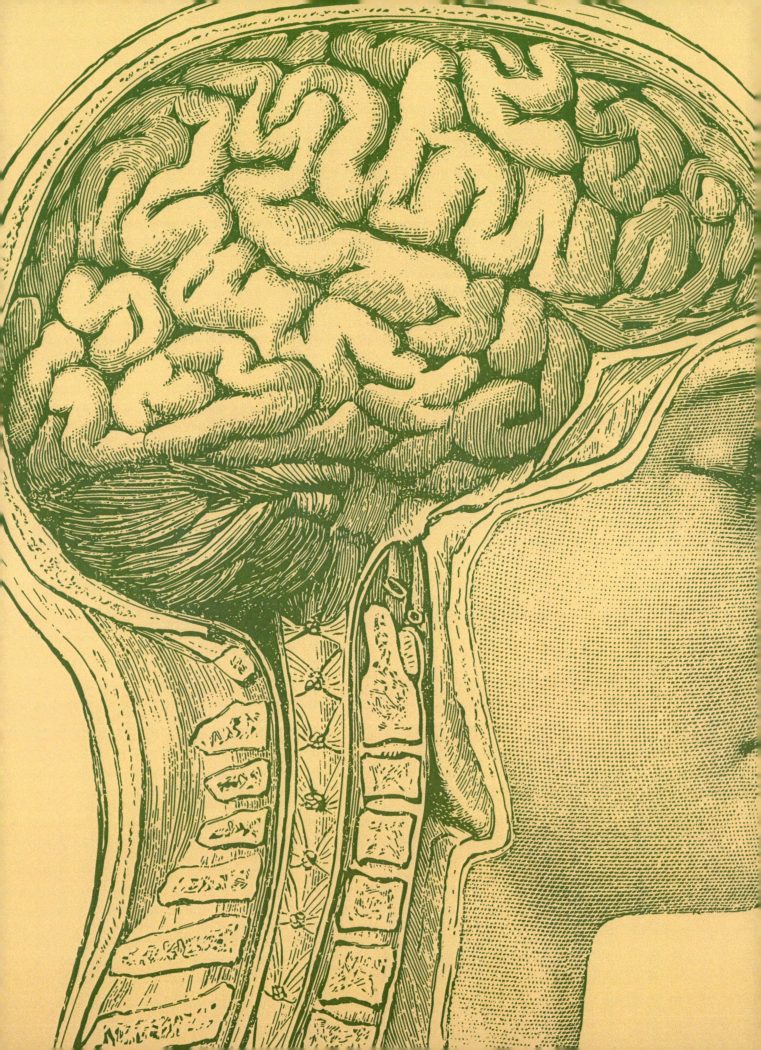

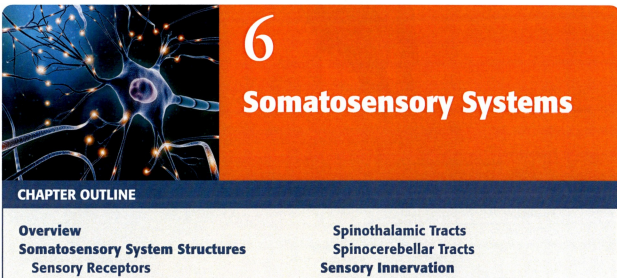

6 Somatosensory Systems

CHAPTER OUTLINE

Overview
Somatosensory System Structures
   Sensory Receptors
      Mechanoreceptors
      Nociceptors
      Proprioceptive Sensory Receptors
   Thalamic Nuclei
   Primary Somatosensory Cortex
   Cortical Association Areas
Sensory Pathways
   Dorsal Column–Medial Lemniscal Pathway

Spinothalamic Tracts
Spinocerebellar Tracts
Sensory Innervation
Damage to Somatosensory System Components
   Spinal Cord Damage
   Thalamic Damage
   Cortical Damage
Summary

Overview

The somatosensory systems carry information about pain, touch, temperature, and proprioception from the body to the brain. Special sensory systems (e.g., vision, hearing, taste, smell) have unique pathways and are discussed individually in the following chapters. Somatosensory information from the head and neck is carried along cranial nerves and is covered in Chapter 11.

Sensory functions are integral to the function of speech and swallowing systems and aid in all forms of communication that rely on movement. Somatosensory functions, particularly proprioception, are crucial inputs for the motor systems. For example, if you are gesturing to show a friend exactly how big the fish was that you caught compared to your brother's fish, your motor system needs to know where your arms are to begin with (e.g., by your side) to move your hands close together to show how small your brother's fish was. That new proprioceptive information about where your hands are will then aid in the motor system moving your hands out a sufficient distance to show how much bigger your fish was compared to your brother's fish. It is even more incredible that you could carry out these gestures with your eyes closed and your arms and hands would know exactly where to be positioned.

Somatosensory System Structures

Sensory Receptors

Somatosensory receptors are embedded in skin, muscles, joints, and even blood vessels. You can think of these receptors as specialized dendrites, sometimes called nerve endings, that respond to specific stimuli (Figure 6–1). **Mechanoreceptors** respond to tactile (touch, pressure, and vibration) and kinesthetic (limb position and movement) stimuli (Table 6–1). **Thermoreceptors** respond only

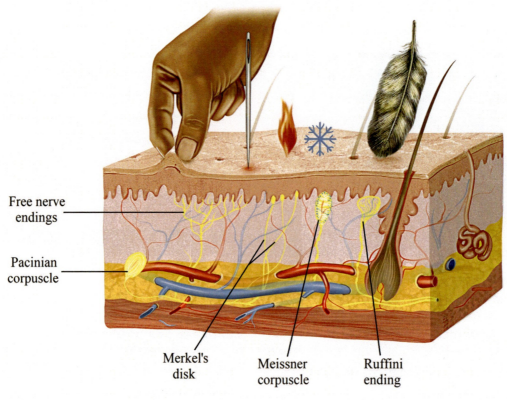

FIGURE 6-1. Somatosensory receptors of the skin.

Table 6-1. Mechanoreceptors of the Skin

Mechanoreceptors	Location	Receptive Field	Adaptation Rate	Sensitivity
Meissner corpuscle	Glabrous skin: palms, fingers, soles of the feet	Small, well-defined	Rapidly adapting	Light touch; vibrations less than 50 Hz; detect texture especially when moved across the skin
Merkel disk	Superficial epidermis; primarily fingertips and lips	Small, well-defined	Slowly adapting	Gentle pressure, rough texture, discrimination of edges and shapes
Pacinian corpuscle	Deep skin (subcutaneous), glabrous and hairy skin	Large, diffuse	Rapidly adapting	Pressure receptor; 200- to 300-Hz vibrations; discrimination of fine surface texture
Ruffini endings	Deep in skin, also ligaments and tendons	Large, diffuse	Slowly adapting	Skin stretching; angle changes of joints
Hair follicles and free nerve endings	Hairy skin; superficial epidermis	Small	Slow or rapid	Respond to movement of hair; temperature, touch, pressure, pain

to temperature. Finally, **nociceptors** (Latin: *noci* = *hurt*) respond to painful stimuli—those that can cause destruction of body tissues.

Two important characteristics of the somatosensory systems are the density of receptors and the size of receptive fields. Combined, these characteristics determine sensitivity and ability to localize sensation. Areas of the body with high density have more somatosensory receptors per square centimeter. The sensory neurons in these high-density areas tend to have small receptive fields, meaning that they respond to stimuli only within a very small region. Fingers and lips are high-density, small receptive field regions, which makes them highly sensitive areas where you can precisely localize touch. In areas of the body with low density and large receptive field neurons, sensation is not as acute and localization is more difficult. Box 6–1 presents a clinical application of these characteristics.

A third characteristic is adaptation of neurons. **Adaptation rates** refer to the pattern of action potentials created from a long-lasting stimulus. At the onset of a stimulus, **rapidly adapting receptors** will fire a large number of action potentials, but as the stimulus remains, the firing rate will decrease dramatically. In contrast, **slowly adapting sensory neurons** will begin firing action potentials at the onset of the stimulus and will continue that same rate of firing for as long as the stimulus is present. Consider sitting in the movies with a significant other who reaches out to hold your hand. When your two hands initially touch, all of your mechanoreceptors will start firing action potentials. Over time, however, the rapidly adapting neurons (Meissner and Pacinian corpuscles) will slow the rate of action potentials so that they fire only occasionally. The slowly adapting neurons (Merkel disks and Ruffini endings) will sustain their rate of action potentials for as long as you continue to hold hands. Essentially, the fast-adapting neurons tell the brain that something new has happened, and the slowly adapting neurons tell the brain that something is continuing to happen. This phenomenon applies to feeling clothing on your skin as well: When you put a shirt on, you feel it initially, but over time, you become unaware that it is there. This does not apply, however, to nociceptors. Pain does not subside but persists, which is why sunburned skin in contact with clothing is so irritating.

Box 6–1. Two-Point Discrimination (Sensory Discrimination)

Sensory receptor fields can be roughly mapped out through a simple process. To orient you to this principle, receptor field density is a reflection of the distance between sensory receptors in a region of the body (in this case, regions of skin). Areas with high receptor field density (e.g., fingertips) have narrow receptive fields, and sensory neurons are closer together. Areas with low receptor field density (e.g., back/trunk) have broader receptive fields, and sensory neurons are spaced farther apart.

Two-point discrimination is used to determine receptor density. Clinically, a calipers would be used (and a neurologist would conduct this test). The calipers has two arms affixed to a moving joint and a sharp point at the end of each arm. In lieu of a calipers, you can use a paper clip (a large paper clip works best), bent in the shape of a "V" with two equal arms. You can bring the tips together to assess two-point discrimination of narrow receptive fields or spread them apart to assess two-point discrimination of broad receptive fields. Choose a partner or you can even map fields on yourself. Let's begin with a location where we expect narrow receptive fields. Simply begin with tips spread slightly apart. Ask your partner to close their eyes and then apply slight pressure to the two tips equally. Ask them, "Do you feel one or two points?" If they indicate two points, narrow the tips in small increments and continue to ask if they feel one or two points. When they feel only one point, you have roughly mapped out the size of that receptor field. Now, move to an area of the body where you expect to see broad receptive fields. Begin again with the tips spread slightly apart. Repeat the procedure. They should indicate feeling only one point, meaning their receptor field is much broader than your starting point. Incrementally spread the tips apart and repeat the question. Eventually, you should reach a point where the tips are far apart (in some cases, you may even need a tip from two separate paper clips to serve as point A and point B). When they indicate "I can feel two points," you have roughly mapped that receptor field.

Mechanoreceptors

There are multiple mechanoreceptors that differ in their location and how they respond to mechanical touch and pressure (see Figure 6–1 and Table 6–1). Additionally, they are distributed differentially in hairy and **glabrous** (nonhairy) skin: The receptors in the palm of your hand will be slightly different from those on your forearm.

Nociceptors

There are several types of nociceptors: mechanosensitive, mechanothermal, and polymodal. Mechanosensitive nociceptors respond to pain caused by touch/pressure, and mechanothermal nociceptors respond to pain related to heat or cold. Polymodal nociceptors respond to touch, temperature, or chemical signals that result in pain. The majority of nociceptor neurons have narrow, unmyelinated axons. This results in relatively slow conduction of signals to the brain (see Chapter 3). This is why you can experience a deep cut that is not immediately painful or do not immediately sense water that is too hot when you wash your hands. In addition, nociceptors tend to have rather large receptive fields, which often makes it difficult to specifically localize pain.

Proprioceptive Sensory Receptors

There are three main types of proprioceptive sensory receptors: **joint receptors**, **Golgi tendon organs**, and **muscle spindle afferents** (Figure 6–2). Each of these receptors provides inputs to the ascending sensory pathways. Joint receptors are low-pressure mechanoreceptors (Ruffini-like receptors and Pacinian-like corpuscles) found within joint capsules and provide rudimentary information about joint compression and position. As shown in Table 6–1, Ruffini-like receptors provide information about muscle tone and

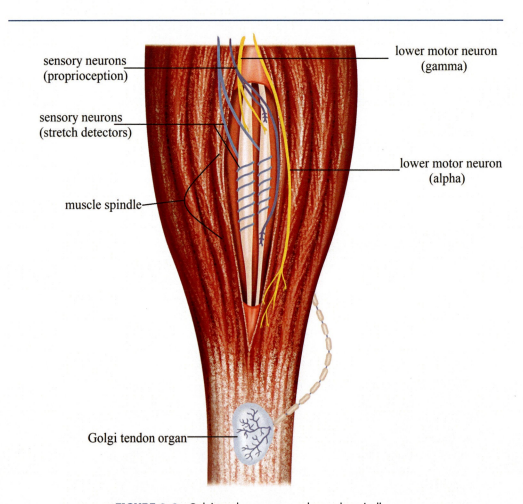

FIGURE 6–2. Golgi tendon organs and muscle spindles.

joint angle. Pacinian-like corpuscles also provide information about joint position. Once thought to be critical for proprioception, their role is now known to be auxiliary because these receptors are removed in joint replacement surgeries without consequence. Golgi tendon organs (GTOs) are found near the tendon/head of muscle attachments to bones. GTOs detect tension created through muscle contraction (shortening). You can also remember this by thinking of GTOs as Golgi *tension* organs. GTOs are involved in some types of reflexes (e.g., autogenic inhibition spinal reflex—causing muscle fibers to relax and redistribute effort across groups of fibers within a muscle) and provide information about the state of muscle contraction that relates to joint position. Spindle afferents are a slinky-like coil that is wrapped around muscle fibers. As the muscle fiber lengthens, the spindle afferent lengthens. It detects muscle stretch (lengthening) and is crucial to stretch reflexes (e.g., patellar tendon stretch reflex). Like GTOs, spindle afferents provide important information about joint position (proprioception). For more information about the action of spindle afferents, see a description of the patellar stretch reflex in Chapter 10.

Thalamic Nuclei

As described in Chapter 5, all somatosensory inputs synapse in the thalamus prior to being sent to the cortex. The synapses occur in the ventroposterolateral (VPL) nucleus. While the signals are relayed to the cortex, some processing occurs in the VPL nucleus, including integration of excitatory signals from corticothalamic neurons and inhibitory signals from interneurons within the thalamus, along with integration of signals from different modalities (touch, pain, and temperature). The two major types of neurons in the VPL nucleus are large multipolar neurons whose axons extend to the cortex and interneurons that facilitate integration and modulation of signals.

The VPL nucleus is precisely organized not only by body region but also by function. The lower body is represented in the lateral portion of the VPL nucleus, and the upper body more medially. Neurons that transmit information from the skin are arranged more centrally, whereas those from the joints are along the edges.

Primary Somatosensory Cortex

The primary somatosensory cortex (S1), or primary sensory strip, is located in the postcentral gyrus of the parietal lobe, immediately posterior to the central sulcus. As with the motor strip in the precentral gyrus, representations of body areas can be precisely mapped onto the sensory strip, creating a sensory homunculus (Figure 6–3). The regions of the body that have the highest density of sensory receptors, such as the hands, tongue, lips, and face, take up the most space in the sensory strip. The vast number of cortical sensory neurons representing these regions, combined with the number of receptors in the periphery, account for the fine discriminative touch of your hands, lips, tongue, and lower face. The regions associated with the trunk, leg, and foot together are no larger than the region associated with the face. Consequently, you have limited sensory discrimination of these large areas of the body.

Other regions of the brain, such as the insula, receive signals related to pain and temperature from the thalamus. Further processing occurs in the frontal lobes and anterior cingulate area, which integrate the sensory signals with feelings, emotions, and motivation.

Cortical Association Areas

Association areas for the somatosensory system lie primarily in the superior parietal lobes. In these regions, signals

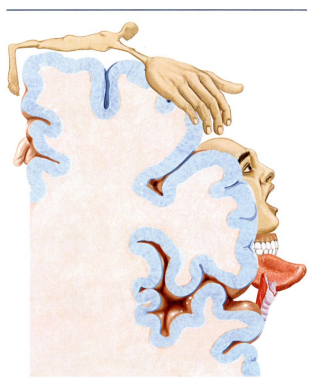

FIGURE 6–3. Somatosensory homunculus in the primary sensory strip.

are analyzed and integrated with other sensations, previous experiences, and memories in order to interpret the sensory signals. In addition, the right parietal lobe is important for one's perception of one's own body—your sense of how tall you are, where your limbs are, and how graceful or coordinated you are.

Box 6–2. Sensory Representations

Graphesthesia is the ability to determine shapes or letters drawn onto the skin solely based on the sensation of touch. Close your eyes and have a friend draw letters onto your palm. You should be able to determine the letters with relative ease because your palm has hundreds of touch receptors with small receptive fields that send precise information about location and direction of touch to the somatosensory cortex. Now have your friend draw letters on your back. You will find that the letters have to be much larger to be correctly discriminated, especially letters that have similar shapes such as O and G. Your back has fewer touch receptors with small receptive fields and so the shapes must be large enough to span across neurons with large receptive fields.

The hundreds of receptors on the palm of your hand convey information to a vast number of neurons in the somatosensory cortex, whereas fewer cortical neurons are required to receive the gross information conveyed from the touch receptors on your back. These patterns of representation contribute to the awkward-looking depiction of the sensory homunculus.

Consider the eloquent complexity of this system. It not only allows you to discriminate between stimuli in two separate receptive fields as in Box 6–1 but also allows you to integrate that information and associate it with orthographic (letter) representations. This speaks to the interconnectedness of sensory regions with not only motor but also language and cognitive areas.

Box 6–3. Disorders of Body Schema

There are a variety of disorders of body schema, and most are related to damage to the parietal lobes.

Finger agnosia (Greek: *agnosia = without knowledge*) is a deficit in localizing or naming fingers (e.g., index finger, pinky).

Autotopagnosia (Greek: *auto = self, topos = place, agnosia = without knowledge*) is the inability to identify body parts. This can be one's own, another person's, or even a picture. It is typically related to left parietal damage and may be associated with lexical–semantic aphasic deficits.

Right–left confusion, as the name suggests, is a problem with confusing right and left directions. It is a symptom of some forms of dementia.

Gerstmann syndrome is a combination of finger agnosia, right–left confusion, impairment in math calculations (acalculia), and a writing disorder (agraphia). A rare syndrome, it is most commonly seen after left posterior parietal lesions that include the angular gyrus. There is some controversy regarding whether the syndrome is truly a unique disorder or if it is a consequence of aphasia or a broader deficit in sequencing and organizing components into a larger whole.

Somatoparaphrenia (Greek: *somato = body, para = beside/next to, phren = mind*; English usage *phrenia = mental disorder*) is the belief that one's own body part belongs to someone else. In his book *The Man Who Mistook His Wife for a Hat*, Oliver Sacks describes a man who found someone's leg in his bed and tried to throw it out. Unbeknownst to him, the leg actually belonged to him, and he threw himself onto the floor. This can occur after right parietal damage.

Sensory Pathways

There are three major sensory pathways: **dorsal column–medial lemniscus (DCML)**, **spinothalamic**, and **spinocerebellar** tracts. Although they differ in the type of sensory information carried, the location of the axons in the spinal cord, the location of the crossover, and the number of neurons in the pathway, there are some general similarities. The DCML and spinothalamic tracts both begin in the periphery and convey signals through a set of three neurons up to the primary sensory strip in the contralateral postcentral gyrus. The **first-order neurons** are pseudounipolar with receptors (dendrites) in the body (e.g., embedded in skin, muscles, joints) and cell bodies in the dorsal root ganglion near the spinal cord. The axons enter the spinal cord through the dorsal root. These neurons remain ipsilateral and synapse onto second-order neurons. The **second-order neurons** decussate (cross the midline) and extend up to the VPL nucleus of the thalamus, where they synapse onto third-order neurons. The axons of the **third-order neurons** extend up to the appropriate location in the sensory strip (depending on body region), where they synapse. The locations of these pathways within the spinal cord are illustrated in Figure 6–4.

Dorsal Column–Medial Lemniscal Pathway

This pathway is named for the location of the axons of the sensory neurons as they extend through the spinal cord and brainstem to the thalamus. There are three neurons within the pathway. The pathway is outlined in Table 6–2 and described here.

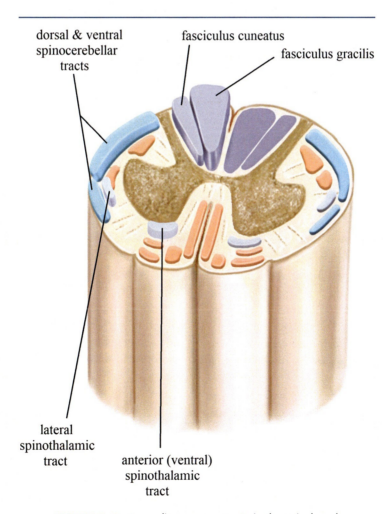

FIGURE 6–4. Ascending sensory tracts in the spinal cord.

Table 6–2. DCML Pathway Carries Localizable Touch, Vibratory Sense, and Proprioception

	Type of Neuron	Dendrites/Cell Body	Axon	Synapse*
First-order neuron	Pseudounipolar	Mechanoreceptors and proprioceptors in the PNS/dorsal root ganglion	Through dorsal root to dorsal column: gracilis (lower body); cuneatus (upper body)	Ipsilateral medulla: nucleus gracilis (lower body) or nucleus cuneatus (upper body)
Second-order neuron	Multipolar	Nucleus cuneatus or gracilis	Crosses over and extends through medial lemniscus	Contralateral thalamus, ventroposterolateral nucleus
Third-order neuron	Multipolar	Thalamus, ventroposterolateral nucleus	Extends through corona radiata	Contralateral postcentral gyrus; primary somatosensory area

Note. *Laterality is in reference to the beginning of the tract; for example, if the first-order neuron begins on the left side of the body, ipsilateral means the left side of the CNS and contralateral means the right side of the CNS.

The first-order neuron is a pseudounipolar sensory neuron with its dendritic extension in the peripheral nervous system. Its dendrites are mechanoreceptors. The cell body of this first-order neuron is in the dorsal root ganglion. The axonic extension enters the spinal cord via the dorsal root and extends superiorly toward the brainstem in the **dorsal column**. The dorsal column is a region of white matter in between the two dorsal horns of the spinal cord. In the lower levels of the spinal cord (below approximately vertebrae T7), the dorsal columns consist only of axons carrying information from the lower body (feet, legs, hips). This is called the **fasciculus gracilis** (Latin: *slender*) and is particularly relevant to physical therapists regarding ambulation. In the midregion of the spinal cord, a second portion of the dorsal columns develops laterally. This is the **fasciculus cuneatus** (Latin: *wedge-shaped*), and it is created by neurons coming from the trunk and upper body. This region is particularly relevant to occupational and physical therapists for arm movement and self-cares activities.

The axons in the dorsal columns synapse in the medulla in either the **nucleus gracilis** or the **nucleus cuneatus**, depending on which fasciculus they travelled in. They synapse onto second-order neurons whose axons cross the midline and then extend superiorly toward the thalamus in a region of the brainstem called the **medial lemniscus**. Axons of these second-order neurons extend to the VPL nucleus of the thalamus, where they synapse onto third-order neurons. Axons from these neurons extend primarily to the primary sensory strip in the postcentral gyrus of the parietal lobe (Figure 6–5). Somatotopic organization is maintained throughout the pathway.

Box 6–4. Dorsal Columns

Discriminative touch and proprioceptive information for the lower body is carried within the fasciculus *gracilis* (Latin: *slender*). You can also remember this as thinking of *graceful* walking. At the lower levels of the spinal cord, the fasciculus gracilis makes up the entire dorsal columns. Touch and proprioception are carried in the fasciculus *cuneatus* (Latin: *wedge-shaped*). The fasciculus cuneatus develops lateral to the gracilis as sensory neurons from the trunk and upper body enter the spinal cord. You can think of them wedging their way into the dorsal column space, taking up the lateral region while squeezing the fasciculus gracilis into a slender region medially. You can also imagine the dorsal columns being created in a caudal–rostral direction, with each successive group of axons adding in laterally so that those from the toes are most medial, then the heels, lower legs, upper legs, etc.

Spinothalamic Tracts

The anterolateral spinothalamic tracts also are three-neuron pathways. They are outlined in Table 6–3. There are two sections—one that lies in the anterior white matter of the spinal cord and the other in the lateral region. Pain and temperature sensations are carried through the lateral spinothalamic tract, and unlocalizable (gross, diffuse) touch is

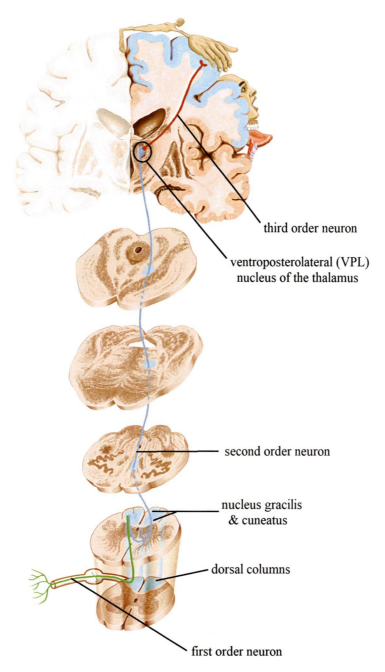

FIGURE 6–5. Dorsal column–medial lemniscus sensory pathway.

carried through the anterior portion of the tract. The first-order neuron, like that of the DCML system, has dendrites in the periphery and a cell body in the dorsal root ganglion. Once the axon enters the spinal cord, it enters the dorsal horn and synapses onto the second-order neuron. This neuron's axon crosses over and then extends up the spinal cord in the contralateral white matter. If it is part of the lateral spinothalamic tract, it will extend up in the lateral spinal cord; if it is part of the anterior tract, it will extend up in the anterior region of the spinal cord (Figure 6–6). Regardless of the tract, the second-order neuron axons extend superiorly through the brainstem to the thalamus, where they synapse in the VPL nucleus onto the third-order neuron. The axon of the third-order neuron extends to the postcentral gyrus.

Table 6–3. Anterolateral Spinothalamic Pathway Carries Pain and Temperature

	Type of Neuron	Dendrites/Cell Body	Axon	Synapse*
First-order neuron	Pseudounipolar	Pain and temperature receptors in the PNS/ dorsal root ganglion	Through dorsal root to dorsal horn	Ipsilateral dorsal horn
Second-order neuron	Multipolar	Dorsal horn	Crosses over and extends superiorly through the anterior or lateral white matter	Contralateral thalamus, ventroposterolateral nucleus
Third-order neuron	Multipolar	Thalamus, ventroposterolateral nucleus	Extends through corona radiata	Contralateral postcentral gyrus; primary somatosensory area

Note. *Laterality is in reference to the beginning of the tract; for example, if the first-order neuron begins on the left side of the body, ipsilateral means the left side of the CNS and contralateral means the right side of the CNS.

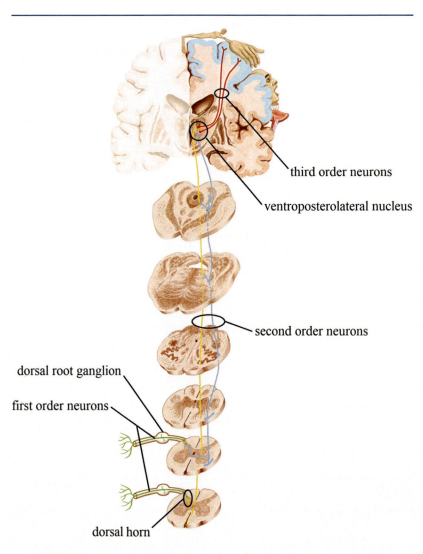

FIGURE 6–6. Anterior (*yellow*) and lateral (*blue*) spinothalamic tracts.

Spinocerebellar Tracts

Spinocerebellar tracts are two-neuron pathways that carry proprioceptive information about the position, range, and direction of limb movements to the ipsilateral cerebellum. Because these tracts end in the cerebellum and not the cerebrum, the information does not reach consciousness. Thus, they are responsible for **unconscious proprioception**. The signals are integrated in the cerebellum with the motor system, and they aid in monitoring and modifying ongoing movements. The cerebellum is discussed in more detail in Chapter 10. What is important to know now is that there are extensive connections between the motor and sensory systems. In order to create a purposeful movement such as picking up a water bottle, you have to know not only where the water bottle is located but also the position of your arm and your hand. If your arm is to the left of the water bottle, the movement will be very different than if your arm is to the right of it. Unconscious knowledge of where your limbs are positioned is critical for planning and carrying out movements.

There are two components of the spinocerebellar tracts: the anterior and the posterior tract (Table 6–4). Remember that anatomical terms are used within a specific context, so having an anterior and a posterior tract tells you that the names highlight that one is located more anteriorly than the other, not necessarily that one is in the anterior and the other the posterior spinal cord. In fact, they both lie along the lateral borders of the spinal cord.

Like the other sensory pathways, the first-order neurons of the spinocerebellar tracts are pseudounipolar neurons with cell bodies in the dorsal root ganglia. They enter the spinal cord and synapse in the dorsal horn onto the second-order neurons. In the anterior portion of the tract, the axons either stay ipsilateral and extend up the lateral spinal cord and enter the cerebellum or they decussate, extend up the contralateral spinal cord, and then decussate again in the brainstem before entering the ipsilateral cerebellum. The reason for and impact of the double crossover is unknown. In the posterior portion of the tract, the axons of the second-order neurons extend up the lateral spinal cord and enter the ipsilateral cerebellum.

Table 6–4. Spinocerebellar Pathways Transmit Signals for Unconscious Proprioception

	Type of Neuron	**Dendrites/Cell Body**	**Axon**	**Synapse***
First-order neuron	Pseudounipolar	Proprioceptive receptors in the PNS/dorsal root ganglion	Through dorsal root to dorsal horn	Ipsilateral dorsal horn
Second-order neuron	Multipolar	Dorsal horn	Anterior: either crosses over and extends superiorly through the lateral edge of the contralateral spinal cord and then crosses back over in the brainstem or extends superiorly through the lateral edge of the ipsilateral spinal cord Posterior: extends superiorly through the lateral edge of the ipsilateral spinal cord	Ipsilateral cerebellum

Note. *Laterality is in reference to the beginning of the tract; for example, if the first-order neuron begins on the left side of the body, ipsilateral means the left side of the CNS and contralateral means the right side of the CNS.

> **Box 6–5.** Clinical Application: Spinal Assessment
>
> After a spinal cord injury, neurologists and nurses will assess the integrity of the DCML and anterolateral spinothalamic tracts. Typically, they begin by assessing the entire length of the tract, from head to toe. Providers often begin at the toes but move toward the head if necessary. Somatosensory assessment is not within the scope of practice of speech–language pathologists or audiologists, but this assessment helps explain the function of these pathways.
>
> To assess the integrity of the DCML, the provider assesses light touch, vibration sense, and proprioception. Light touch is assessed by asking the patient if they can feel a cotton ball brushed against the sole of their foot or toes on either side. Similarly, vibration sense is addressed by striking a tuning fork, placing it on the great toe, and asking the patient if they can feel it. Proprioception can be assessed (assuming there is some sensation to the feet) by moving the great toe upwards and downwards, asking the patient about the position (up or down).
>
> Assessing the integrity of the anterolateral spinothalamic tract involves assessment of pain, deep touch, and temperature. Pain is assessed through a pin prick on the great toe or sole of the foot. Deep touch is addressed as the provider exerts deep pressure, squeezing the great toe between their thumb and index finger. Finally, temperature is assessed by placing a cold metal object on the sole or great toe.
>
> The spinocerebellar tract is not typically assessed in this context because it requires the person to ambulate or at least sit upright. Proprioceptive inputs from the spinal cord (body) to the cerebellum have a role in sitting balance, posture, and standing/walking.

Sensory Innervation

Each spinal nerve innervates a section of the body. These sections, called dermatomes, are horizontal "stripes" across the trunk and vertical regions down the arms and legs (Figure 6–7A). As noted in the beginning of this chapter, sensation from the head is carried through the cranial nerves (see Chapter 11). The corresponding segments innervated by motor neurons are called myotomes. Dermatomes are clearly indicated by the shingles virus, which tends to infect a single dorsal root ganglion, causing a painful rash that extends unilaterally along a single dermatome. As shown in Figure 6–7B, there is slight overlap of regions innervated such that three consecutive spinal nerves have to be treated to anesthetize one dermatome.

Damage to Somatosensory System Components

Spinal Cord Damage

Damage to the spinal cord that interrupts the somatosensory pathways will reduce the perception of pain, touch, and/or temperature depending on the location of the damage. A complete transection (cut) of the spinal cord will result in loss of all sensation below the level of the lesion. All sensation above the lesion will remain intact because the axon pathways above the lesion can still send signals to the brain. Due to Wallerian degeneration, neurons will die back approximately one spinal segment above the level of damage.

A hemisection (one-half of the cord, either right or left to the midline) creates an interesting pattern of sensory deficits known as Brown–Séquard syndrome. Although this is rare and is not directly relevant to speech-language pathology or audiology, it illustrates the consequences of the separation of somatosensory modalities into different pathways (Figure 6–8).

The first-order neurons of the DCML pathway, carrying information about fine touch, extend ipsilaterally up the spinal cord until they synapse in the medulla, where the second-order neurons then cross over and extend to the thalamus. Damage to the right side of the spinal cord would cause a loss of touch sensation ipsilaterally—on the right side of the body. (Note: Although the motor pathways are not discussed until Chapter 10, they cross over in the medulla on their way down to the spinal cord, and thus run down the contralateral cord. A spinal hemisection

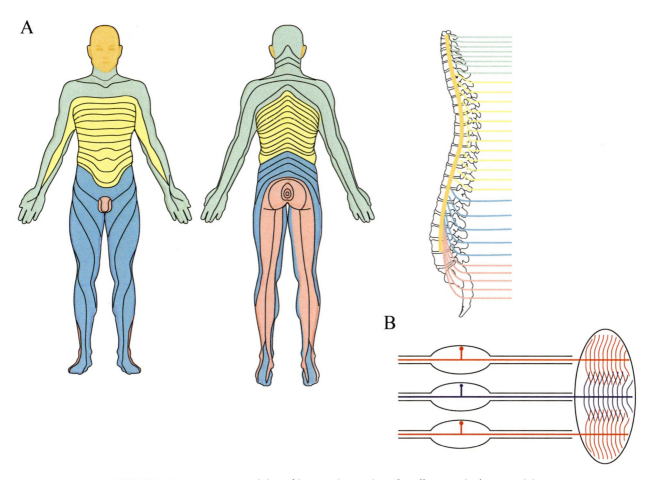

FIGURE 6–7. Dermatomes (**A**) and innervation regions for afferent spinal nerves (**B**).

would cause ipsilateral paralysis, so the loss of touch would be accompanied by paralysis of that side of the body.)

The first-order neurons of the spinothalamic tracts, carrying information about pain and temperature, synapse immediately upon entering the spinal cord onto second-order neurons that cross over and then extend to the thalamus. Damage to the right side of the spinal cord would cause loss of pain and temperature sensation for the left side of the body. If you placed an ice cube on the left leg of someone with a right hemisection, they would feel the touch of the ice cube but not the cold temperature. If you put the ice cube on the person's right leg, they would feel a cold sensation with no accompanying touch of the cube.

Thalamic Damage

Because of the variety of functions of the thalamus, the site of lesion will determine the symptoms that occur. Disorders of sensation are discussed here; other effects of thalamic damage are covered in the relevant chapters.

Damage to the thalamus, such as due to a small stroke, can result in a central pain disorder (sometimes called **thalamic pain syndrome**, although similar disorders can occur with damage to spinal cord or brainstem regions of the spinothalamic tracts). The disorder is called a central disorder because pain is "created" in the central nervous system as opposed to in the periphery. There are several potential components of the syndrome. One is **allodynia**, or the perception of touch as pain. Another is **hyperalgesia**, when painful stimuli are experienced as much more painful than is typical. Temperature perception also is affected so that cold stimuli are perceived as a burning pain. The **dysesthesia** (disordered sensation) can be localized to specific regions (e.g., hand, foot) or multiple regions, all contralateral to the thalamic damage. Whereas some patients may experience the pain syndrome immediately, for others it

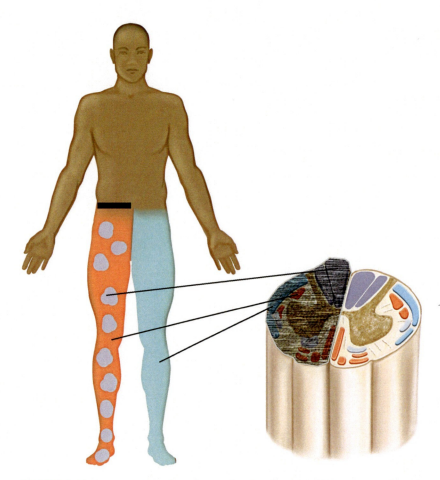

FIGURE 6–8. Brown–Séquard syndrome due to a hemicord lesion. Loss of touch sensation ipsilaterally (*blue dots*) due to cutting the DCML pathway that ascends in the ipsilateral spinal cord; loss of pain and temperature sensation contralaterally (*light blue shading*) due to damage to the anterolateral spinothalamic tracts that ascend the spinal cord contralaterally; and loss of movement (paralysis) ipsilaterally (*red*) because the lateral corticospinal tracts cross over in the medulla, so any spinal cord lesion will result in motor deficits on the same side as the lesion.

does not appear until months after a thalamic stroke. Emotions, stress, or situational factors can exacerbate centralized pain, whereas distraction and relaxation can reduce it.

Remember that the thalamus is not only a relay station but also an integration station with extensive two-way connections with the cortex as well as motor system. Disruption of corticothalamic loops can alter the balance of excitatory and inhibitory signals, resulting in not enough inhibition. Without the balancing "no-go" signals, thalamic neurons that typically relay pain signals can create and send too many action potentials to the cortex, resulting in the perception of pain.

Cortical Damage

Damage to the primary somatosensory strip will result in sensory loss in the contralateral body. All modalities (pain, touch, temperature, proprioception) will be affected. The region of the body impacted is based on which areas of the somatosensory strip are affected: face, hand, arm, leg, or a combination of consecutive areas. Loss that affects the entire half of the body is called **hemisensory loss**. Typically, hemisensory loss is accompanied by **hemiparesis** (half-weakness) because the primary motor and sensory areas are adjacent to each other.

Reduced sensation in the face and laryngeal areas can affect swallowing and increase the risk of penetration of food and liquid into the respiratory system because without the sensory signal, the cough reflex will not be triggered. Speech production also may be affected because the rapid, precise movements of the articulators rely on integration of motor and sensory signals. Studies of speech production after local anesthetic to regions of the tongue or mouth indicate that some people experience minor changes in articulatory precision, whereas others do not. Either way, the changes have minimal impact on speech intelligibility. Dysarthria resulting from middle cerebral artery strokes (see Chapter 13) is likely due to a combination of weakness and reduced somatosensory signals.

tracts that convey signals to the ipsilateral cerebellum for integration with motor systems, all somatosensory axons cross over and synapse in the contralateral thalamus from where signals are then sent to the appropriate regions of the cortex.

Somatosensation is critical for safe swallowing and has a role in speech production. In addition to those direct connections to speech-language pathology, somatosensory deficits can play a role in aspects of communication. Hemisensory loss can impair writing and possibly gesturing (due to reduced sensory feedback) on the affected side. Inability to feel a tap on the shoulder or spilling a cup of coffee can impact social communication.

Box 6–6. Everyday Consequences of Reduced Somatosensory Perception

A 75-year-old male with a stroke in the right middle cerebral artery described the effects of his hemisensory loss. When he picked up a Styrofoam cup full of coffee, he could not feel the cup in his hand and thus could not sense how tightly to grasp the cup. This resulted in either dropping his coffee because he did not grasp the cup tight enough or crushing the cup because he grasped too tightly. His compensatory strategy was to use only ceramic mugs and to grasp tightly. That way, he could minimize the risk of either crushing or dropping it.

Key Concepts

- Somatosensory systems process pain, touch, temperature, vibratory sense, proprioceptive, and kinesthetic signals.
- Specific sensory receptors selectively process each type of information.
- Touch and proprioception are carried together; pain and temperature are carried by a separate pathway.
- In the three-neuron pathways (dorsal column–medial lemniscus and anterolateral spinal thalamic), the first-order neuron remains entirely ipsilateral, the second-order neuron decussates, and the third-order neuron is entirely contralateral.
- The spinocerebellar pathway carries sensory signals to the ipsilateral cerebellum for integration with the motor system.
- Damage to the pathways can differentially affect the two systems (pain/temperature versus touch), whereas cortical damage typically affects all modalities.

Summary

Somatosensory receptors are designed to register and respond to specific stimuli: pain, touch, temperature, and proprioception. With the exception of the spinocerebellar

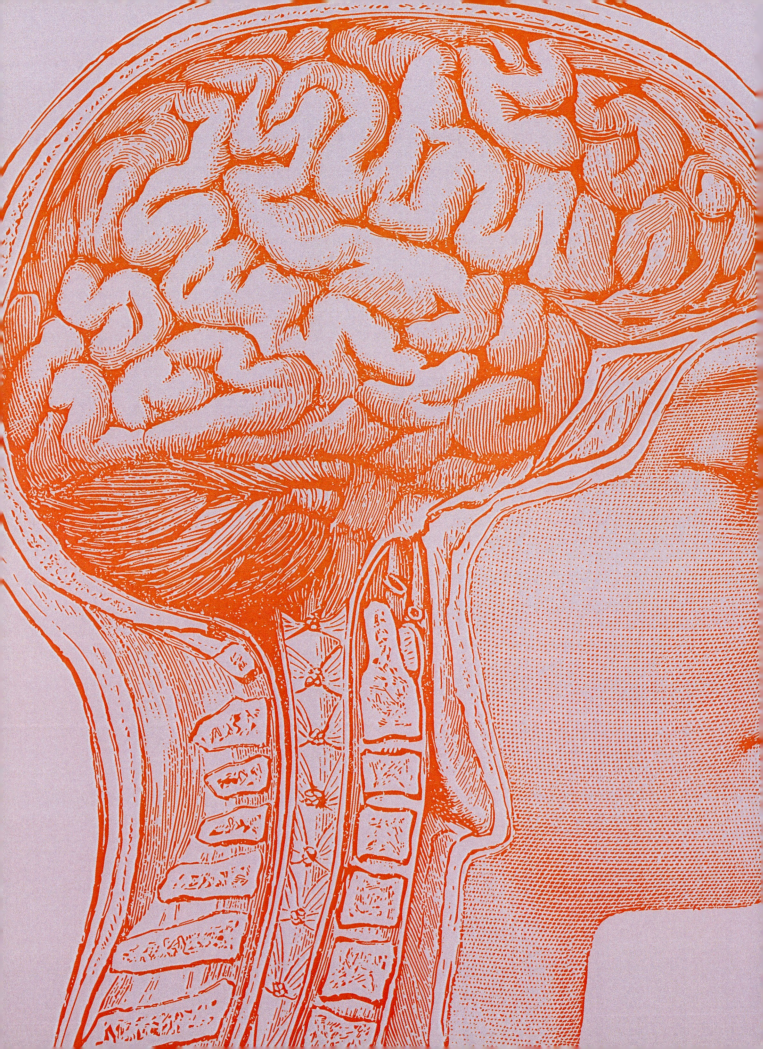

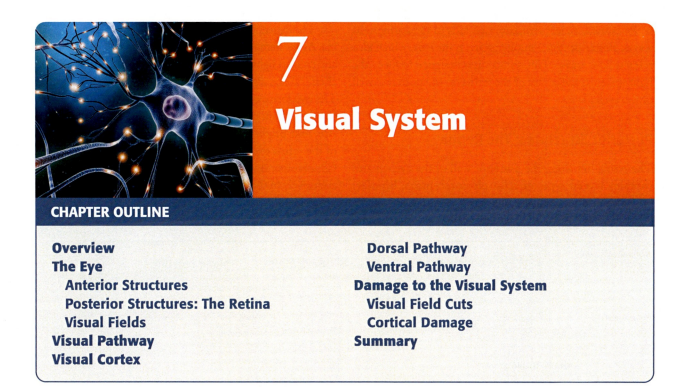

7
Visual System

CHAPTER OUTLINE

Overview
The Eye
   Anterior Structures
   Posterior Structures: The Retina
   Visual Fields
Visual Pathway
Visual Cortex

Dorsal Pathway
Ventral Pathway
Damage to the Visual System
   Visual Field Cuts
   Cortical Damage
Summary

Overview

The visual system has an enormous role in communication. Most obviously is the role of vision in reading and writing. Even for people who do not explicitly lip read (speech read), visual information helps us process what we hear. If you have ever tried to listen to a television program when there is a lag between audio and video, you recognize that it is more difficult to understand speech without the correct visual cues. Likewise, when listening to a less intelligible client, we rely more heavily on visual information. This visual information comes in the form of lip movement, facial expressions, and gestures. Augmentative alternative communication systems also often rely heavily on visual systems, including eye gaze, tracking, and direct selection.

The visual system is designed to convert light waves into representations of the items in our environment. Image processing begins in the retina, a group of cells on the posterior wall of the eyeball. The processing continues at multiple stages along the pathway to the occipital lobe and then to the parietal and temporal lobes. Interestingly, one-third of cortical tissue in the brain is involved in processing visual images.

A few characteristics of the visual system are repeatedly illustrated in this chapter. First is that the system is designed to have the best, most efficient processing of images in the center of the visual field. Several structural and processing features ensure that this is the case. Second, there is parallel processing such that the same information can be conveyed through different cells. Third, there is fractionation of the visual image. Different neurons respond best to different features of a visual image (e.g., brightness, color, shape, or orientation), and these features are integrated in the cortex. Fourth, there is contralateral sensory control as with the somatosensory system; however, the contralateral control involves the right and left visual fields of each eye and not simply the left versus right eye.

The Eye

Anterior Structures

The anterior eye includes the **cornea**, **lens**, **pupil**, and **iris**. The pupil is an opening in which light waves enter the eye. The size of the pupil is controlled by **ciliary muscles** in the iris, the colored region surrounding the pupil. Constriction of the pupil decreases the amount of light that can enter, and dilation increases it. The ciliary muscles that change pupil size are innervated by cranial nerves, which are discussed in Chapter 11. Anterior to the pupil and iris is the cornea, a clear structure that aids in refracting light waves. Posterior to the pupil and iris is the lens, which also refracts light waves. This refraction is designed to focus the light waves in the center of the retina on the posterior wall of the eyeball.

Posterior Structures: The Retina

The retina lies along the posterior wall of the eyeball and contains several types of cells: **photoreceptors**, **bipolar**, **amacrine**, **horizontal**, and **ganglion cells** (Figure 7–1).

Photoreceptors are in the most posterior layer of the retina. As the name suggests, these cells respond to light (photo-) and convert light signals into electrical (action potentials) and chemical signals (neurotransmitter release at the synapse). The two forms of photoreceptors are **rods** and **cones**, named for their shapes. Rods are responsible for detecting shape, size, and brightness and are distributed throughout most of the retina except for the central region called the **fovea**. Cones respond to color and fine detail and are found almost exclusively in the central portion of the retina. Specific characteristics of photoreceptors are listed in Table 7–1.

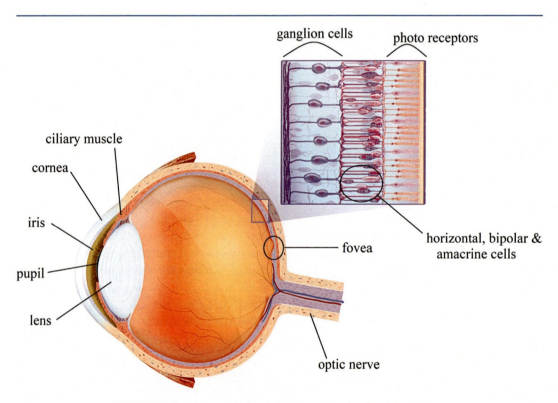

FIGURE 7–1. Anatomy of the posterior eye and cells of the retina.

Table 7–1. Characteristics of Photoreceptors

	Rods	**Cones**
Types of cells	One type	Three types (red, green, blue responders)
Best function	Primarily nighttime or low light	Primarily daytime or strong light
Feature detection	Shape, size, brightness	Color, fine detail
Location	Located in periphery of retina (none in central retina)	Located primarily in central retina
No. in retina	92 million	5 million

Box 7–1. Viewing the Night Sky

Cones, found in the central retina, do not process signals well in low light. Rods respond well in both bright and low light. This is why, when looking at the night sky, it is often difficult to identify dim stars when you're looking directly at them—because the cones do not process the dim light well. Shifting your gaze slightly to one side puts that image on to the rod-dense region of the retina, where you can perceive it.

The rods and cones synapse onto bipolar cells. As described in Chapter 3, these bipolar cells have two extensions from the soma: a single dendrite stalk and the typical single axon. The bipolar cells in turn synapse onto ganglion cells (which are also bipolar in shape). The axons to the ganglion cells exit the retina as the optic nerve. As shown in Figure 7–1, there is a "hole" in the retina for the optic nerve to exit (this is also where blood vessels enter/exit the eye). The absence of photoreceptors in this region creates a blind spot. Although all humans have a blind spot in each eye, these do not affect everyday life because of binocular (two-eye) vision and because the brain will fill in parts of the image that are not detected.

Box 7–2. Finding Your Blind Spot

There are various ways to find your blind spot. Some quick and easy tasks can be found at Neuroscience for Kids at https://faculty.washington.edu/chudler/ch vision.html

The fovea appears as a depression in the center of the retina and serves as a landmark for dividing superior versus inferior and lateral (called temporal) from medial (called nasal) sections of the retina (Figure 7–1). In the fovea, the bipolar and ganglion cells are displaced so that the light waves directly hit the photoreceptors. This enhances processing of images that are in the central region of the visual field.

Image processing begins in the retina, where the neurons respond to differences in intensity of light. Somewhat counterintuitively, photoreceptors' preferred stimulus is darkness. They are hyperpolarized in the light and depolarize when light is removed. Depolarization results in release of glutamate at the synapse with bipolar cells.

The horizontal and amacrine cells provide connections between photoreceptors and ganglion cells. This allows adjacent cells to "know" what their neighbors are doing. As described in more detail later, this feature is important for distinguishing borders and edges of images. There is also convergence of signals in the retina. The approximately 97 million photoreceptors synapse onto approximately 1 million ganglion cells. In the central retina, only a few photoreceptors synapse onto each ganglion cell, whereas in the periphery many photoreceptors converge onto each ganglion cell. This, in addition to the fovea and the concentration of cones in the central retina, results in enhanced visual processing in central vision in comparison to peripheral vision.

Throughout the entire visual pathway, beginning with the retina, there is **visuotopic organization**. This means that the neurons are organized in relation to the signals they receive and carry; those that carry information from the upper portion of the visual field are located in a slightly different location than those that carry/receive information from the lower visual field (Figure 7–2). There is also parallel processing in the visual system, in which the same information is sent via different cells and pathways and reconstructed or compared at later stages in the pathway.

Visual Fields

One critical distinction in understanding the visual system is the difference between **visual fields** and **retinal fields**. Visual fields are what you see around you. Close your right eye, and what you can see is the visual field of your left eye. Retinal fields are the images represented on your retina. The retinal fields have the same images as those you see in your visual fields except that they are upside down and the right and left halves are reversed (Figure 7–3). The fact that it is upside down has little consequence for the pathways and disorders of vision, so you can set that aside for now. The reversal of left and right visual fields, in contrast, is very important. In the retina, the right and left sections are referred to as temporal and nasal fields. Temporal fields are more lateral, near the temples; nasal fields are more medial, near the nose. In the left eye, the temporal retinal field is lateral, close to the temple, and on the left side. In the right eye, the temporal retinal field is lateral, close to the temple, but this time on the right side. The nasal fields, as you may have guessed, are the retinal fields close to the nose. For the left eye, the nasal retinal field is on the right side of the eye, and for the right eye, the nasal retinal field is on the left side of the eye.

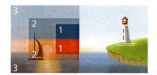
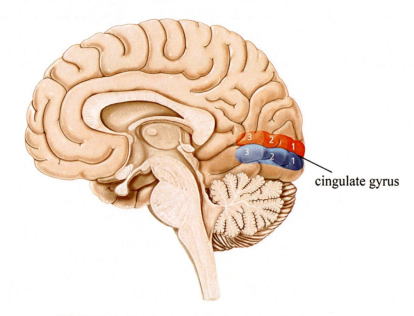

FIGURE 7–2. Visuotopic organization in the visual cortex.

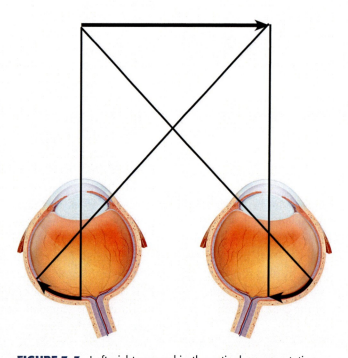

FIGURE 7–3. Left–right reversal in the retinal representation.

Given the way light waves are refracted by the lens of the eye, images from the left side of space (left visual field) will hit the right side of the retina and vice versa. Importantly, this happens separately for each eye. The result is that things in the left visual field of the left eye end up on the nasal retinal field of that eye, and things in the left visual field of the right eye end up on the temporal retinal field of that eye.

Visual Pathway

The visual pathway extending from the retina changes names several times. The name changes are important because different information and different axons are contained in each segment (Table 7–2; Figure 7–4). The pathway beyond the retina is sometimes referred to as the **retinofugal** pathway. Given the etymology of the word (Latin: *fugal = to flee*), the retinofugal pathway contains all the axons and neurons extending away from the retina.

The **optic nerves** (one each from the right and left eye), containing ganglion cell axons, extend from the retina to the optic chiasm. Each optic nerve carries all of the signals from a single eye.

The **optic chiasm** is the point of crossover. Just as in other sensorimotor systems in which the right side of the brain is responsible for the left side of the body, there is a crossover in the visual system. It is not, however, a simple right eye–left brain switch. Approximately half of the axons in each optic nerve cross over at the chiasm (Figure 7–5). Axons from the nasal retinal fields of each eye cross over in the chiasm, whereas those from the temporal retinal fields remain ipsilateral. Remember that the retinal fields contain images from the opposite visual field: The left visual field of the left eye projects onto the nasal retinal field; this is what crosses over. The result is that for each eye, images from the left visual field end up on the right side of the brain and vice versa.

The pathway extending posteriorly from the chiasm is called the **optic tract**. Due to the partial crossover, the optic tract contains some axons from each eye. In fact, the right optic tract contains axons carrying signals from the right temporal and left nasal retinal fields. These represent the left visual field of each eye. The majority of optic tract axons extend to the lateral geniculate nucleus (LGN) of the thalamus, where they synapse onto thalamic neurons. Approximately 10% of the optic tract axons extend to the midbrain in and around the superior colliculus. These

Table 7–2. Segments of the Visual Pathways With Retinal and Visual Field Contents

Pathway Segment	Retinal Field		Visual Field	
	Left	Right	Left	Right
Optic nerve	Axons from both retinal fields of the left eye	Axons from both retinal fields of the right eye	Entire visual field of the left eye	Entire visual field of the right eye
Optic chiasm	Crossover of axons from nasal retinal fields; axons from temporal retinal fields remain ipsilateral	Crossover of axons from nasal retinal fields; axons from temporal retinal fields remain ipsilateral	Left visual field (periphery) crosses over; right visual field remains ipsilateral	Right visual field (periphery) crosses over; left visual field remains ipsilateral
Optic tract	Axons from right nasal retina and left temporal retina	Axons from left nasal retina and right temporal retina	Right visual field from each eye	Left visual field from each eye
Optic radiations (geniculocalcarine fibers)	Axons from right nasal retina and left temporal retina	Axons from left nasal retina and right temporal retina	Right visual field from each eye	Left visual field from each eye

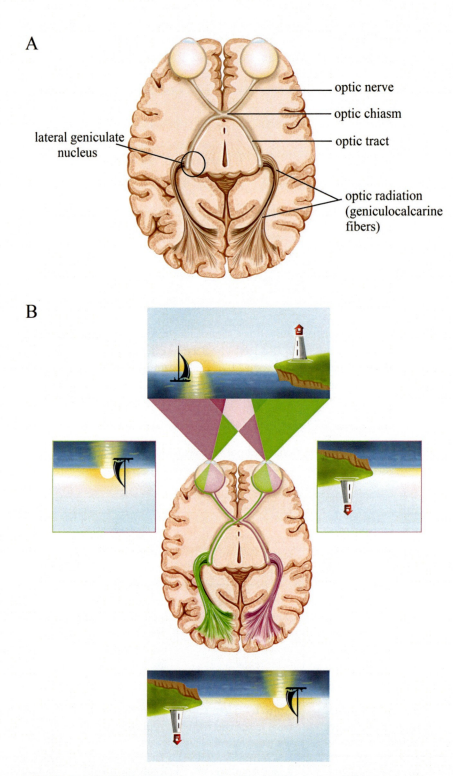

FIGURE 7–4. **A.** Segments of the visual pathway. **B.** Segments of the visual pathway color-coded to show information carried.

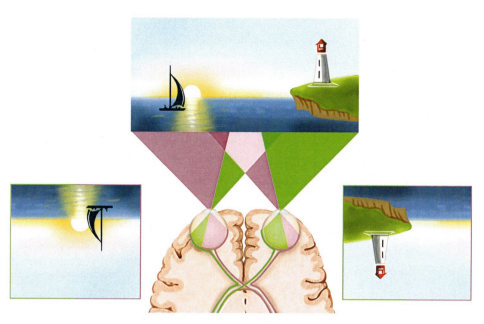

FIGURE 7–5. Crossover of nasal versus temporal fields at the optic chiasm. The images from the nasal visual field of each eye (left eye—sailboat, highlighted in *pink*; right eye—lighthouse, highlighted in *green*) each cross over at the optic chiasm. In the optic tract, after the crossover, the images from the right visual field of each eye (left eye—ocean, highlighted in *green*; right eye—lighthouse, highlighted in *green*) all are in the left optic tract.

neurons influence pupil size and eye movement, including orientation of the eyes and head to visual stimuli. Finally, a small portion of the optic tract axons synapse in the hypothalamus and influence circadian rhythms and sleep–wake cycles.

Each LGN consists of six layers of cells that are arranged retinotopically but also by which eye the inputs come from. Thus, in the left LGN, neurons in layers 1, 4, and 6 connect with ganglion cell axons from the right eye, and the remaining layers (2, 3, and 5) receive signals coming from the left eye. In addition to the inputs from the optic tract, the LGN also receives signals from regions of the visual cortex. These inputs are not well understood but could be involved in the attentional control of vision, in which people do not "see" things that they are not focusing on, even though the images are being detected on the retina and signals are sent through the visual pathways.

The final segment of the pathway to the brain is called either the **optic radiation** (because the axons appear to fan out from the LGN before converging on the occipital lobe) or the **geniculocalcarine** fibers. The latter name describes the location of the pathway—from the lateral *geniculate* nucleus to the region of the occipital lobe surrounding the *calcarine* sulcus. The optic radiation is made up of LGN axons, and because there was no additional crossover after the optic chiasm, the optic radiation carries the same information as the optic tract: The left radiation carries information from the right visual field of each eye and vice versa. These axons synapse onto neurons in the occipital lobe, which is the final stop in getting signals from the periphery to the brain but not the final stop for visual processing.

Visual Cortex

Visual signals reach the occipital lobe by way of the geniculocalcarine fibers (or optic radiation). The axons from the LGN synapse in Brodmann area 17, at the posterior-most extent of the occipital lobe. Brodmann area 17 is also known as the primary visual cortex (V1) or the striate cortex, so named because when it is dissected out, it has a striped appearance. The calcarine sulcus along the medial surface of the occipital lobe separates this region into superior and inferior sections. Remember that there is a retinotopic representation maintained throughout the pathway (neurons/axons organized by region of the retina where the signal began) and that the image is upside down and backwards. Thus, axons carrying signals from the inferior retina will synapse in the area superior to the calcarine sulcus, and those carrying signals from the superior retina will synapse inferior to the sulcus. There is additional distortion of the retinotopic image such that the portion of the image that hits the central retina is larger and more detailed than the part of the image that was more peripheral. This is yet another component of the pattern described all along that emphasizes images in the central region of the visual field. The organization also includes ocular dominance columns, in which images from the right and left eye are organized in distinct regions. Many occipital neurons in these columns receive signals only from one eye, although some receive signals from both left and right eyes. Neurons in the occipital lobe also have selectivity, meaning that they respond best to certain stimuli. Some have orientation selectivity and respond best to lines oriented in a specific direction (e.g., horizontal, vertical, diagonal). Others respond best to a specific direction of movement.

Brodmann areas 17–19 are considered the initial visual processing areas. From this point, signals are sent via cortical neurons to association areas in the temporal and parietal lobes, in which signals are processed further and visual signals are integrated with other sensory and cognitive systems.

Dorsal Pathway

Extending from the occipital lobe is a dorsal pathway that ends in the parietal lobe (Figure 7–6). This is known as the "where" pathway and is important for putting items within the broader context of the environment, so you know where, for example, your pencil is in relation to your notebook, both of which are on the desk in front of you. This pathway also is important for detecting and processing motion and using visual input to direct action. Neurons in this pathway respond not only to actual movement but also to perceived movement, as in visual illusions in which an image appears to move even though the lines and colors are stationary. Cells in this pathway selectively respond to linear, radial, or circular motion.

Ventral Pathway

There is also a ventral pathway that extends into the inferior temporal lobe (Figure 7–6). This is known as the "what" pathway and is responsible for processing shape, color, and size. These three features are processed separately and only combined at a later stage of processing. Additional processing through connections to other areas of the temporal and parietal lobes is necessary to assign meaning to

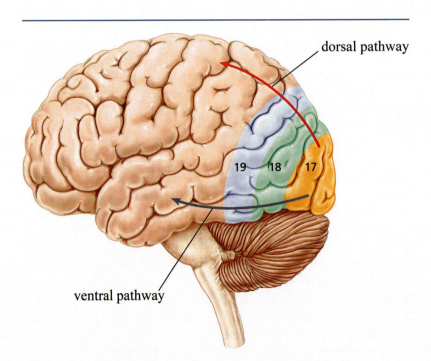

FIGURE 7–6. Dorsal and ventral visual pathways.

shapes for object or image recognition. The fusiform gyrus in the inferior temporal lobe is specialized for recognition of faces, whereas other temporal regions aid in recognition of other objects. In the left hemisphere, further connections with the temporo-parieto-occipital lobe regions such as the angular and supramarginal gyrus are important for reading and writing.

Damage to the Visual System

Damage to or degeneration of the peripheral components such as the cornea and retina result in visual loss called blindness. Damage to the pathways causes partial visual loss depending on the region of the pathway that is affected. Most of these are referred to as visual field cuts as opposed to blindness because there is often a substantial proportion of the visual fields that remains intact.

Visual Field Cuts

Knowledge of the visual pathways, the axons contained in each segment, and the representations carried in each segment is critical for understanding the types of visual field cuts that result from damage to the pathways. A breakdown of the naming conventions will help with the discussion. First, visual field cuts are named for what is lost: the region that the person can no longer see. Thus, they refer to the visual field, not the retinal field. The suffix *-anopsia* (sometimes seen as *anopia*) refers to loss of vision (Greek: *an-* = *without; -opsia* = *seeing*). The loss rarely affects the whole visual field and thus can be a **hemianopsia** (loss of half of the visual field) or **quadrantanopsia** (loss of a quarter of the visual field). In some cases, the same visual field of each eye is affected (e.g., the right visual field of each eye), which is called **homonymous** (same-sided). In other cases, the opposite visual fields are affected, such as the left visual field of the left eye and the right visual field of the right eye; these are labeled **heteronymous**. Knowing how to break down the names will go a long way in understanding visual field cuts. Figure 7–7 illustrates the visual field cuts that result from damage to various areas of the visual pathway.

Damage to either optic nerve will result in ipsilateral **monocular blindness**, or blindness in one eye. It will be ipsilateral because each optic nerve contains all the axons from the retina in a single eye.

Damage to the center of the optic chiasm will cause a **bitemporal heteronymous hemianopsia** (Figure 7–7A). Breaking apart the name, it is bilateral and affects the temporal visual field of each eye. This means it will affect the

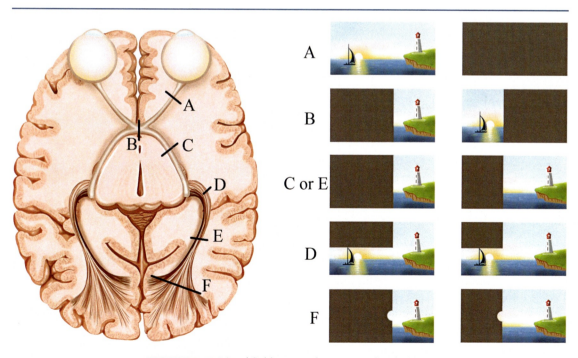

FIGURE 7–7. Visual field cuts and corresponding lesions.

left visual field of the left eye and the right visual field of the right eye; these are opposite visual fields, thus "heteronymous." The person loses only half of the visual field in each eye, and thus it is a hemianopsia. Remember which axons cross over in the optic chiasm—the fibers from the nasal retinal field, which represent the temporal visual fields. When these are cut, the person can no longer perceive the images in the periphery—the temporal visual fields.

Damage to the lateral portion of the optic chiasm is almost always unilateral. It would be extremely unlikely to incur damage to both right and left edges of the structure while sparing the middle. Damage to the left lateral optic chiasm would result in an ipsilateral **nasal hemianopsia** —loss of the nasal (right) visual field in the left eye (Figure 7–7B) [the opposite would occur with damage to the right side—loss of the nasal (left) visual field in the right eye].

After the partial crossover in the optic chiasm, all of the pathways contain axons from the same visual field in each eye (e.g., left visual field of both right and left eyes). Because of this, all of the post-chiasmic visual field cuts will be homonymous (same visual field in each eye).

Damage to the optic tract will cause a contralateral **homonymous hemianopsia** (Figure 7–7C). It is contralateral because damage to the right optic tract will affect vision in the left visual field of each eye.

Damage to the optic radiations will also cause a hemianopsia, but because the axons fan out over a broader region, most damage affects only part of the tract. In many cases, this will result in a contralateral **homonymous quadrantanopsia** (Figure 7–7D).

Unilateral damage to the occipital lobe results in a contralateral **homonymous hemianopsia with central sparing** (Figure 7–7F). This means that the central portion of the visual field remains intact despite loss of the rest of the visual field. This is due to duplicate representations of the focal point of the eye in both occipital lobes.

Cortical Damage

As described previously, unilateral damage to the posterior occipital lobe (Brodmann area 17; V1) will result in a homonymous hemianopsia with central sparing. Bilateral occipital lesions result in a deficit called **cortical blindness**. People with cortical blindness often can sense and follow light but cannot process any other visual information. Anton syndrome, or **visual anosognosia** (Latin: *lack of knowledge of deficit*), is a rare disorder in which a person has cortical blindness but believes that they can see and will deny any loss of vision. Such patients will attempt to walk or otherwise move around their environments and bump into walls, doors, or furniture. Visual anosognosia is likely due to damage not only to the bilateral occipital lobes but also to the pathways to the temporal or parietal lobes.

Damage to the dorsal "where" pathway can cause difficulty locating items within the visual field. A person may be able to recognize an object, name it and describe it, but may not be able to point to the location or to grab the object without searching with their hand. Visual disorientation or difficulty with topographical orientation, such as reading a map or navigating within the environment, can also be affected. Alzheimer disease often causes degeneration of superior temporal and parietal lobes, which can contribute to patients' disorientation and way-finding difficulties.

Damage to the ventral "what" pathway can result in an **agnosia**, which is a deficit of recognition. There are several forms of agnosias. **Apperceptive agnosias**, as the name suggests, have to do with a perceptual deficit: The person has trouble perceiving an item and thus cannot recognize it. It results in the person being unable to read letters, copy simple shapes and line drawings, and objects appear as a blurry mass without distinctive characteristics.

Associative agnosias are more interesting because they affect the ability to recognize an item even though it is perceived accurately. **Prosopagnosia** is difficulty recognizing familiar faces. People with prosopagnosia can recognize that a picture is that of a human face (and if you mix it up, putting the eyes where the mouth should be, they will know that it is wrong), but they cannot recognize familiar faces. Imagine being at an event with a lot of people—for example, a concert or ballgame—and scanning the crowd looking for a friend. You know that all the faces you see are human faces, and you can tell that each one is different from the others, but none of them stand out as familiar. People with prosopagnosia deal with this phenomenon every day, even in a room of family members or friends. In some cases, they cannot even recognize their own face in the mirror. When they are in public places with multiple people in front of a mirror, they may reach up and touch their hair or make some other movement in order to determine which face in the mirror belongs to them. Prosopagnosia can be congenital or acquired as a result of brain injury. People with prosopagnosia learn to identify other people by other characteristics, such as their voice, idiosyncratic gestures, or even their gait. Although these strategies help in the "real world," they do not help identify

> **Box 7–3.** Prosopagnosia
>
> Janice was a 65-year-old woman who developed prosopagnosia following a stroke in the left middle cerebral artery. She presented with mild fluent aphasia and no significant motor deficits, so she was released from acute care and transitioned to outpatient care after only a few days of hospitalization. She had difficulty navigating novel environments and her pathfinding was poor, particularly outside of her home. When her speech–language pathologist (SLP) greeted her in the waiting room prior to sessions, Janice often appeared fearful or apprehensive (much like you may react to a total stranger saying "Hi, let's leave this public area and go to my office"). The prosopagnosia was so severe that even though her husband would say "We're here to see Jerome," she did not recognize the SLP or make the connection that he was coming to get her for her session. Each session began the same way, with Janice being fairly reserved and cautious with her interactions. A few minutes into the sessions, she would interrupt to exclaim "Why you're Jerome!" Her ability to recognize voice, prosody, and other physical cues improved, allowing her to connect with others more quickly, but she never reached a point where she recognized others solely by vision. In fact, if you were walking by her and waved, she would not recognize you, as if you were just a friendly stranger.

photographs of people. Dementias or other degenerative diseases that impact neurons in the inferior temporal lobe can cause difficulties with recognizing familiar people.

Visual agnosia is an impairment in recognition of an object just by sight. A person may be able to describe or draw an object but cannot name it or attach meaning to it—such as what it is used for. A classic example is provided by Oliver Sacks in his book, *The Man Who Mistook His Wife for a Hat*. The man was given a glove and asked to name it. He couldn't, although he described it accurately (made of leather, has five "pockets" extending from a central region) and even suggested what it could be used for—holding coins, with separate pockets for quarters, dimes, and pennies. At the end of the interview when he got up to leave, he pulled his own gloves out of his pocket and put them on his hands. He had no trouble using them appropriately but still would not have been able to name them.

As mentioned previously, different components of a visual signal are processed in separate areas of the brain. Given that the visual system is represented bilaterally (left visual field of each eye in the right hemisphere and vice versa), unilateral damage to the association areas typically does not cause significant visual processing impairments. However, in rare cases, people may lose the ability to process movement, a disorder called **akinetopsia**. This impairment has been described as having a strobe light on constantly. You can see incremental changes in placement of items, but you do not see the actual movement from one place to another. This can affect various aspects of daily life. Pouring coffee into a cup, for example: The liquid from the coffee pot appears as a frozen waterfall, and without being able to see the actual movement, it is difficult to judge when the coffee mug is full. Crossing a street can be very dangerous, as oncoming vehicles become incrementally closer but it is very difficult to judge the speed of movement to determine if it is safe to cross.

Another rare disorder is **achromatopsia** or loss of color vision. This is very different from color blindness, which is a genetic condition in which a person does not have the full complement of cones for color detection but is able to distinguish some colors—just not all of them. In achromatopsia, the person sees only shades of gray.

One final rare disorder that involves the visual system is **alexia without agraphia**. This is an impairment in reading (alexia) without an impairment in writing (agraphia). You can ask a person to write a sentence about their family and later ask them to read it to you, and they will be unable to read it. This, too, is rare, and it is attributed to damage to both the occipital cortex and the posterior corpus callosum.

Box 7–4. Aphasia, Alexia Without Agraphia, and Poetry

Desiree is a 75-year-old female who developed nonfluent aphasia, acalculia, and alexia without agraphia following a cardioembolic stroke (shower clot). This resulted in diffuse lesions in the left cerebral hemisphere, with greatest concentration in the left middle cerebral artery distribution. During her initial recovery, her nonfluent aphasia was the prominent issue, but in the chronic phase, as verbal communication improved, her reading impairments became more evident. In addition, her ability to complete math calculations remains severely impaired. She was a lawyer prior to her stroke, but she states that because she is not returning to work, she does not have any desire to work on her math. When reading for pleasure, she uses a Kindle with audio because she says it helps if she can see it and hear it.

During the chronic phase of her recovery, Desiree joined a poetry group, which really brought her alexia without agraphia to the forefront. Although she can write, she is completely unable to read her own writing. Despite her impairments, her writing is quite profound and beautiful. Given her ongoing, mild nonfluent aphasia, she shifts back and forth between telegraphic use of nouns and verbs to more integrated, syntactically complete, and eloquent written descriptions. From an artistic stance, it reads/sounds as if she is doing it intentionally. She notes that outside of poetry group, she sometimes uses her tablet's dictate function to help with writing. Although she can write without it, Dictate helps her get words written, and then she can use the text-to-speech function to hear what she wrote. Her husband typically reads poetry during sessions, which is necessary when she uses handwriting. Editing her own writing requires use of text-to-speech or collaboration with a partner to read it out loud.

Summary

The visual system is highly complex given the reversals of visual fields, fractionation of images, and parallel processing. This complexity is reflected in the amount of cortical real estate dedicated to visual processing. On the flip side, the retinotopic organization throughout the system results in very clear-cut differentiation of deficits caused by damage to discrete regions of the pathways and cortical processing areas. As with all sensory systems, there is contralateral cortical control, but in this case it refers to contralateral visual fields as opposed to simply contralateral organs (eyes).

Key Concepts

- The visual system converts light into representations of the environment.
- Both damage to and degeneration of peripheral components of the eyes such as the cornea and retina result in blindness.
- Special photoreceptors (rods and cones) begin to process specific elements of lightness/darkness, colors, shapes, size, and fine details.
- Visual fields are what you see around you. Retinal fields are the images on the retina, which are reversed, upside-down representations of the visual fields.
- The visual system is visuotopically (retinotopically) organized, mapping visual representations from the retinas to the cortex.
- Due to the partial crossover at the optic chiasm, segments of the visual pathway anterior to the chiasm carry information from the ipsilateral eye, whereas segments posterior to the chiasm carry information about the contralateral visual field.
- Damage to various points along the visual pathways results in specific types of visual field cuts.
- Damage to visual processing areas can result in cortical blindness and a variety of visual agnosias.

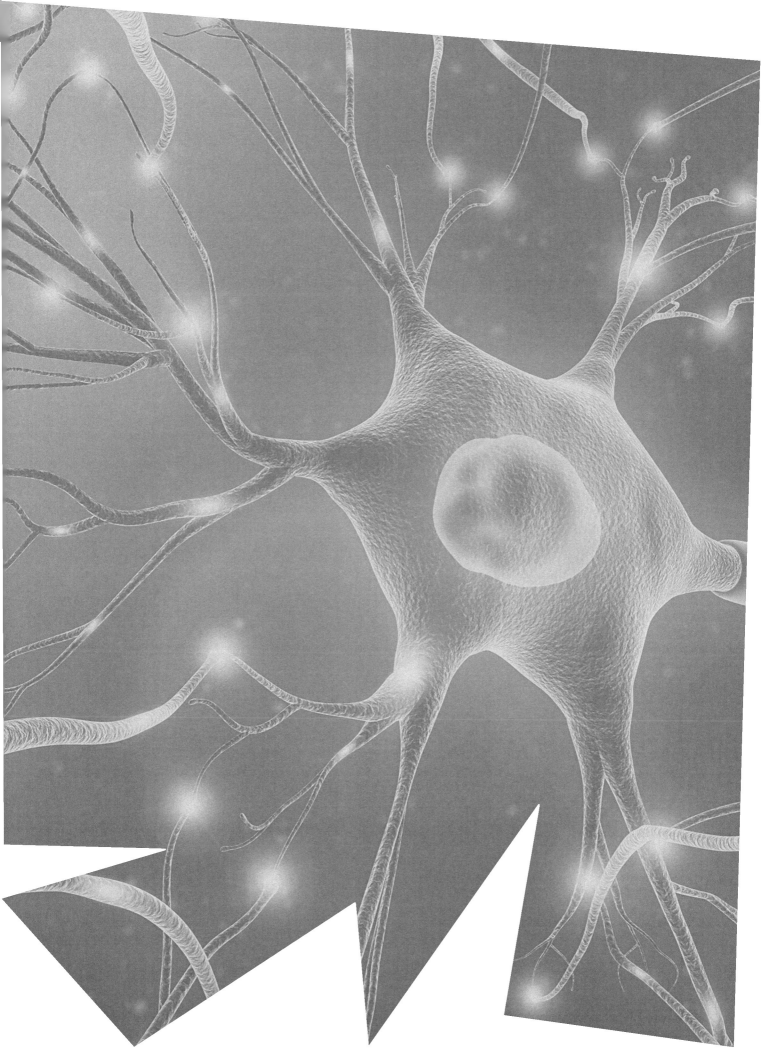

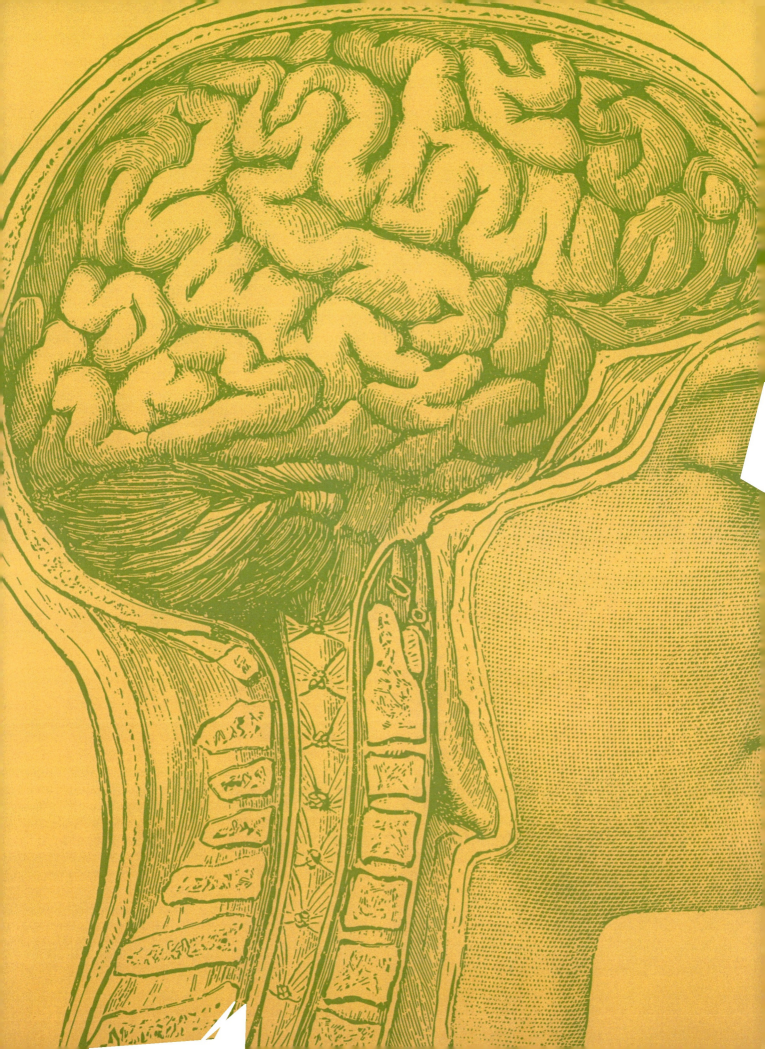

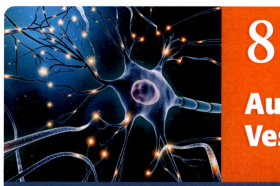

8
Auditory and Vestibular Systems

CHAPTER OUTLINE

Overview
Auditory System
   The Cochlea
      Converting Sound Waves Into Neural Signals
   Auditory Pathway
   Frequency and Intensity Coding in the Auditory System
   Localization of Sound

Auditory Processing in the Cortex
Hearing Impairment and Damage to the Auditory System
   Conductive Hearing Loss
   Sensorineural Hearing Loss
Vestibular System
   Vestibular Pathways
Summary
Reference

Overview

Perhaps there is not a need to convince you of the relevance of the auditory and vestibular systems to our disciplines, particularly for those of you on the audiology path. Regardless, it is important to make several key connections. Our language and cognitive systems are dependent on input systems such as the sense of hearing or some functional equivalent like visual comprehension of signs, gestures, lip movements, and written forms of communication. It is not only important from a sensory, comprehension standpoint but also critical to self-monitoring and motoric adjustments to the phonatory, articulatory, and resonance systems. Along with balance, the vestibular system works closely with the visual and proprioceptive systems to provide inputs to motor systems. Although they have quite different functions, the auditory and vestibular systems share structure, physiology, and location: Both involve hair cells that transduce mechanical energy into action potentials, and both are located in the inner ear.

Auditory System

The function of the auditory system is to transform sound waves into action potentials that code the frequency, intensity, and other characteristics of the sound waves. The process actually involves several energy transformations, from mechanical to hydraulic, electrical, and neurochemical.

A brief overview of the anatomy of the auditory system will set the stage for the processes (Figure 8–1). The cartilaginous outer ear is called the **pinna**. The various ridges and grooves serve a distinct purpose: to reflect sound waves into the outer ear canal, known as the external auditory meatus. As noted later, this reflection is important for localizing sounds on the vertical plane. The outer ear canal, called the **external auditory meatus**, extends medially into the skull and terminates at the eardrum or **tympanic membrane**. This section of the auditory system is known as the **outer ear**. Acoustic energy enters the outer ear in the form of sound pressures, which are amplified in the external auditory meatus and displace the tympanic membrane.

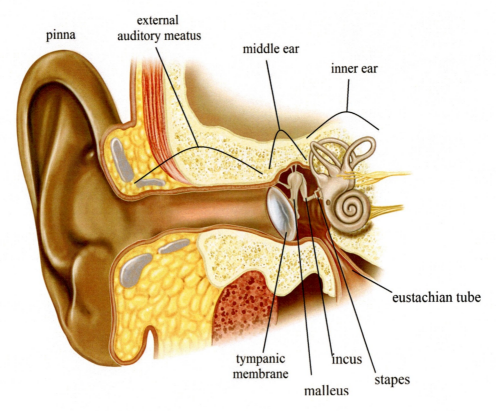

FIGURE 8–1. Outer, middle, and inner ear structures.

On the medial side of the tympanic membrane is the air-filled **middle ear** cavity. Here, you find the **ossicles**, the three smallest bones in the body: the **malleus** (hammer), **incus** (anvil), and the **stapes** (stirrup). The inferior portion of the malleus is attached to the center of the tympanic membrane, and the superior end is connected to the incus, which is in turn connected to the stapes. Together, the ossicles form a bony chain (the **ossicular chain**) from the tympanic membrane to the **inner ear** that houses the organs of hearing and vestibular function. Displacement of the tympanic membrane and thus the ossicular chain transforms acoustic energy into mechanical energy. As the stapes pistons into and out of the oval window of the cochlea, energy is transformed again, into hydraulic energy. In this transformation, the source frequency and amplitude/intensity are passed along.

A narrow canal called the **eustachian tube** connects the middle ear to the **nasopharynx** [the region between the posterior nasal cavity and the upper throat (pharynx)]. The bony region of the tube near the middle ear is permanently open, whereas the cartilaginous portion near the pharynx is normally closed but opens during swallowing and yawning and otherwise when necessary to equalize the pressure between the middle ear and the environment. When you "pop" your ears, you are opening the eustachian tube.

The inner ear consists of the **cochlea**, the **vestibule**, and the **semicircular canals**. The latter two are part of the vestibular system and are discussed later in this chapter. The cochlea is the organ of hearing. The bony exterior (**bony labyrinth**) of the inner ear is embedded in the temporal bone of the skull and lined with a membrane called the **membranous labyrinth**. The membranous labyrinth is filled with fluid and houses the organs of the vestibular and auditory systems.

The footplate of the stapes in the middle ear covers an oval-shaped hole in the lateral cochlea called the **oval window**. When sound waves enter the external auditory meatus, they create vibrations of the tympanic membrane. These vibrations are mechanical energy and are conducted through the ossicular chain ending in movement of the footplate of the stapes on the oval window. Sound pressure is amplified again in the ossicular chain in order to overcome acoustic impedance (essentially overcoming the pressure differential between air conduction and fluid conduction in the inner ear, thus maintaining information about the source frequency and intensity). This movement displaces the fluid within the cochlea, and the conversion of mechanical energy to hydraulic energy is complete.

The Cochlea

The membranous labyrinth divides the cochlea into three fluid-filled ducts separated by two membranous partitions (Figure 8–2). From superior to inferior, these are the **scala vestibuli**, **scala media**, and **scala tympani**. The **Reissner membrane** divides the scala media from the scala vestibuli; the **basilar membrane** divides the scala media from the scala tympani. The scala media is filled with a fluid called **endolymph**, which has a high concentration of potassium. The other two ducts are filled with **perilymph**, which has a high sodium concentration. Along the external wall of the scala media is a layer of cells called the **stria vascularis** that actively absorbs sodium and excretes potassium to maintain the correct proportions of these ions within the endolymph.

The scala tympani and vestibuli are connected at the apex of the cochlea in a region called the helicotrema, creating a continuous structure. The oval window of the cochlea is at the base of the scala tympani, and the round window is at the base of the scala vestibuli. When the stapes moves as a result of sound waves hitting the tympanic membrane and vibrating the ossicular chain, it puts pressure on the oval window and the perilymph on the other side. The resulting movement of the perilymph is conveyed up through the cochlea to the upper tip (called the apex or apical end) and back down to the round window, where the membrane covering the window bulges out in response to the movement of the fluid. Movement of the perilymph also displaces the basilar membrane. The basilar membrane (Figure 8–3) has two important characteristics: (1) It is narrow at the base and wider at the apex, and (2) the narrow base is stiffer than the wide apex. Because of these characteristics, different regions of the basilar membrane will be displaced by vibrations of different frequencies. High frequencies will cause displacement of the base of the basilar membrane, mid frequencies affect the middle portion, and low frequencies have the largest impact on the apex. The resulting vibration of different regions of the basilar membrane related to the frequency of the sound wave results in a phenomenon called **place coding** because the place or location of greatest movement serves as a code for the frequency of the sound.

Conversion of the hydraulic energy to neural signals occurs within the **organ of Corti**, which sits on the basilar membrane within the scala media (Figure 8–4). The structure of the organ of Corti is created by two rods of Corti that form two sides of a triangle. The basilar membrane creates the base. On the medial side of the organ of Corti

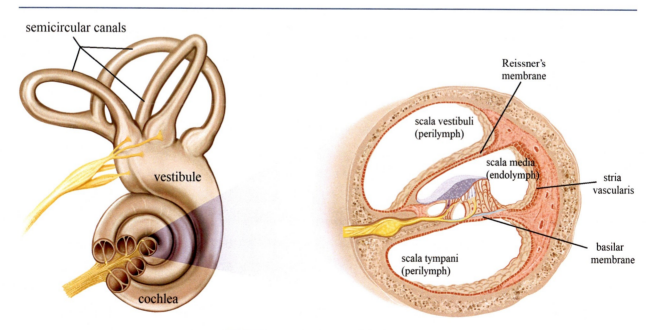

FIGURE 8–2. Structures of the inner ear.

124 Clinical Neuroscience for Communication Disorders: Neuroanatomy and Neurophysiology

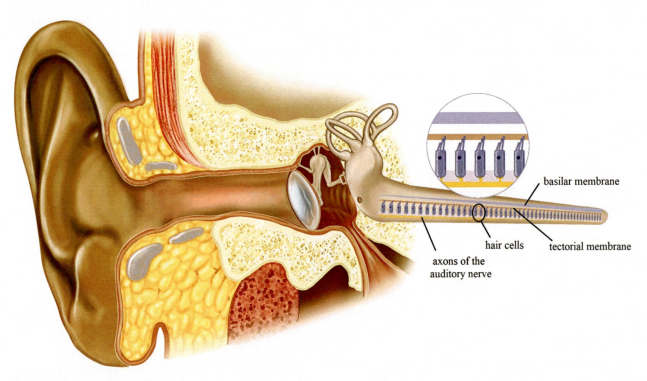

FIGURE 8–3. Basilar membrane and hair cells in an unrolled cochlea. Note the basilar membrane (shown in *blue*) is narrow at the base and wide at the apex.

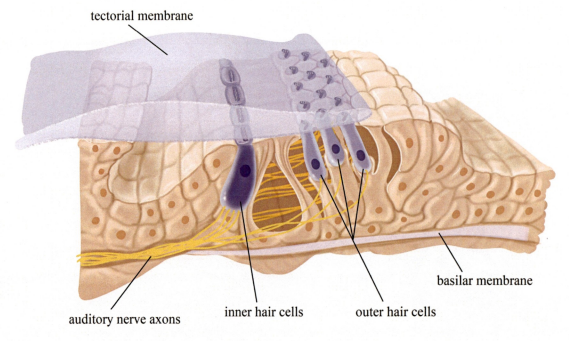

FIGURE 8–4. Organ of Corti.

is one row of **inner hair cells (IHCs)**, and on the lateral side are three rows of **outer hair cells (OHCs)**. These cells have a resting intracellular charge of –70 mV and contain synaptic vesicles filled with glutamate. Despite these characteristics that sound a lot like the neurons described in this book, cochlear hair cells are not actually neurons but are specialized epithelial cells. For our purposes, they function like neurons. As the name suggests, the hair cells have cilia —called **stereocilia**—that extend superiorly. Each hair cell can have 10 to 300 stereocilia that are arranged from tallest to shortest and are connected by tip links (imagine a thread from the tallest connecting to the nearest cilium, and from that cilium to the next one, and on and on). The tallest cilium on each cell is called the **kinocilium**.

Originating from the medial core of the cochlea is a gelatinous structure called the **tectorial membrane**. It extends out over the hair cells. Cilia of the outer hair cells are embedded into the tectorial membrane while inner hair cell cilia come in close proximity to the tectorial membrane (White & Peterson, 2020). Movement of the basilar membrane causes the cilia of the hair cells to move in relation to the tectorial membrane. This affects ion channels in the cilia, leading to movement of ions into the cell and depolarization or hyperpolarization of the hair cells.

Converting Sound Waves Into Neural Signals

As described previously, sound waves travel through the outer ear canal to the tympanic membrane. Vibrations of the membrane are conveyed through movement of the ossicular chain, resulting in movement of the footplate of the stapes against the oval window. The positioning of these bones and the size difference between the tympanic membrane and the oval window both serve to amplify the pressure from the sound waves, increasing the efficiency of the auditory system.

Movement of the perilymph in the scala vestibuli and scala tympani displaces the basilar membrane. Upward movement of the basilar membrane causes the kinocilium to bend in relation to the tectorial membrane. When the kinocilium is bent away from the other cilia, the tip links open potassium channels. Remember that potassium has a single positive charge (K+), and when channels are open, it will flow down the electrical gradient into the cell and depolarize the hair cell. This depolarization causes opening of voltage-gated calcium channels in the base of the hair cell. Just as with typical central nervous system (CNS) neurons, the influx of calcium triggers the release of neurotransmitters—in this case, glutamate—from synaptic vesicles. The glutamate then binds to receptors on bipolar neurons whose cell bodies are in the spiral ganglion just outside of the cochlea and whose axons create the cochlear portion of the VIIIth cranial nerve (the other portion arises from the vestibular system), which extends to the brainstem (Figure 8–5). These neurons are called **spiral ganglion neurons**, named for the location of their cell bodies. Movement of stereocilia away from the kinocilium will cause closure of K+ channels and result in hyperpolarization of the hair cells.

Inner and outer hair cells differ in several important ways. First, although there are approximately 4500 inner and approximately 20,000 outer hair cells, 95% of the spiral ganglion neurons are connected to inner hair cells. In other words, each inner hair cell synapses with multiple spiral ganglion neurons while multiple outer hair cells synapse onto a single spiral ganglion neuron. The IHCs are purely afferent and are responsible only for the transmission of signals representing sound waves. OHCs send afferent signals but also receive efferent signals that have an important role for enhancing detection of low-intensity sounds (Figure 8–6). The cell membranes of OHCs contain motor proteins that can elongate the shape of the cells. Motor signals from the brain activate these proteins to lengthen the cell bodies. This change in shape can enhance the effect of the basilar membrane up to 100-fold. A very quiet sound will have small-amplitude sound waves. Although these are amplified in the middle ear due to the size difference between the tympanic membrane and the oval window, the movement of the basilar membrane will still be minimal. If the OHCs elongate to create greater movement of the stereocilia in relation to the tectorial membrane, there will be a resulting increase in the amount of K+ influx, depolarization, and release of glutamate.

Box 8–1. Ototoxicity

A relatively large number of drugs have an ototoxic effect, meaning they can damage the auditory system. Some antibiotics, cancer drugs, and even nonsteroidal anti-inflammatory drugs such as aspirin can be ototoxic. These drugs damage or destroy OHCs. The loss of OHCs decreases the amplifying effect of these cells in the cochlea. Although inner hair cells are not affected, the sensitivity of those cells appears to decrease noticeably due to the loss of the amplification from OHCs, resulting in hearing loss.

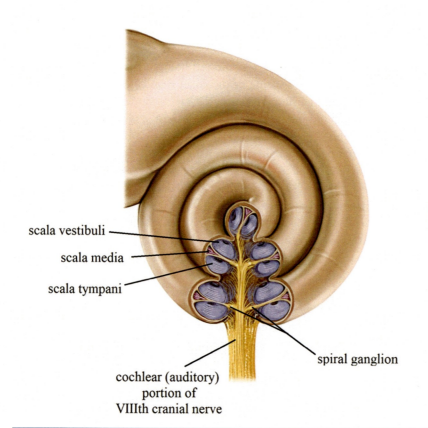

FIGURE 8–5. Spiral ganglion neurons forming the cochlear portion of the VIIIth cranial nerve.

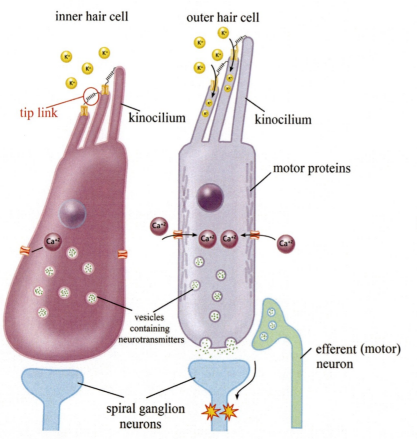

FIGURE 8–6. Auditory hair cells.

Auditory Pathway

The auditory pathway (Figure 8–7) begins with the bipolar spiral ganglion neurons, whose axons form the cochlear or auditory portion of the VIIIth cranial nerve. The axons from these bipolar cells travel through the internal auditory meatus and split near the brainstem to synapse in both the **dorsal** and **ventral cochlear nuclei**. From the ventral cochlear nucleus, the next set of neurons extend their axons to synapse in the **superior olivary complex** (SOC; also called the superior olive or superior olivary nucleus). The SOC is the first site of binaural processing (crossover that carries the sound information on both sides of the pathway). Axons from SOC neurons extend through a region called the **lateral lemniscus** (remember that *lemniscus* is a name for an axon tract) up to the **inferior colliculus** located on the dorsal midbrain. The inferior colliculus is the second point of binaural processing, achieved by crossover of fibers to the opposite side of the ascending pathways.

Axons from neurons in the dorsal cochlear nucleus bypass the SOC and synapse directly onto neurons in the inferior colliculus. There are several pathways from the inferior colliculus. One extends to the cerebellum, another to the superior colliculus for integration of visual and auditory sensations, and another to the medial geniculate nucleus (MGN) of the thalamus. MGN neurons then

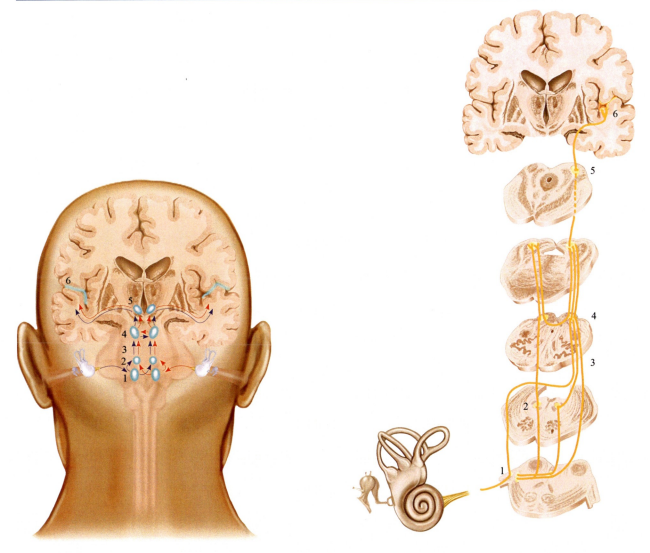

FIGURE 8–7. Auditory pathway. *Red*, from right ear; *blue*, from left ear; 1, cochlear nuclei; 2, superior olivary complex; 3, lateral lemniscus axon tract; 4, inferior colliculus; 5, medial geniculate nucleus of the thalamus; 6, auditory cortex (A1, Heschl gyrus).

extend to the primary auditory cortex located in the superior temporal lobe. The primary cortical area responsible for auditory processing (A1) is **Heschl gyrus**, a portion of the superior temporal gyrus that corresponds with Brodmann area 41 (Figure 8–8).

Box 8–2. C-SLIMA

The C-SLIMA mnemonic may help you remember steps on this pathway. There is a synapse at each point except the lateral lemniscus, which is an axon tract.

C = cochlear nucleus

S = superior olivary complex

L = lateral lemniscus

I = inferior colliculus

M = medial geniculate nucleus

A = A1, auditory cortex

The cochlear nuclei are the only components of the auditory system in which there is unilateral (or monaural—one ear) representation of sound in the CNS. Approximately 80% of the cochlear nuclei axons cross over and synapse onto to the contralateral SOC or inferior colliculus. The remaining 20% stay ipsilateral. The crossover and resulting bilateral (binaural) representation is critical for localization of sound, as described later.

In addition to these afferent, ascending pathways, there are also descending feedback systems. Neurons from the auditory cortex synapse onto the MGN and the inferior colliculus. These systems modulate signals from the inner ear and aid in plasticity and learning. As discussed previously, there are also efferent neurons extending from the cochlear nuclei out through cranial nerve (CN) VIII to the hair cells.

Frequency and Intensity Coding in the Auditory System

Two primary characteristics of sound are **frequency** and **intensity**. Frequency, the number of cycles of a sound wave that occur within a period of time, is perceived as pitch. Intensity, or the amplitude of the sound waves, is perceived as loudness (Figure 8–9).

Sound frequency is coded in several different ways, in several different regions of the auditory system. First is the location of hair cells along the basilar membrane. Because the basilar membrane vibrates in different regions depending on the frequency of the sound, only those hair cells in the region of a specific frequency will be stimulated/depolarized. Second, hair cells respond best to their individual **characteristic frequency** (also referred to as the centering or resonant frequency). They will not respond, or have only a limited response, to frequencies outside of their small characteristic range. Third, there is **tonotopic organization** of neurons at each stage of the pathway (e.g., cochlear nuclei, MGN, auditory cortex). The axons in the

Box 8–3. Tonotopy

A 260-Hz tone will create vibrations near the apical end of the basilar membrane, triggering depolarization in a specific group of IHCs resulting in action potentials in a specific group of spiral ganglion cells that synapse onto cochlear nuclei neurons in a specific region of the nuclei and in turn synapse onto neurons that extend to the SOC, IC, and the MGN, each time synapsing on neurons in a region populated with neurons receiving signals from approximately 260-Hz tones. The MGN neurons extend to the region of A1 representing approximately 260 Hz, where the signals are perceived as the musical note middle C.

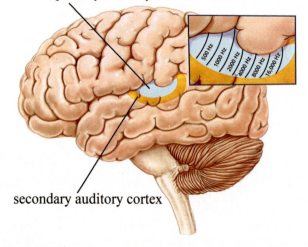

FIGURE 8–8. Primary auditory area in Heschl gyrus in the superior temporal lobe.

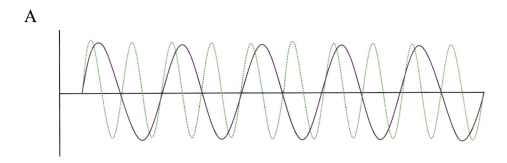

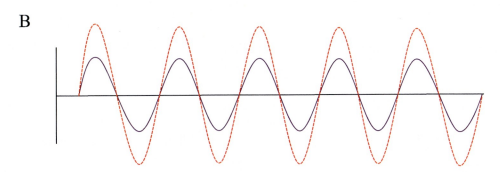

FIGURE 8–9. **A.** Two sounds: *purple*, lower frequency (pitch); *green*, higher frequency. Both are the same intensity (loudness). **B.** Two sounds: *purple*, lower intensity (loudness); *red*, higher intensity. Both are the same frequency (pitch).

pathways and the cell bodies in the nuclei are arranged according to their frequency response. This tonotopy is mapped onto the primary auditory cortex in the superior temporal gyrus (Heschl gyrus, Brodmann area 41), with low-frequency sounds represented more anteriorly and laterally and high-frequency sounds more posteriorly and medially (Figure 8–10).

A fourth method of coding for frequency is **phase locking**, or the timing of action potentials in relation to sound waves. Neurons with characteristic frequencies in the low- and mid-pitch ranges fire at the same phase in the sound wave, creating a match between the frequency of the sound and the frequency of action potentials. In Figure 8–11, the yellow bars represent action potentials. You can see that the neuron is firing at the same point in the sound wave each cycle so that the timing of action potentials reliably represents the frequency of the sound wave. This phase locking is the primary mechanism for coding low-frequency sounds.

Tonotopy is the primary method of coding high-frequency sounds (>5000 Hz) because the speed of action potentials in the CNS is not fast enough to code high frequencies by phase locking: Auditory system neurons can fire up to 200 times per microsecond, whereas CNS neurons can only fire 2 times per microsecond. Midrange frequencies are coded by a combination of phase locking and tonotopy.

Intensity coding provides a representation of the loudness of sounds. The two mechanisms for intensity coding are the number of action potentials and the number of neurons involved. Imagine the vibration of the basilar membrane for soft versus loud sounds. A loud sound (high-intensity, high-amplitude sound wave) will cause greater deflection of the basilar membrane, creating more displacement of stereocilia, greater depolarization, and more action potentials. It also will affect more hair cells than a smaller deflection, so not only is each hair cell creating more action potentials but also there are more hair cells creating action potentials.

Localization of Sound

Two different mechanisms are used for localizing sounds in the vertical (superior/inferior) and horizontal (left/right) planes. For vertical localization, sound waves are reflected

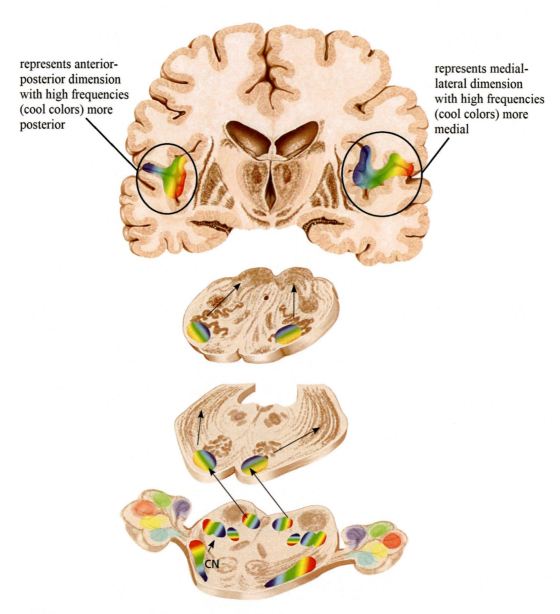

FIGURE 8–10. Tonotopy throughout the auditory pathway. Warm colors (*red, orange*) represent lower frequencies, and cool colors (*blue, green*) represent higher frequencies.

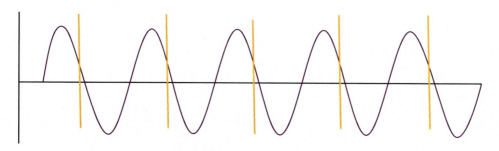

FIGURE 8–11. Phase locking.

off the structures in the pinna (outer ear cartilage). Horizontal localization is based on differences in the timing and intensity of signals from the left and right ears. As noted previously, there is binaural (bilateral) representation at all levels beyond the cochlear nuclei. Because of this, the timing and intensity of signals received in each ear can be directly compared. One cue is the timing of the sound waves (and subsequent action potentials) that hit the left and right ears, called the interaural time delay. A sound coming directly from the left will impinge on the left tympanic membrane approximately 6 msec prior to hitting the right tympanic membrane. The signal from the left will arrive in the superior olivary complex prior to the one from the right. The SOC contains neurons specifically tuned to interaural delays and will respond to timing difference between signals. Figure 8–12 depicts the signals arriving at the neurons in the SOC from the left and right. The yellow lines illustrate signals created by an auditory signal from the left side of space. Because the sound had a "head start" from the left cochlea, the signal reaches the right-most SOC neuron at the same time as the signal from the right ear reaches that same neuron. The convergence of the two signals in this spot is interpreted as a sound from the left. As you might guess, signals from the right and left that converge on the middle neuron at the same time indicate the sound is coming from the midline region, and so arrive at the left and right tympanic membranes at the same time. The auditory system is sensitive enough to detect sounds that are 2 degrees apart, which differ by 11 msec.

A second localization cue is the phase differential. A sound wave will hit the left and right tympanic membranes at different phases of its cycle. This difference too will be compared and used for localization. This is particularly useful for continuous sounds that do not have a distinct onset that would provide interaural time delays.

A third cue is the interaural intensity difference. For mid- to high-pitched sounds, the head creates a "sound shadow": Sounds coming from the left will be louder in the left ear than in the right ear. Again, this differential will be noted in direct comparisons between the signals at the superior olivary complex, inferior colliculus, and A1.

Auditory Processing in the Cortex

Auditory processing occurs in both right and left hemispheres in A1 (Heschl gyrus), with additional processing in Brodmann area 42, on the lateral surface of the superior temporal gyrus and the **planum temporale**, a region on the superior surface of the superior temporal gyrus that is hidden in the lateral sulcus (sylvian fissure). The planum temporale is thought to contribute to language processing in part because it is typically larger in the left than the right hemisphere. In the left hemisphere, Brodmann area 22 in the middle temporal gyrus immediately inferior to BA 41 and 42, is called **Wernicke area**. This region is the primary site for language comprehension. The Wernicke homolog area in the right hemisphere may be linked to processing speech prosody, but its function is not precisely known.

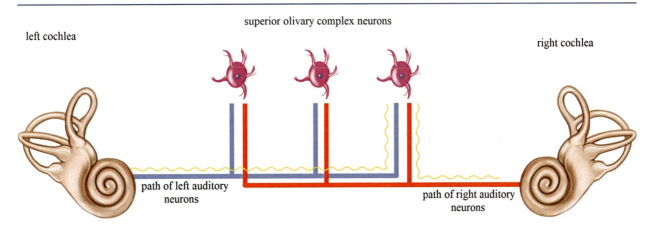

FIGURE 8–12. Interaural time delay coded by neurons in the superior olivary complex. *Blue*, path of auditory neurons from left ear; *red*, path of auditory neurons from right ear. The yellow line represents a sound that came from the left side of space. It had a "head start" in the left auditory pathway because the sound hit the left ear first. By the time it reached the right-most superior olivary complex neuron, the signal from the right ear was just arriving. The timing of the arrival of signals from the left and right at that particular neuron will be interpreted by the brain as a signal coming from the left side of the head.

Hearing Impairment and Damage to the Auditory System

Conductive Hearing Loss

Conductive hearing loss is a result of impediments to the conduction of sound waves through the outer or middle ear. Buildup of cerumen (ear wax) reduces the diameter or patency of the external auditory canal. If the cerumen impinges on the tympanic membrane, it will reduce the vibratory capacity of that tissue. A torn or ruptured tympanic membrane also will not vibrate properly. Ear infections in which fluid builds up in the middle ear space will restrict the movement of the tympanic membrane and the ossicular chain. Damage to the bones in the middle ear, such as ossicular chain disruption or disarticulation, also will interrupt the transmission of sound waves. For instance, ossicular dislocations or fractures sometimes occur with traumatic brain injuries. Conductive hearing loss is typically treatable (e.g., removing ear wax, healing of tympanic membrane, or treatment of infection).

Sensorineural Hearing Loss

Sensorineural hearing loss is a result of damage to the cochlea (sensory organ) or the auditory nerve (neural structure). The most common form of sensorineural hearing loss is **presbycusis**, a reduction in hearing acuity associated with aging. Normal wear and tear over a lifetime of exposure to noise affects the health of the hair cells. Because high-frequency sounds are represented in the base of the cochlea where they are more exposed, those hair cells and thus those frequencies are affected earlier than mid and low frequencies. Exposure to loud noises, especially extended exposure, hastens damage to those hair cells (Figure 8–13). Once the cilia are damaged, the hair cells can no longer depolarize in response to movement of the basilar membrane, and the result is a reduced ability to hear the frequencies represented by the affected hair cells.

Damage to the auditory nerve will reduce the efficiency of action potential conduction through the nerve to the brainstem. The most common cause is tumors, specifically **acoustic neuromas** or **vestibular schwannomas**. The axon fibers from the cochlea and the vestibular system run together through the **internal auditory meatus** on their way to the brainstem, and thus a tumor on one will put pressure on both. In addition, the facial nerve (CN VII) also travels through the internal auditory meatus, so a growth on CN VII will often impact the function of CN VIII and vice versa (see Chapter 11 for more details about the cranial nerves).

Given the binaural representation of the auditory pathway beyond the cochlear nuclei, brainstem or tha-

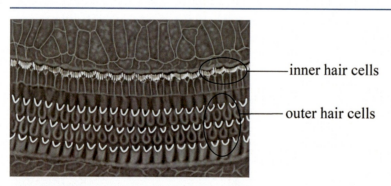
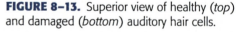
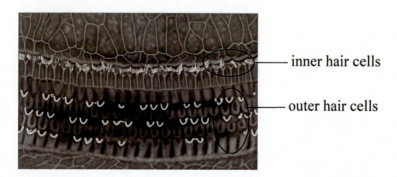

FIGURE 8–13. Superior view of healthy (*top*) and damaged (*bottom*) auditory hair cells.

lamic lesions rarely result in significant loss of auditory processing. Cortical damage can result in a variety of issues, although not loss of acuity.

Damage to Wernicke area in the left hemisphere results in a form of aphasia in which the primary impairment is reduced auditory comprehension. Recall that the right hemisphere is less clearly organized and more interconnected. Because of this, damage to the right superior temporal lobe does not consistently affect a single cognitive-communication process. Some individuals may have difficulty interpreting emotional speech prosody, a disorder called **aprosodia**. Types of aphasia and aprosodia are discussed in more depth in Chapter 14.

Pure word deafness is a rare disorder in which the left hemispheric primary auditory area is intact but isolated from the association areas by lesions in the white matter. Due to the preservation of the peripheral system and auditory nerve and brainstem regions, the sound signals are still processed, but the cortical processing that aids in identifying and interpreting speech sounds is disrupted. Thus, speech is uninterpretable, and patients report that it sounds like meaningless noise. Interestingly, recognition of nonspeech noises (e.g., a police siren, the ring of a phone, or the zipping sound of a zipper) remains intact.

A final rare disorder is cortical deafness, caused by bilateral damage to the Heschl gyrus. Akin to cortical blindness, it is the inability to hear despite intact peripheral auditory systems and pathways. In this case, none of the auditory signals that reach the cortex are processed, resulting in the inability to consciously perceive sounds.

Vestibular System

The vestibular system develops alongside the auditory system, and the two systems have several physical similarities in terms of organs and pathways. The vestibular system has two different types of organs that sense and respond to head movement: the **cristae** in the **semicircular canals**, which respond to head rotation, and the **otolith organs** in the vestibule, which respond to vertical and horizontal head movements (Figure 8–14).

The semicircular canals are a set of three near-circular tubes. As with the cochlea, they are embedded into the

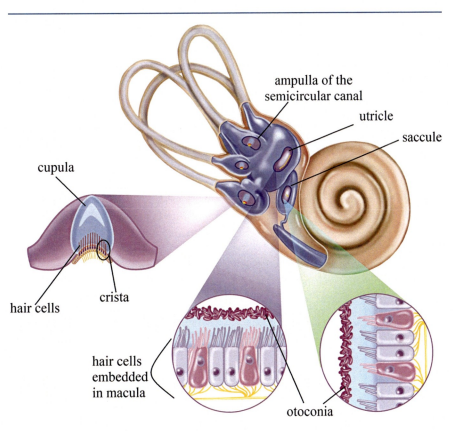

FIGURE 8–14. Vestibular organs.

temporal bone of the skull, and within the bony structure is a membranous labyrinth. The semicircular canals extend out from a central structure called the vestibule, in which the otolithic organs are found. There are three canals on each side of the head: the anterior, posterior, and lateral canals, each set at right angles to each other (along X, Y, and Z axes). All are filled with endolymph, which has a high concentration of potassium (K^+). At the base of each canal near where they connect to the vestibule is an enlarged area called the **ampulla** (plural: ampullae). This is where the vestibular organs, the ampullae crista, are found. The crista is a sheet of sensory cells into which hair cells are embedded. Cilia from the hair cells extend into a gelatinous structure called the **cupula** that forms a cone shape in the ampulla. Just as in the auditory system, the cilia are arranged by height and are connected via tip links. When you move your head, the endolymph inside the canals moves in response and will put pressure on the cupula. This causes displacement of the cupula and the cilia embedded into it. Again, like in the auditory system, deflection of the cilia toward the kinocilium will result in opening of potassium channels, allowing the potassium to flow in and depolarize the hair cells. The depolarization in turn will signal the opening of calcium channels, and the influx of calcium triggers the release of glutamate from the hair cells. The glutamate binds to receptors on the vestibular neurons of CN VIII to create an action potential that travels up the axons to the brainstem.

Box 8–4. Perception of Motion

Due to the principle of inertia, movement of the endolymph lags behind movement of the head. Thus, there is a slight delay in the sensation of movement—or of stopping movement. Think about when you would spin in circles as a child or the sensation of getting off a roller coaster. For a brief time after the movement stops, you feel dizzy or off-balance and may feel as if you are still spinning. This is due to the lag in movement of the endolymph.

Imagine turning your head to the right. The fluid in the right and left lateral semicircular canals will begin to move. Due to the positioning of the semicircular canals, fluid in the left and right lateral canals will cause opposite effects: One will move the cilia toward the kinocilium and cause depolarization, whereas the other will move the cilia away from the kinocilium causing hyperpolarization. Thus, the signals being sent to the brainstem will be an increase in the number of action potentials from one side and a decrease from the other side. This pattern of signals will be interpreted by the brain to determine which direction your head is moving.

Within the vestibule are two otolithic organs called the **utricle** and the **saccule** (Figure 8–14). Each has three components: the **macula**, which is sensory epithelium containing hair cells; a gelatinous structure into which cilia are embedded; and calcium carbonate crystals called **otoconia** (Greek: *ear stone*) on top of the gelatinous portion. Movement of the head will cause the otolithic membrane to shift in the direction of movement. The weight of the otoconia will add additional movement. As with the hair cells in the cochlea and the semicircular canals, the cilia are arranged by height. Movement of the otolithic organ in one direction will result in cilia bending toward the kinocilium, opening K^+ channels to allow K^+ to flood in, causing depolarization that opens calcium (Ca^{2+}) channels, allowing Ca^{2+} to flood in and trigger the release of neurotransmitters. The utricle is positioned horizontally and the saccule vertically in order to detect linear movements in multiple planes.

Vestibular Pathways

The glutamate released from the vestibular hair cells binds to dendrites of bipolar vestibular neurons. Cell bodies of these neurons are found in the **Scarpa ganglion** outside the vestibule, and axons extend through the internal auditory meatus (along with axons from the cochlea and CN VII) to the brainstem.

The first synapse in the brainstem is in the vestibular nuclei in the pontomedullary region. From the vestibular nuclei, there are multiple pathways. One extends through the medial longitudinal fasciculus to the midbrain, where the axons synapse onto cranial nerve nuclei for the oculomotor, trochlear, and abducens cranial nerves, which control movement of the muscles of the eyes (see Chapter 11). These connections serve several purposes. One is to aid in conjugate eye movement (the synchronous movement of both eyes as if they were tied together). A second is to coordinate head and eye positioning and movement. The close connection between the eyes and the head allows you to fixate on an object and move your head while maintaining eye contact. This is called the vestibulo-ocular reflex, which helps keep the world in focus while your body and head are moving. Another phenomenon associated with the connections between the vestibular and ocular systems is **nystagmus**. This is an oscillating or beating movement of the eyes in which they move swiftly in one direction and then more slowly return to midline. Many of you may have induced nystagmus by spinning around multiple times. When you stop, because the fluid in the semicircular canals continues to move although your head is stationary, the vestibular system continues to send signals to your ocular control system, resulting in the eye movement. Once the fluid stops moving, the nystagmus resolves. Nystagmus also can be stimulated by putting either warm or cold water into the ear canal (the caloric test); the temperature change stimulates the horizontal semicircular canal, and because the head is not moving, nystagmus will occur. The caloric test can be used to test the function of the vestibular system.

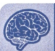

Box 8–5. Vestibulo-Ocular Reflex

It can be difficult to appreciate the importance of the vestibulo-ocular reflex because it is so common as to be overlooked. To illustrate how important (and omnipresent) it is, next time you're outside, take a video as you're walking down the sidewalk. As you watch the video, notice how "bouncy" the world looks. You don't see the bouncing without the camera because all of that movement is compensated for by your vestibulo-ocular reflex, making it appear to your brain as if you are moving smoothly through space.

A second pathway extends to the cerebellum, specifically the flocculonodular lobe and vermis. These connections influence the cerebellovestibular and spinocerebellar tracts to coordinate movement and maintain balance. Due to these pathways, damage to the cerebellum can result in nystagmus. A third pathway is the vestibulospinal pathway, which extends inferiorly through the spinal cord to influence axial (trunk) muscles; this pathway contributes to muscle tone needed to withstand the pull of gravity. A fourth pathway extends to the reticular formation and reticular activating system. These connections facilitate visceral–autonomic activities. It is these connections that lead some people to develop seasickness or feel nauseous after spinning or riding roller coasters.

Finally, there are pathways to the cerebrum. As with all other sensory pathways, there is a synapse in the thala-

Box 8–6. Astronaut Training

Spinal meningitis (infection of the meninges) can spread to the inner ear and cause labyrinthitis (infection of the membranous labyrinth) and damage the cochlea and vestibular organs.

In the 1960s, while NASA was preparing humans for space flight, it enlisted the help of 11 men whose inner ears were damaged by spinal meningitis, leaving them both deaf and immune to motion sickness. Recruited from Gallaudet University, these men underwent a variety of experiments designed to mimic the weightlessness of space travel. The results provided a wealth of knowledge about how the body responds when there is limited gravity to signal body movement and orientation in space. One experiment on a ship in choppy waters had to be canceled because the researchers were so sick they could not finish the study. The Gallaudet 11, in contrast, had no negative physical effects.

Source: https://www.nasa.gov/feature/how-11-deaf-men-helped-shape-nasas-human-spaceflight-program.

mus—in this case, the ventral posteromedial nucleus. From there, it is not entirely clear where projections end in the cortex. Some likely extend to the regions of the motor system; others may extend to the frontal eye fields in the middle frontal gyrus that control volitional eye movements. Still others may extend to the parietal lobes to aid in perception of body schema.

Summary

The auditory and vestibular systems share spaces and mechanisms but perform strikingly different functions. The auditory system is clearly linked to communicative function, although as seen from a vibrant and productive Deaf community, it is not necessary for human communication. The vestibular system has a major role in daily activities as mundane as moving around in one's familiar environment and as fantastic as being an elite gymnast or dancer. The integration of vestibular, visual, and proprioceptive systems is crucial for carrying out those basic and complex movements.

Key Concepts

- The auditory and vestibular systems both rely on hair cells that convey signals to the auditory–vestibular nerve (CN VIII).
- Movement of cilia in one direction results in depolarization and release of neurotransmitters, and movement in the other direction will cause hyperpolarization.
- Localization of sound and determination of the direction of movement are coded by comparison of signals from the left and right inner ears in the brainstem.
- Tonotopic organization is present throughout the entire auditory system.
- Conductive hearing loss is caused by impediments to the conduction of sound waves to the cochlea; sensorineural hearing losses are caused by damage to the cochlea or pathways extending from there to the brain.
- Damage to the superior temporal lobes can affect comprehension of language (left hemisphere) or emotional prosody (right hemisphere).
- The vestibular system has two sets of organs that detect rotational and linear movements of the head.
- Through its widespread connections, the vestibular system influences eye movements, body movement, coordination, body schema, and visceral responses to movement.

Reference

White, H. J., & Peterson, D. C. (2020, March 9). Anatomy, head and neck, ear organ of Corti. *StatPearls*. Available from https://www.ncbi.nlm.nih.gov/books/NBK538335

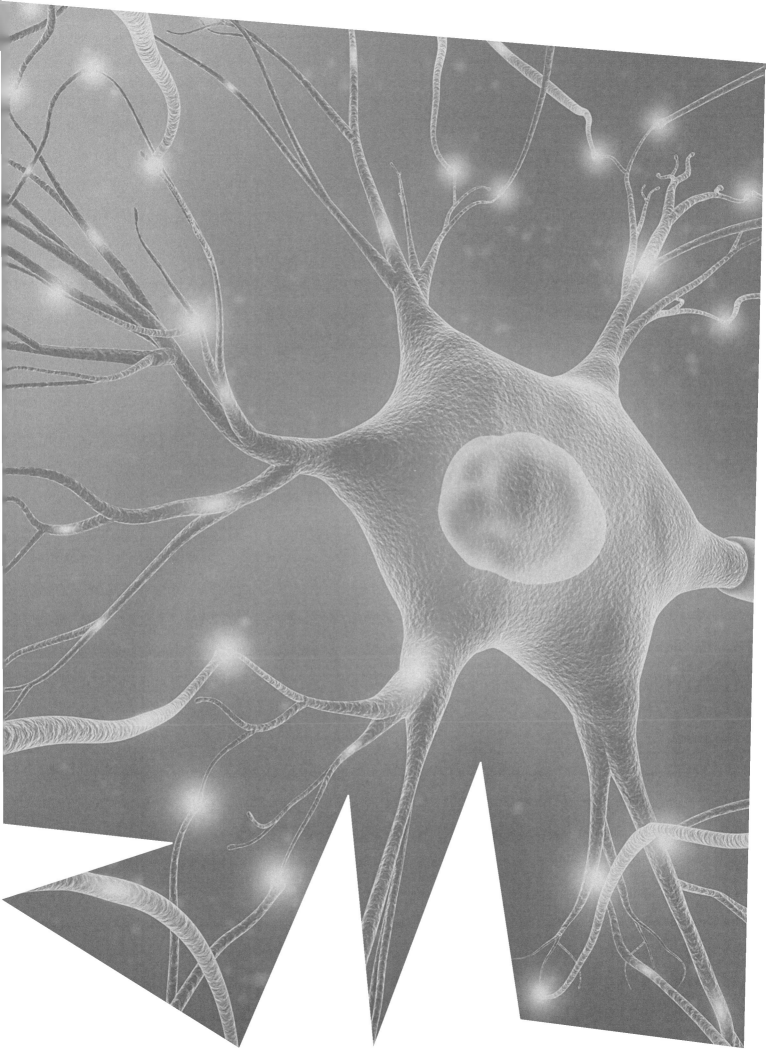

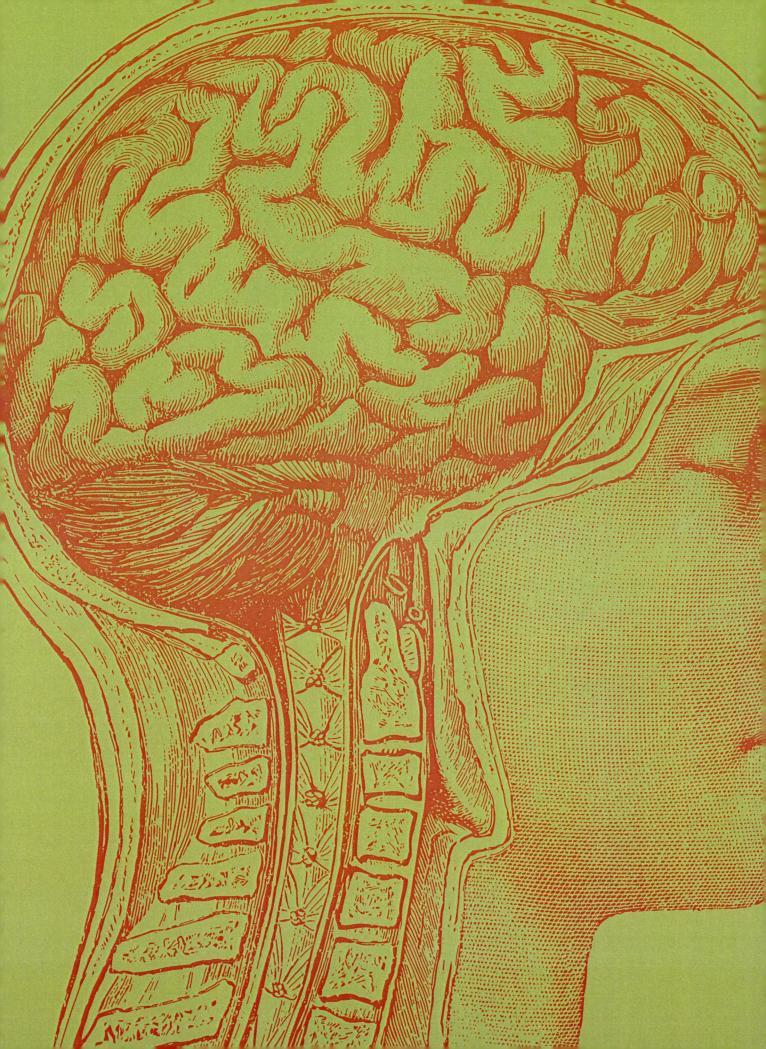

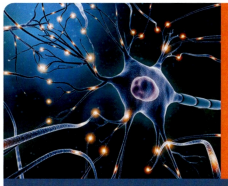

9
Chemical Senses: Smell and Taste

CHAPTER OUTLINE

Olfaction
Olfaction: The Sense of Smell
  Olfactory Pathway
  Impairments of Olfaction
Gustation: The Sense of Taste

Gustatory Pathway
Factors Influencing Taste Perception
Impairments of Gustation
Summary
Reference

Olfaction

The chemical senses, **olfaction** (smell) and **gustation** (taste), are, evolutionarily speaking, the oldest of the senses. They are of importance for speech–language pathologists because of their function in eating and drinking, and thus swallowing disorders. Both of these senses have chemoreceptors that transform chemical stimuli into neural signals. When combined together, taste and olfaction lead to what we perceive as different flavors.

Olfaction: The Sense of Smell

The olfactory epithelium, approximately 10 square centimeters, is located along the superior nasal cavity. It consists of olfactory receptors and basal cells that facilitate regeneration of the olfactory neurons throughout their 4- to 8-week life cycle. In additions, there are supporting cells (similar to glial cells) that continually secrete mucus and replenish a thin mucous sheet approximately every 10 minutes. This is a critical component as **odorants** (compounds that have an odor) dissolve in the mucus and then bind to cilia on the olfactory neurons.

Humans have approximately 350 different odorant receptors, each of which has a different level of receptivity to specific odorants. The responses from any single neuron are ambiguous, but specific smells can be identified by a

 Box 9–1. Follow Your Nose

The human sense of smell is relatively poor compared to that of animals. Dogs' epithelial surface area is 1,600% larger than humans, and they have 100 times more receptors. Their olfactory bulbs also are significantly larger, and they have an additional organ to aid in olfactory processing. Rats have approximately 1,000 different odorant receptors compared to 350 in humans. However, even with this rather limited capacity, humans are still able to detect more than 1 trillion combinations of odorants.

population coding system. In other words, each odorant will create a unique pattern of responses from a large number of neurons. The pattern is based not only on action potentials from specific groups of receptors but also on the timing of the action potentials. These patterns are identified as specific odors.

Olfactory Pathway

Each first-order olfactory neuron has a single receptor. Multiple odorants can bind to the receptor, but each creates a specific pattern of response. Receptors are organized into different zones within the olfactory epithelium, which contributes to the pattern of responses.

The olfactory nerve does not look like a typical cranial nerve. It consists of all of the first-order olfactory neurons whose cilia are embedded in the mucous sheet with axons that extend through the cribriform plate of the ethmoid bone (Figure 9–1) into the ipsilateral **olfactory bulb** (Figure 9–2). In the bulb, they synapse onto one of

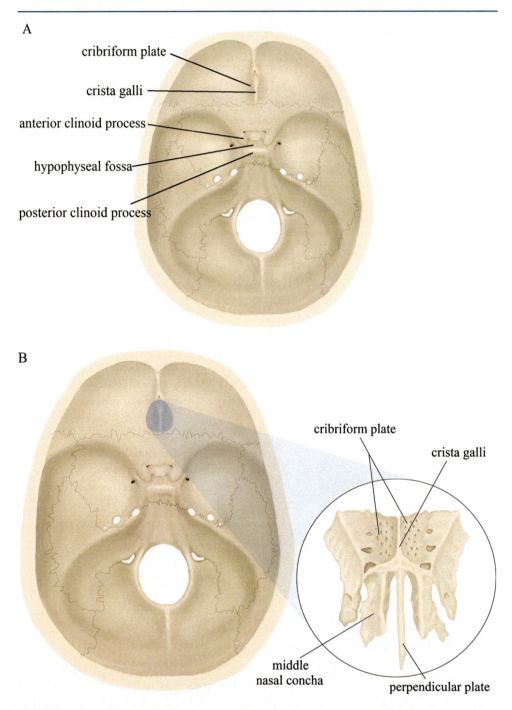

FIGURE 9–1. A. Superior view of the ethmoid bone in the ventral cranium. **B.** View of the cribriform plate and the crista galli on the superior ethmoid bone. The middle nasal concha and perpendicular plate create the walls of the nasal cavities. Illustration by Mariah Hoepner.

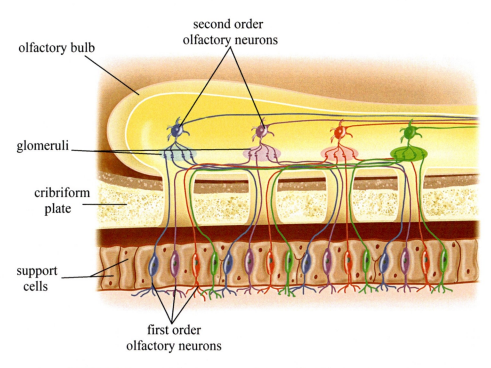

FIGURE 9–2. Olfactory receptors and glomeruli within the olfactory bulb.

approximately 200 **glomeruli** (clusters of nerve endings). There is extensive convergence at this point, with more than 25,000 first-order neurons synapsing onto approximately 100 second-order neurons. The first-order neurons each synapse onto a specific glomerulus depending on the receptor type. Glomeruli are organized systematically both within and across individuals. It is not clear whether this spatial organization has a role in type of odor processing or if the arrangement is related to efficiency of processing.

When odorants bind to the cilia on olfactory neurons, they trigger G protein-coupled receptors that in turn trigger cAMP to bind and open sodium and calcium channels. This allows influx of sodium and calcium, which begins depolarization. Interestingly, the increase in intracellular calcium triggers the opening of chloride (Cl^-) channels, and the resulting efflux of chloride (moving out of the cell, down its concentration gradient) adds to the depolarization. As with other neurons, once a threshold is met, an action potential is created that travels down the olfactory axon to the point of synapse in the glomeruli. Action potentials stop when odors diffuse away or scavenger enzymes within the mucous sheet destroy the odorants. In addition, olfactory neurons habituate or adapt to a constant odor so that they stop responding after a period of time. Ever had this experience? You smell the aroma of dinner cooking but by the time dinner is finished, the odor is gone (or at least that's what you think). Then you step outside for a moment (perhaps to walk the dog), and when you come back inside, much to your surprise the rich aroma of the meal remains.

Interneurons within the glomeruli are both inhibitory and excitatory and likely aid in initial processing or sorting the responses. There are also descending projections that synapse in the glomeruli. These are suspected to play a modulatory role, such as enhancing the response to food odors when one is hungry.

Box 9–2. Key Definitions

G protein-coupled receptors are membrane proteins that cells use to convert extracellular signals into intracellular responses. They are crucial in mediating vision, olfaction, gustation, and pain.

Cyclic adenosine monophosphate (cAMP) is a derivative of adenosine triphosphate (ATP) and has key roles in intracellular communication.

The axons of the second-order neurons form the olfactory tract that synapses in the olfactory cortex on the inferior surface of the brain, including the piriform cortex on the medial edge of the uncus and the entorhinal cortex posterior to the uncus (Figure 9–3). As noted in Chapter 5, olfaction is the exception to the rule that all sensory information passes through the thalamus prior to reaching the cortex.

Crossover between the right and left olfactory pathways occurs through the anterior commissure (a bundle of neurons connecting the left and right hemispheres that interconnects the temporal lobes and amygdalae). From the olfactory cortex, there are connections to the orbitofrontal cortex, insula, amygdala, hippocampus, and the mediodorsal nucleus of the thalamus (Figure 9–4). Integrating what you know about functions of various structures within the olfactory network, you can develop an appreciation for the impact of the sense of smell on many different functions. As listed in Table 9–1, the hippocampus and frontal lobe structures associated with memory are part of the olfactory network. These connections explain why smells can be powerful triggers for memories. For example, the scent of the aftershave your grandfather used to use can take you back to fond memories of summers spent at his house. Or the odor of burning wood and plastic can bring up bad memories of a house fire. Connections to the hypothalamus drive the relationship between odors and eating. Delicious smells can make you hungry, whereas disgusting odors can turn your stomach and make you lose your appetite.

Impairments of Olfaction

Sensitivity to odors is quite variable across humans, but there is a range beyond which reduced sensitivity is considered a deficit. Deficits of the sense of smell take several forms and have a variety of etiologies. **Anosmia** is the loss of the sense of smell, whereas **hyposmia** is a reduced sensitivity to odors. Some people have specific anosmia in which they have a reduced sensitivity to specific odors. **Dysosmia** refers to alterations in olfactory perception, including **parosmia**, in which the perception is distorted, and **phantosmia**, in which a smell is reported in the absence of any stimulus (i.e., olfactory hallucination). One specific form of phantosmia is **cacosmia**, the perception of a foul smell. This has been linked to epilepsy in some people, particularly those in whom seizures begin in the uncus. For people without epilepsy, the cause of olfactory hallucinations remains a mystery.

There are both **conductive** and **sensorineural** forms of anosmia, just as for hearing loss (see Chapter 8). Anything that blocks the transmission of odorants to the primary olfactory neurons creates a conductive anosmia. This includes respiratory infections, colds, or allergies that cause increased production of mucus that blocks the olfactory receptors. Tumors or other growths within the nasal cavity

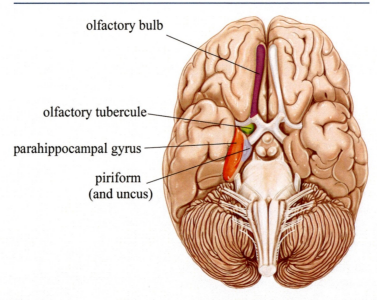

FIGURE 9–3. Structures of the olfactory cortex seen on inferior surface of the brain.

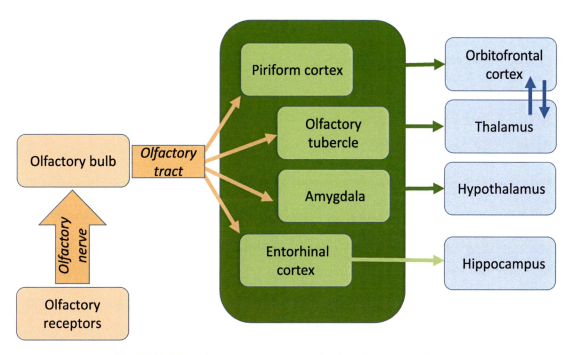

FIGURE 9–4. Schematic of regions involved in olfactory processing.

Table 9–1. Functional Role of Structures in the Olfactory Processing Network

Connection	Physiological/Behavioral Importance
Hypothalamus	Appetite, eating/drinking behaviors
Orbitofrontal cortex	Odor discrimination Impact motivation, emotion, memory
Mediodorsal nucleus of thalamus	Integration of cognition, emotion, memory
Limbic system	Emotion, motivation
Hippocampus	Memory, recall triggered by smells

also can cause conductive loss of smell. As with hearing loss, in most cases conductive losses are transient or can be treated relatively easily.

Sensorimotor anosmia is caused by damage to the nervous system and is more likely to be permanent. Many people with Parkinson or Alzheimer disease report a reduced sense of smell. Traumatic brain injury is another common cause. In Figure 9–2, take a close look at the axons of the primary olfactory neurons that extend up through the cribriform plate in the ethmoid bone. In a traumatic brain injury, the brain moves in relation to the skull (see Chapter 14). It is not difficult to see that the olfactory axons can be sheared as the brain and the olfactory bulbs move in relation to the cranium. Although olfactory neurons can regenerate, after a traumatic injury this regrowth can be impeded by scar tissue. A reduction in the sense of smell also can occur as part of the aging process. As might be surmised, reduced sense of smell affects the perception of taste and often will lead to reduced food intake. Older adults are at risk for malnutrition because when food does not smell or taste good, they reduce the amount they eat.

Gustation: The Sense of Taste

There are five basic tastes perceived by the human system: sweet, sour, salty, bitter, and umami (Japanese for "delicious"), which is the taste of glutamate. Our perceptions of flavors are a combination of the taste as well as smell, temperature, and texture. Each person has some inborn preferences and instincts that can be shaped by experiences, such as learning to love coffee that originally was perceived as bitter and yucky or developing an aversion to the smell or taste of a food that once caused food poisoning.

The majority of taste receptors, called **papillae**, are on the tongue, but others are located in the pharynx, palate, and even the epiglottis. There are three major forms: **foliate**, **vallate**, and **fungiform**. Foliate papillae have a ridged structure and are found primarily on the anterior two-thirds of the tongue. Vallate papillae, which look like a smattering of pimples, are found on the lateral and posterior tongue. Fungiform papillae, with a mushroom shape, are located on the superior surface of the posterior tongue. Inside each papillae are hundreds of taste buds (Figure 9–5), which in turn house 50 to 150 taste receptors.

Tastants, the chemicals that stimulate taste receptors, have several mechanisms for transducing the environmental stimulus (food/drink) onto the neural response (Table 9–2). Salty and some sour tastants pass through ion channels. Other sour tastants bind to and block ion channels. For bitter, sweet, and umami, the tastants trigger G protein-coupled receptors that open ion channels via a second-messenger mechanism.

Taste cells respond to multiple tastants but are tuned to respond best to specific tastes; those that respond primarily to sour and salty tastants release serotonin (5-HT), whereas sweet, bitter, and umami release ATP, which creates an excitatory postsynaptic potential in the postsynaptic cell. Representation of specific flavors or tastes is created by patterns of action potentials. Slight differences in the patterns code for differences in flavors.

Gustatory Pathway

As discussed in Chapter 11, taste is carried through three different cranial nerves. Taste from the anterior two-thirds of the tongue is carried through the facial (VIIth) cranial nerve, whereas the posterior one-third is innervated by the glossopharyngeal (IXth) cranial nerve. Taste from the pharyx is carried through the vagus (Xth) cranial nerve (Figure 9–6).

Regardless of the cranial nerve, all primary afferents carrying taste information synapse in the **gustatory nucleus**, part of the **solitary tract** in the medulla. From

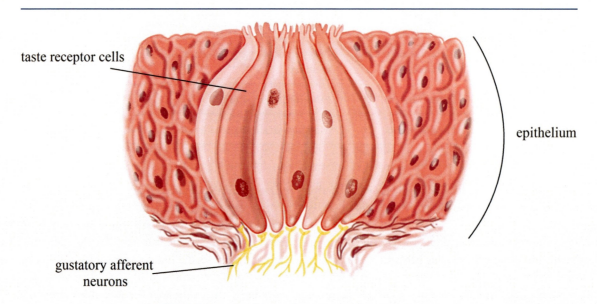

FIGURE 9–5. Taste bud and gustatory first-order afferents.

Table 9-2. Functional Differences in the Five Categories of Taste

	Signaling	Mechanism of Depolarization	Result of Depolarization
Sweet	High caloric content	Trigger G protein-coupled receptors	Release ATP
Salty	Aids in electrolyte balance	Tastants flow through Na^+ ion channels	Release 5-HT
Sour	Acidic; protection against spoiled foods	Tastants flow through Na^+ and K^+ channels or block ion channels	Release 5-HT
Bitter	Caffeine, nicotine, alkaloids; often toxins are bitter	Trigger G protein-coupled receptors	Release ATP
Umami	Amino acids; protein	Trigger G protein-coupled receptors	Release ATP

Note. ATP, adenosine triphosphate; 5-HT, serotonin.

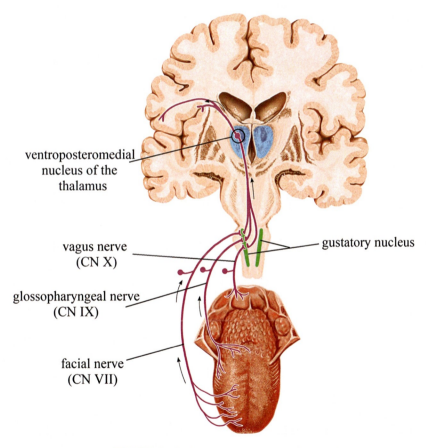

FIGURE 9-6. Taste pathways through cranial nerves.

this nucleus, some signals are transmitted to the ipsilateral ventroposteromedial nucleus of the thalamus and then to the gustatory cortex in the region of the anterior insula and frontal operculum. Other signals follow pathways to the hypothalamus and limbic system and impact palatability and motivation to eat. Still other connections send signals to nuclei in the brainstem involved in swallowing, salivation, gagging, vomiting, digestion, and respiration. Identification of specific tastes or flavors is accomplished through patterns of action potentials coming from a variety of taste buds. Small differences in the patterns are interpreted by the brain as different flavors.

Factors Influencing Taste Perception

As noted previously, what we perceive as "taste" is actually a combination of olfaction, gustation, and somatosensation, primarily texture and temperature. It is also influenced by hunger: Food tastes better when you are hungry than when you are not. Other contexts, such as access to food, also matter; after being deprived of a certain food (e.g., chocolate), your first taste may be pure heaven, or it may not be as good as you had been anticipating it would be.

You experience the role of olfaction in the sense of taste when you have a cold and your nose is stuffed up (a conductive taste impairment). Nothing tastes quite right because your olfactory receptors are blocked by mucus, eliminating that component of the sense of taste. Temperature can also affect taste, as coffee/tea drinkers can attest. The first sip of a hot cup of your morning beverage tastes much different from the last lukewarm swallow left at the bottom of the mug. Texture is also a component of taste: Raw vegetables (e.g., carrots or potatoes) taste different than their soft, cooked versions. One reason for the combination of these sensory systems is to aid in rapid identification of foods that have gone bad and have the potential to make you sick (or even kill you if they are toxic).

In addition to the behavioral differences, studies have demonstrated that responses of neurons in the gustatory cortex can be generated in response to nonfood stimuli. Drinking tasteless beverages can result in responses in the gustatory cortex, and there are beverages that, depending on temperature or viscosity, result in different cortical responses. Similarly, pictures of food can elicit neuronal responses in the gustatory cortex. Finally, cognitive expectations can alter both perceived taste and cortical responses. When given a bitter drink, responses from gustatory neurons will be less if the person is told it is not very bitter than if the person is told it is very bitter. Or maybe you have had the experience of drinking a beverage such as water when you were expecting lemon-lime soda or vice versa.

Impairments of Gustation

Ageusia is the term for loss of the sense of taste. **Dysgeusia** refers to a reduced or altered sense of taste. Taste cells regenerate on a regular basis, approximately every 2 weeks. The cranial nerves that carry taste information, however, do not; thus, damage to the VIIth, IXth, or Xth cranial nerve can cause ageusia, or permanent loss of taste. Loss of taste can occur with normal aging or as a result of neurological damage. Whatever the etiology, ageusia often precipitates a loss of interest in food and subsequent weight loss. It is difficult to maintain interest in eating when everything tastes the same.

Box 9–3. Smell/Taste in Space and With COVID-19

Astronauts experience a reduction in sensitivity of smell and taste. On the International Space Station, there is a high demand for spicy foods and hot sauce because foods that taste just fine on Earth are rather bland in space. This is because the absence of gravity results in mucus and other fluids pooling in the nasal cavity and sinuses. This impacts the function of the olfactory cells and results in a reduction in the ability to smell and taste in space.

While there is still much to be learned and understood about the effects of the coronavirus, the resulting disease COVID19 is thought to damage support cells in the olfactory epithelium. These cells (called sustentacular cells) have a variety of functions including providing structure and nutrients to olfactory neurons and clearing out odorants. When these cells are damaged the olfactory neurons are unable to respond as efficiently. Sustentacular cells regenerate within several days, restoring the sense of smell (Butowt & vonBartheld, 2020).

Source: https://www.scientificamerican.com/article/why-covid-19-makes-people-lose-their-sense-of-smell1

> **Box 9–4.** That'll Make You Pucker
>
> Individuals with Alzheimer dementias experience a number of changes in addition to the well-known memory losses, including less sensitivity to tastes and smells. Coupled with frequent presence of oral agnosias (failure to recognize food in the mouth as food), it is common for individuals with Alzheimer disease to either hold food in their mouth or ruminate on it (essentially chewing on it with no intent to swallow). Gustatory stimulation, in the form of a sour bolus, can help them become aware of food in their mouth and to subsequently swallow.
>
> Similarly, individuals with impairments to oral sensation also benefit from gustatory stimulation (sour boluses) for similar reasons. Whenever we can employ multiple modalities (taste, texture, temperature, etc.), it increases the likelihood of a stronger and more timely swallow.

Summary

The chemical senses of olfaction and gustation are similar not only because they are chemical senses but also because the perception of taste is highly influenced by the sense of smell. Much like audition, there can be conductive and sensorineural impairments to these senses.

Key Concepts

- Although the human sense of smell is limited compared to that of other mammals, it still allows for distinction between trillions of odors.
- Odors are distinguished by spatial and temporal patterns of signals along the olfactory pathway.
- The variety of structures in the olfactory pathway allows for the sense of smell to impact memories, motivation, cognition, as well as intake of food and drink.
- Traumatic brain injury can cause shearing of the olfactory afferents and result in anosmia.
- The perception of taste is a combination of taste, smell, temperature, and texture.
- Taste signals from various areas of the tongue and pharynx are carried through three different cranial nerves (VII, IX, and X).
- Connections along the gustatory pathway include the insula, frontal operculum, hypothalamus, and limbic system.
- Brainstem connections in the taste pathway affect swallowing, salivation, and even gagging and vomiting.
- Ageusia can lead to disinterest in food and weight loss.
- The perceptions of smell and taste are influenced by descending cortical input that allows expectations to alter perceptions.

Reference

Butowt, R., & vonBartheld, C. S. (2020). Anosmia in COVID-19: Underlying mechanisms and assessment of an olfactory route to brain infection. *The Neuroscientist*, 1–22. https://doi.org/10.1177%2F1073858420956905

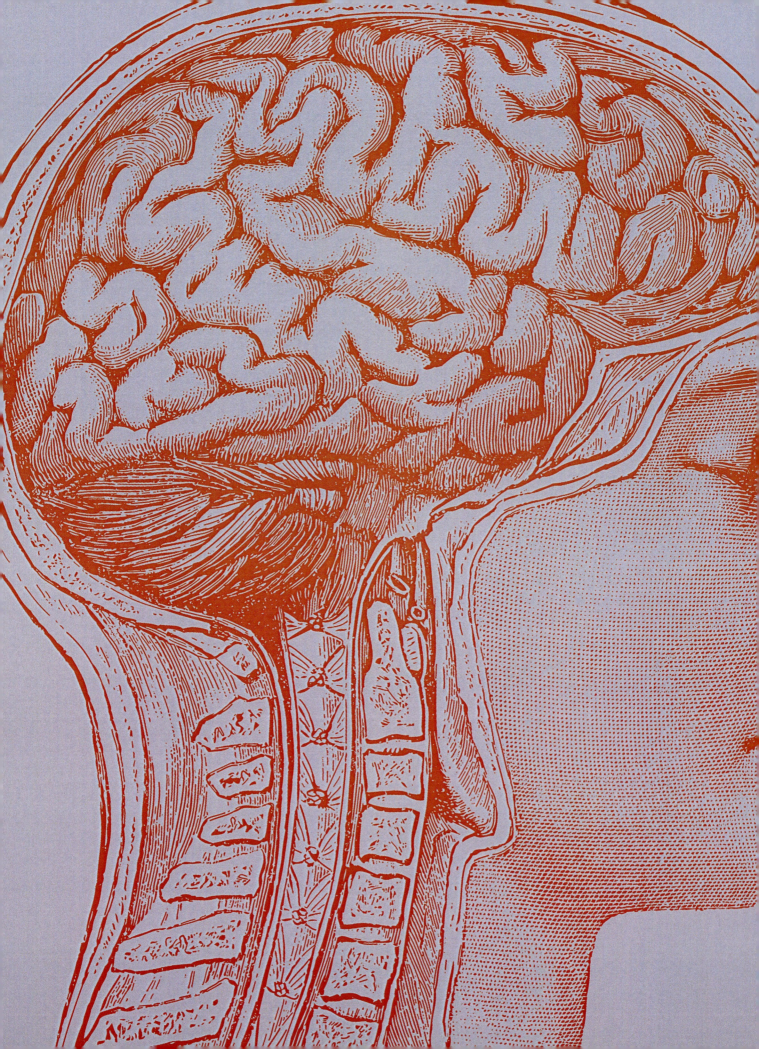

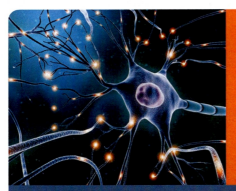

10
Motor Systems

CHAPTER OUTLINE

Overview
Motor System Structures
   Primary Motor Strip
   Premotor and Supplementary Motor
     Areas
   Basal Ganglia
   Cerebellum
Motor Pathways
   Pyramidal Tracts
     Cranial and Spinal Nerves
     Corticospinal Tracts
     Corticobulbar Tract
   Extrapyramidal Tracts

     Rubrospinal Tract
     Tectospinal Tract
     Vestibulospinal Tract
     Reticulospinal Tract
Motor Units and Muscle Innervation
Clinical Implications
   Motor Cortex
   Motor Pathways
   Neuromuscular Junction
   Basal Ganglia
   Cerebellum
Summary

Overview

Several structures in the central nervous system (CNS) have primary roles in movement. These interconnected structures and the pathways between them and the muscles of the body are responsible for all voluntary skeletal movements. Although somatosensory and motor systems are discussed in separate chapters, it is important to understand that the two systems are extensively interconnected and in constant communication. In order to begin a movement such as raising your hand, you need to know where your arm is to start with to know which muscles to contract and how strongly to contract them. As the movement is occurring, sensory feedback from the muscles and joints is sent to the CNS for comparison between the planned movement and the actual movement. This relationship is particularly relevant to speech-language pathologists who are concerned with muscle and joint movements that cannot easily be observed. Movements of oral, velar, pharyngeal, laryngeal, and esophageal structures in the context of speech and swallowing are complex. Coordinating movement and timing of that movement is crucial for accurate and safe movement sequences. All of this depends on a system to plan movements, initiate gross motor movements, and refine or modulate those movements. Implicitly knowing where your tongue is in conjunction with where your velum is positioned and the shape of your pharynx is crucial to accurate production of sounds and is thus highly dependent on sensory systems.

    Motor system control is arranged in a hierarchy. Starting from the most complex, strategizing occurs in the frontal lobes and the basal ganglia, tactics are controlled by the motor cortex and cerebellum, and the execution is directed by brainstem and spinal cord structures. There is a **direct** motor system, also known as the **pyramidal** system, which includes upper motor neurons that originate from the primary motor strip and project toward the body (Figure 10–1). Those that serve the lateral motor systems decus-

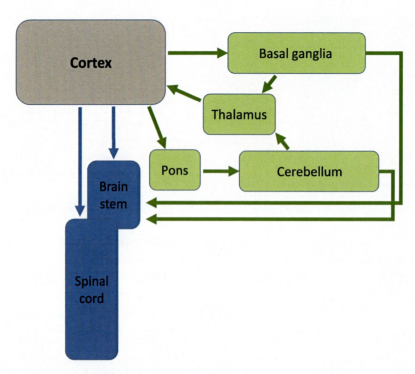

FIGURE 10–1. Direct (pyramidal, in *blue*) and indirect (extrapyramidal, in *green*) motor systems.

sate (cross over) in the medulla and innervate contralateral body structures. Those that serve the medial motor system remain ipsilateral and/or have bilateral outputs such as the bilateral outputs to trunk muscles. Damage to the direct or pyramidal motor system results in disorders characterized primarily by weakness (e.g., paresis or paralysis). There is an **indirect** motor system, also known as the **extrapyramidal** system, that includes structures such as the basal ganglia and cerebellum, which refine and modulate movements initiated in the direct motor system (Figure 10–1). Damage to the indirect or extrapyramidal system results in disorders characterized primarily by abnormal movement (e.g., Parkinson disease).

Motor System Structures

Primary Motor Strip

The primary motor strip (also called M1) occupies the precentral gyrus [Brodmann area (BA) 4] in the posterior frontal lobe of both the right and left hemisphere. Neurons on each side are arranged by body area to create a **homunculus** (Latin: *little man*) or map of the body (Figure 10–2). As noted in Chapter 1, the areas of the body with greater fine motor control (hands and articulators) take up more space in the motor strip. Humans have contralateral sensorimotor control, meaning that the motor strip in the right hemisphere sends signals to the left side of the body and vice versa.

Premotor and Supplementary Motor Areas

The **premotor area** (BA 6) is anterior to the motor strip in the dorsal frontal lobe. Once considered a single region, more recent work on functional distinctions has led to separating this into multiple areas, including the dorsal and ventral premotor areas and the **predorsal premotor area**. Just anterior to the premotor area is the **supplementary motor area** (SMA) proper and the **pre-SMA** (BA 8) (Figure 10–3). These areas have somatotopic maps similar to, but less detailed than, the maps in the primary motor strip. Inputs to the premotor area and SMA come from the primary motor area and various somatosensory regions in the parietal lobes. Together, they aid in selecting, planning, and generating movement.

Neurons in the ventral premotor area fire when movements are imagined and also when observing another person's movements. The latter are referred to as mirror neurons. Some fire even in response to the sound of a

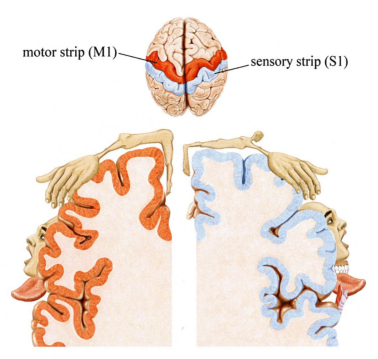

FIGURE 10–2. Superior view of primary motor (*red*) and somatosensory (*blue*) areas and coronal slice showing homunculi.

movement (e.g., hearing a zipper close) even without seeing the action.

The pre-SMA and the predorsal premotor area receive inputs primarily from cognitive processing areas of the frontal lobes, with limited somatosensory input. Most of the output is to subcortical motor regions. This allows movements to be influenced by internal and external needs as well as the context in which movement takes place. For example, neurons in the pre-SMA begin to fire when an object that can be grasped comes into sight, but only if it is close enough to grab. Neurons in the SMA are active prior to the beginning of any movement, suggesting that the role of this area includes intention to move. Indeed, lesions to the SMA result in reduced initiation of movement, a condition called **abulia** (Greek: *boule* = *the will*). In addition to the many connections to other areas of the motor system, the SMA has connections to the limbic system that contribute to its role in motivation or intention to move.

Basal Ganglia

The basal ganglia have the broad role of refining or fine-tuning motor functions. As described in Chapter 1, the basal ganglia consist of several deep subcortical structures made up of cell bodies (thus the name ganglia) (Figure 10–4). Key structures include the **striatum**, composed of the caudate and putamen, and the **globus pallidus** (internal and external), **substantia nigra**, and **subthalamic nucleus** (Figure 10–5).

These structures have extensive connections to each other, to areas of the motor cortex, and to the brainstem and thalamus. Although their primary function is to influence movement, the basal ganglia also play a role in cognition, affect, and language processing.

The **caudate nucleus** is a C-shaped structure that lies alongside the lateral ventricles. The **putamen** and **globus pallidus** are egg-shaped structures that lie lateral to the thalamus inside the curve of the caudate. The internal and external segments of the globus pallidus are separated by white matter tracts. On a frontal (coronal) slice, these three structures look like a tilted candy corn—triangular shaped with three segments (Figure 10–5). The **subthalamic nucleus**, as the name suggests, is located inferior to the thalamus. Inferior to that, in the upper midbrain, is the **substantia nigra** (Latin: *black substance*). This structure gets its name from its dark/black coloring. The substantia nigra has two segments: the pars compacta and the pars reticulata. The pars compacta has a high concentration of dopaminergic neurons and plays a critical role in basal ganglia functioning. The pars reticulata, in contrast, houses

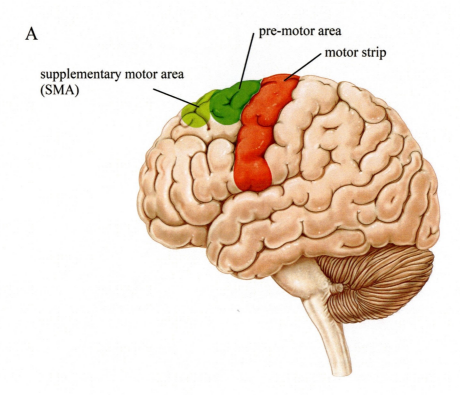

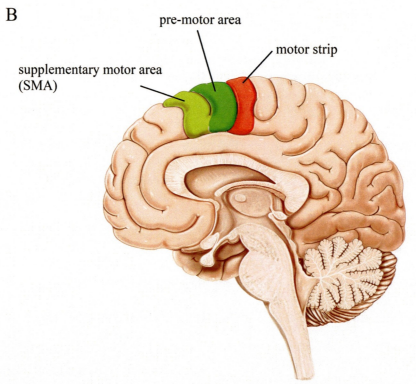

FIGURE 10–3. Premotor and supplementary motor areas on lateral (**A**) and medial (**B**) surfaces.

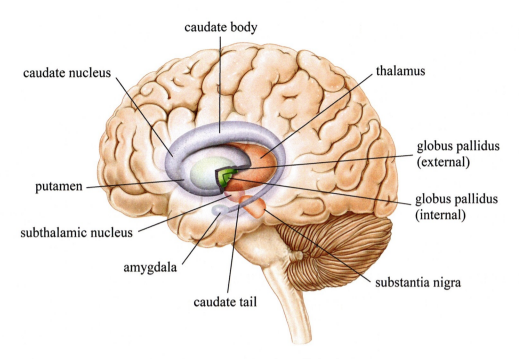

FIGURE 10–4. Basal ganglia in situ.

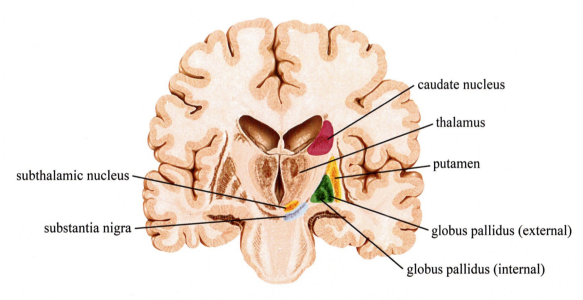

FIGURE 10–5. Coronal section of the basal ganglia.

primarily γ-aminobutyric acid (GABA)-ergic neurons that connect to a variety of CNS structures.

The caudate and putamen are connected by a series of gray matter segments. Together, they are called the striatum, due to the striped appearance of the connectors. The striatum is the primary input structure, receiving signals from the brainstem, thalamus, and various areas of the cortex. The globus pallidus internal and the reticular portion of the substantia nigra are the major outputs from the basal ganglia, sending signals to the thalamus, brainstem, frontal lobes, and cerebellum. The remaining components—the globus pallidus external, pars compacta of the substantia nigra, and the subthalamic nucleus—are components of the basal ganglia circuitry and send/receive signals to and from the other basal ganglia structures.

There are several cortico-basal-thalamo-cortical circuits (Figure 10–6). The functions are determined by the cortical regions from which they originate: the motor, oculomotor, executive/associative, and emotional. Motor circuits typically have two components—a direct circuit that serves to facilitate signals (and thus movement) through the primary motor cortex and an indirect circuit that inhibits or dampens motor function. The connections can be either excitatory or inhibitory. In a simplified example of the direct circuit (Figure 10–6A), the motor cortex sends excitatory signals to the striatum, which in turn has an inhibitory influence on the globus pallidus (GP) and substantia nigra (SN). These structures also have inhibitory connections to the thalamus, which generally sends excitatory signals to the motor cortex. Walking through the circuit, a signal from the motor cortex will send excitatory postsynaptic potentials to the striatum, causing it to send an action potential to the GP and SN. Because the signal here is inhibitory, the GP and SN then do not send a signal to the thalamus. The result, then, is that the thalamus is not inhibited (as it would be if a signal was sent from the

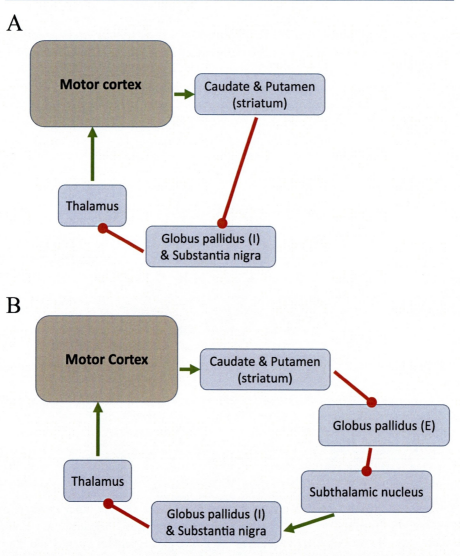

FIGURE 10–6. A. Direct cortico-basal-thalamo-cortical circuit. **B.** Indirect cortico-basal-thalamo-cortical circuit.

GP/SN). Then, because the thalamus has not been inhibited, it will send an excitatory signal back to the motor cortex, thus facilitating or enhancing motor signals.

The indirect circuit is slightly more complicated (Figure 10–6B). The circuit starts out the same, with excitatory signals from the motor cortex to the striatum. The outputs are inhibitory signals to the external component of the GP, which in turn inhibits the subthalamic nucleus. From the subthalamic nucleus, excitatory signals are sent to the internal portion of the GP and SN, which then inhibit the thalamus. The thalamic projections back to the cortex are excitatory. Walking through the circuit, you have excitation of the striatum, which inhibits the external GP. Because it is inhibited, it does not then inhibit the subthalamic nucleus, which will then send excitatory signals to the internal GP and SN. Because these structures have received excitatory signals, they will then inhibit the thalamus, which prevents it from sending signals to the motor cortex. Thus, the overall impact is to reduce movement because the motor cortex does not receive excitatory signals that would stimulate additional motor output.

These circuits illustrate not only the cortico-basal-thalamo-cortical loops but also how the specific pattern of excitatory and inhibitory signals can result in opposite functions.

Disorders involving the basal ganglia are discussed in the final section of this chapter on clinical implications. Such applications can be useful in understanding the ramifications of disruptions to this complex set of structures.

Cerebellum

The cerebellum has the broad motor functions of targeting and smooth tracking. These are applied to movements of the eyes, trunk, limbs, and speech/swallowing structures. Functionally, the cerebellum can be divided into the vestibulocerebellum, spinocerebellum, and cerebrocerebellum.

The **vestibulocerebellum**, made up primarily of the flocculonodular lobe, is the most primitive portion of the structure. It is connected to vestibular and visual nuclei in the brainstem and is responsible for balance, vestibular reflexes, and eye movements that contribute to initiation, planning, and timing of movements.

The **spinocerebellum**, consisting of the vermis and the intermediate regions of the two cerebellar hemispheres, receives somatosensory and proprioceptive information coming up from the spinal cord. In the vermis, inputs from visual, auditory, and vestibular systems as well as somatosensory inputs from the head and proximal body structures are integrated to control posture, locomotion, and eye movements. The intermediate hemispheres receive signals from the distal limbs and digits. Input signals carried along the dorsal spinocerebellar tracts (see Chapter 6) contain information about muscles and joints that is used as feedback regarding the consequences of both active (voluntary) and passive movements. Signals within the ventral spinocerebellar tracts are corollary discharges (also known as efference copies) from motor neurons. These are sent only during active movements and represent the planned movements. Outputs from the cerebellum can modulate actions of descending motor systems to adjust posture and balance during movements. This accounts for proprioception, vestibular sense, and eye movements, which collectively keep us upright and able to adjust for changes in position. We can remain upright when at least two of the three senses are functioning.

Box 10–1. Cerebellar Coordination and Motor Learning

Due to the cerebellum, we have the remarkable ability to coordinate precise movements without looking. Furthermore, the motor learning propensities of the cerebellum allow us to learn and adjust movements to context. One of the buildings at a university in the upper Midwest was built at the time of the Americans With Disabilities Act. As a result, the doorknobs were installed approximately 3 inches below the standard doorknob height. Ask anyone who enters the building for the first time and they will likely tell you that they miss the doorknob as they implicitly reach for it. Interestingly, after just a few days of visiting the building regularly, we adjust and establish a new implicit reach for this building. Cool, right? Here is another good one: A carpenter miscalculates the cut-out size for the top and bottom stair treads. Whereas the middle 12 steps are a standard 7¼ inches, the bottom step is 8¼ inches and the top step is 6¾ inches. The homeowners struggled with this initially, stepping "through" the top step as they descended and feeling like they were going to fall into an abyss as they navigated the final, extra-large step down. Although it may remain a cruel joke for irregular visitors, through repeated use the homeowners unconsciously adjust their first and final steps as they ascend and descend the stairs without a thought.

Box 10–2. Clinical Application of Cerebellar Function

KayLea was a 17-year-old female who was involved in a high-speed motor vehicle crash. Prior to her accident, KayLea was a gifted runner and a member of a cross country team that was poised to capture the state cross country title. It took years of hard work, but KayLea would eventually return to running. Central to her ability to run was the spinocerebellar system. The accident had damaged cerebellar inputs from the medial lemniscal pathway that provided crucial information about proprioception. She could compensate well given intact vestibular and ocular function. It was a bit of an effort to coordinate, but KayLea began to regain her passion for running. One hot August morning, she learned a lesson about the spinocerebellar system: "You've got to have at least two out of three" sensory inputs. In an attempt to beat the heat, she got up before dawn to tackle her morning run. Absent a reliable visualization of her surroundings, she stumbled and earned some short-term road rash that served as evidence for what happens when you only have your vestibular sense to help you remain upright. (See Case 16–4 in Chapter 16 for an expanded version of this case.)

The **cerebrocerebellum** is made up of the lateral portions of the cerebellar hemispheres and is evolutionarily the most recent region. It receives input from the cerebral cortex and sends outputs to the cerebral hemispheres, primarily the premotor, motor, and prefrontal areas where the signals influence movement planning, programming, timing, and execution. Interestingly, in addition to regulating timing of movements, this region influences cognitive processing of time, such as judging elapsed time. Due to the connections with the frontal lobes, the cerebrocerebellum also has a role in some cognitive processes, including working memory, social cognition, and language. These functions have been alternately described as modulating cognitive function or increasing efficiency, the latter of which allows us to perform more complex tasks. The cerebellum's role in communication and cognition is discussed further in Chapter 14.

Despite the variety of functions in the various regions of the cerebellum, the neural architecture (organization of neurons) is remarkably similar throughout. The deepest layer is made up of approximately 100 billion **granule cells** that receive inputs coming into the cerebellum. Some of these inputs come from **mossy fibers**, the axons of neurons in the spinal cord that carry sensory information from the body as well as from cortical neurons. Mossy fibers are important for carrying out learned movements. Granule cell axons extend to the most superficial layer, where they are called **parallel fibers** and synapse onto the dendritic trees of **Purkinje cells** (Figure 10–7). Deep cerebellar nuclei (called fastigial, globose, emboliform, and dentate) are located centrally, embedded in the white matter of the cerebellum. Axons extend out from these nuclei through the superior and inferior peduncles on their way to the cerebra and spinal cord.

A single layer of Purkinje cell bodies creates the output layer. The vast dendrites extending from the cell bodies extend into the molecular layer. Purkinje cells have a broad but rather flat (nearly two-dimensional) dendritic tree. When lined up, the dendritic trees appear similar to folders in a file cabinet (Figure 10–8). Purkinje cells receive inputs from **climbing fibers** and interneurons. Each Purkinje cell has one climbing fiber that originates from the inferior olivary nucleus in the brainstem and carries either sensory information from the body or signals from the cortex. Signals sent through climbing fibers allow detection of new events and are important for motor learning. Climbing fibers can have multiple axon collaterals so that one climbing fiber can affect multiple Purkinje cells. Purkinje cell axons extend deep into the cerebellum to synapse onto deep cerebellar nuclei or vestibular nuclei in the brainstem. At the synapses, GABA is released and has an inhibitory effect on the nuclei.

The molecular layer can be considered the processing layer. As noted previously, axons from the granular layer form parallel fibers that run perpendicular to the Purkinje dendritic trees. In this way, each Purkinje cell receives input from up to 1 million granule cells. The signals from the parallel fibers combine to create information about the magnitude and duration of a stimulus. Amidst the Purkinje dendritic trees are basket and stellate cells.

As with the basal ganglia, there are various cerebellar circuits that provide input to the motor system. These circuits influence the sequence and timing of muscle coordination and have an important role in motor learning because the connections provide comparisons about intended movements and actual movements. Disorders involving the cerebellum are discussed in the final section of this chapter on clinical implications. Such applications can be useful in understanding the ramifications of disruptions to this complex structure.

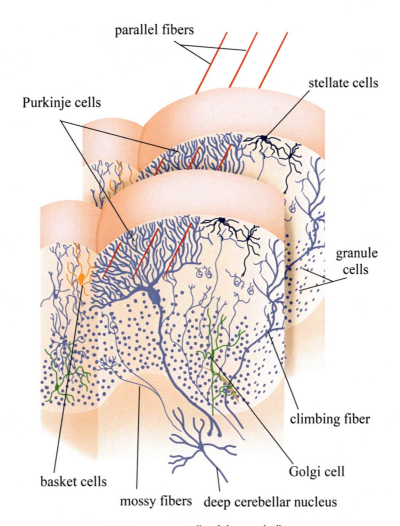

FIGURE 10-7. Cells of the cerebellum.

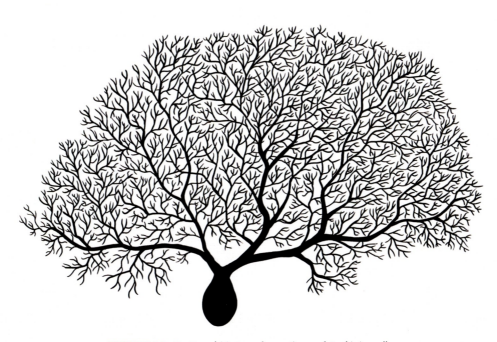

FIGURE 10-8. Dendritic tree formations of Purkinje cells.

Motor Pathways

The major motor pathways provide a link between the motor cortex and skeletal muscles. They can be divided into two major systems: the pyramidal and extrapyramidal tracts. The **pyramidal tracts** create direct connections between the brain and the body and are responsible for innervation of muscles and thus executing movements. The **extrapyramidal tracts** provide connections between various structures within the motor system and between the motor system and brainstem nuclei that serve to modify and adjust movement. The spinal components of the motor pathways are in the lateral or anterior regions of the spinal cord (Figure 10–9).

Pyramidal Tracts

The pyramidal tracts are named for the pyramidal-shaped motor neurons in the cortex. Also, a cross section through the tract reveals a pyramidal shape. This is also called the direct pathway because signals are sent directly from the motor strip to a neuron that carries a signal to the muscle. The signals are sent through a sequence of only two types of neurons: **upper motor neurons (UMNs)** synapse onto **lower motor neurons (LMNs)**, which in turn synapse onto skeletal muscles. This pathway is called **monosynaptic** because there is a single synapse between the brain and the body. Recall that damage anywhere along this pathway results in weakness. The pyramidal tracts can be subdivided into corticobulbar and corticospinal tracts, named for the beginning and end of the pathways within the CNS, respectively. **Corticobulbar tracts** extend through the CNS only to the brainstem. Bulbar refers to the medulla and pons, which look like a bulb on top of the spinal cord. Broadly, bulbar refers to the brainstem (although technically, bulbar includes the medulla, pons, and cerebellum but not the midbrain). In the corticobulbar tracts, signals are sent through cranial nerves to innervate muscles of the head and neck. **Corticospinal tracts**, in contrast, extend down into the spinal cord and innervate muscles of the body via spinal nerves.

Many of the pyramidal motor neurons have excitatory connections to extensor muscles and axon collaterals that provide inhibitory input to flexor muscles. This combination of opposite signals to opposing muscles aids in coordination. There are hundreds or thousands of neurons in the primary motor strip that fire to signal the force and direction of voluntary movement.

Cranial and Spinal Nerves

As described in Chapter 1, the peripheral nervous system is made up of the nerves that branch off from the brainstem (cranial nerves) and spinal cord (spinal nerves). Putting this together with what you just learned about the pyramidal tracts, you see that the motor components of cranial and spinal nerves are LMNs. LMN cell bodies for the 31 pairs of spinal nerves can be found in the ventral horn of the spinal cord, and the axons exit to form the motor portion of the spinal nerves (the sensory component is discussed in Chapter 6). LMNs innervating shoulder and arm muscles exit from the cervical region, those innervating trunk and abdominal muscles exit from the thoracic region, and those innervating leg/foot muscles exit from the lumbar and sacral regions.

The 31 pairs of spinal nerves are all essentially the same—they each contain both motor and sensory axons and innervate skeletal muscles. In contrast, the cranial nerves can contain only motor, only sensory, or a combination of motor and sensory axons. There are 12 pairs of cranial nerves, denoted by roman numerals. In this text, the abbreviation CN is used along with the appropriate

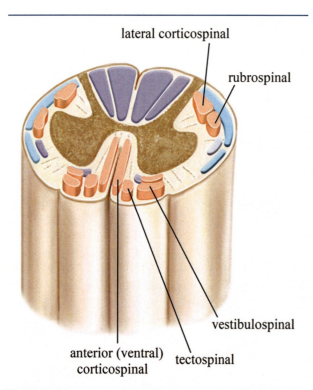

FIGURE 10–9. Location of motor pathways in the spinal cord.

roman numeral to refer to the cranial nerves (e.g., facial nerve is CN VII). Because of their unique innervation and function and the fact that they control the sensorimotor components of speech and swallowing, the cranial nerves are covered only briefly here and discussed in much greater detail in Chapter 11.

Corticospinal Tracts

Labeled by its origin and path, the corticospinal tracts carry motor impulses from the cortex (precentral gyrus) to the spinal outputs (spinal nerve roots with ultimate innervation of corresponding muscles in the body). Corticospinal tracts are made up of two kinds of neurons introduced previously: upper and lower motor neurons. The UMNs synapse onto LMNs, whose cell bodies are in the CNS and whose axons leave the CNS through spinal nerves to innervate skeletal muscles. This seems simple enough—two neurons creating a direct connection from brain to muscle—but there are some important landmarks along the way.

The corticospinal tract is divided into two pathways called the **lateral corticospinal tract** and the **anterior (ventral) corticospinal tract**. They differ in terms of (1) where they cross over, (2) where the UMN axons lie in the spinal cord, and (3) the region of the body they innervate. For the corticospinal tract as a whole, the UMN cell bodies are in the motor strip. The axons of these UNMs extend down from the motor strip all the way into the spinal cord. Mapping this out step by step, the axons course through the white matter region of the **corona radiata** (just deep to the cortex). They then converge as they pass in between the GP and the thalamus in a region called the **internal capsule**. From there, the UMN axons course within a tight group down through the midbrain, pons, and medulla. At this point, there is separation of the lateral and anterior tracts. Axons in the lateral tract, which make up 90% of the corticospinal tract, cross over in the inferior medulla. The remaining 10% of axons stay ipsilateral down to the lower cervical and upper thoracic regions of the spinal cord. These latter axons make up the anterior corticospinal tract.

Lateral Corticospinal Tract. The lateral corticospinal tract innervates muscles in the limbs (Figure 10–10). Thinking about the motor homunculus and the target regions of the lateral corticospinal tract, you can figure

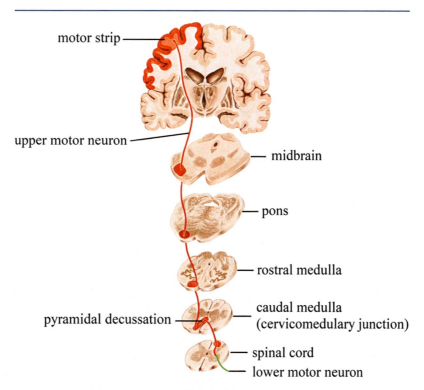

FIGURE 10–10 Lateral corticospinal tract.

> **Box 10–3.** Divisions of the Corticospinal Tract
>
> Corticospinal tracts provide a direct connection between the brain and muscles of the body below the neck.
>
> - Lateral corticospinal tract: UMN axons cross over at the pyramidal decussation in the medulla and continue through the contralateral spinal cord; axons extend down in lateral regions of the spinal cord; UMN axons synapse onto LMN cell bodies in the ventral horn; LMN axons innervate muscles in the limbs.
> - Anterior (ventral) corticospinal tract: UMN axons do not cross over in the medulla but continue through the ipsilateral spinal cord; axons extend down in anterior/ventral regions of the spinal cord; UMN axons cross over prior to synapsing onto LMN cell bodies; LMN axons innervate muscles of the trunk.

> **Box 10–4.** Following the Corticospinal Path
>
> Imagine the entire pathway a signal must travel to get from the brain to your hand to wiggle your right index finger: UMN cell body in the mid-lateral region of the motor cortex in the left hemisphere; axon extends through the left corona radiata, left internal capsule through the left side of the brainstem; then shifts over to the right side of the spinal cord at the pyramidal decussation; extends down to the cervical region of the spinal cord and ends in the right ventral horn. Here, the UMN axon terminal synapses onto the cell body of an LMN residing in the ventral horn. The LMN axon extends out from the spinal cord in a cervical spinal nerve that courses through the right arm and to the muscles of the index finger. Now imagine the pathway traveled to wiggle your right big toe. The UMN cell body lies in the motor strip along the sagittal sulcus. The axon extends through the same regions of the cerebrum. However, once the UMN axon reaches the spinal cord, it continues down the lateral spinal cord until it reaches the lumbar region of the cord, where it ends and synapses in the ventral horn onto the LMN cell body of one of the sacral spinal nerves that then extends all the way down the leg to the foot.

out that the UMN cell bodies are in the mid and superior regions of the motor strip that represent the hands/arms and legs/feet. The axons follow the route described previously—through the corona radiata and internal capsule to the lower medulla. The somatotopy (organization by body area) is preserved throughout the pathway. As shown in Figure 10–11, there is precise organization of UMN axons in the internal capsule. At the inferior extent of the medulla, the axons cross over to the opposite side of the medulla. This region is called the **pyramidal decussation**. Thus, if the UMN cell bodies lie in the right motor strip, their axons will extend through the right corona radiata, right internal capsule, and right side of the brainstem until the inferior medulla, where they shift over to the left side of the medulla and continue extending down the contralateral (in this case, left side) spinal cord. As per the name of the tract, the axons lie in the lateral region of the spinal cord (Figure 10–9). The UMNs in the lateral corticospinal tract end in the ventral horn of the spinal cord, where they synapse onto the cell bodies of LMNs. The axons of those LMNs leave the spinal cord through the nearest spinal root and make up the motor component of the spinal nerves. Those LMN axons end at a neuromuscular junction to synapse onto skeletal muscles of the limbs.

Each spinal nerve innervates a section of the body. In the motor system, these are called **myotomes** (remember from Chapter 6 that the sensory equivalents are called dermatomes). Each thoracic spinal nerve, instead of innervating a specific muscle or muscle group, innervates a variety of muscle fibers along a strip of the body. Due to this arrangement, damage to a spinal nerve will not cause paralysis of a single muscle or muscle group.

Anterior Corticospinal Tract. The anterior corticospinal tract innervates muscles of the trunk. In the previous description, 90% of the UMN axons in the corticospinal tracts cross over at the pyramidal decussation. The remaining 10% of the UMN axons do not cross over in the medulla but, rather, remain ipsilateral until just prior to synapsing. This latter group of axons makes up the anterior corticospinal tract. There is no single point of crossover as for the lateral tract; the axons cross over immediately prior to synapsing onto LMN cell bodies in the ventral horn (Figure 10–12). This group is called the anterior corticospinal tract because the UMN axons lie within the anterior region of the spinal cord.

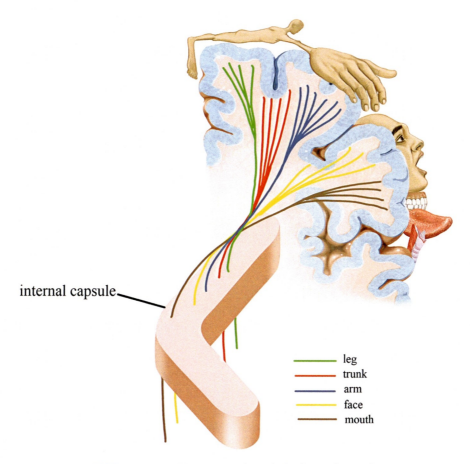

FIGURE 10-11. Motor tracts through the internal capsule.

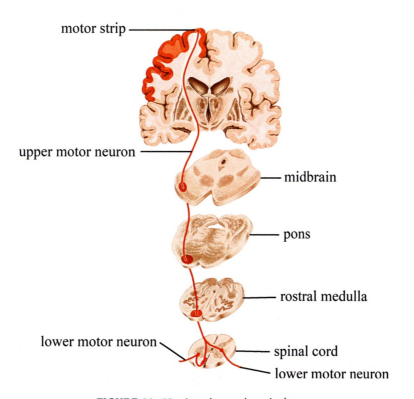

FIGURE 10-12. Anterior corticospinal tract.

Corticobulbar Tract

The corticobulbar tract, as described previously, is monosynaptic (one synapse between two neurons), and the UMN ends in the brainstem. Cell bodies of the UMNs reside in the inferior region of the motor strip, where the larynx, tongue, and facial structures are represented. As in the corticospinal tracts, the axons course through the corona radiata and internal capsule. Differences arise once the axons reach the brainstem. Each paired cranial nerve has paired (bilateral) nuclei that house cell bodies of motor and sensory neurons. UMN axons extending down into the brainstem cross over immediately prior to synapsing on the appropriate nucleus. For example, UMNs innervating muscles of mastication via the trigeminal nerve (CN V) will cross over in the pons and synapse onto trigeminal LMN cell bodies in the trigeminal nuclei. UMNs innervating muscles of facial expression via the facial nerve (CN VII) will extend down to the superior medulla before crossing over and then synapsing in the facial nucleus. From the cranial nerve nuclei, LMN axons extend out within the appropriate CN to innervate the target muscles.

Although the corticobulbar tract innervates only regions of the head and neck, it contains approximately 70% of all the neurons within the pyramidal tracts. This suggests that extensive innervation is required to achieve the necessary level of fine motor control of articulators (larynx, tongue, and soft palate) and muscles of facial expression. Chapter 11 provides a detailed description of the cranial nerves.

Extrapyramidal Tracts

Extrapyramidal tracts provide indirect influences on skeletal muscles. Signals from the motor cortices are sent to the basal ganglia or nuclei in the brainstem before influencing LMN signals to the muscles. These tracts are all named for their locations.

Rubrospinal Tract

The rubrospinal tract is named for the red nucleus (Latin: *rubrum* = *red*) located in the midbrain region of the brainstem. Inputs come from the frontal cortex, and axons from neurons in the red nucleus immediately cross over in the pons and extend down into the contralateral spinal cord to synapse onto LMNs (Figure 10–13). Lesions to this pathway cause impairments in fine, fractionated movements that are performed with few muscle groups. This results

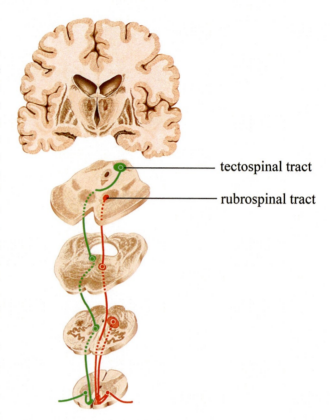

FIGURE 10–13. Rubrospinal (*red*) and tectospinal (*green*) tracts.

in behaviors such as using the whole hand for a movement that requires only a single finger. In contrast to other mammals, in humans the rubrospinal tract is relatively small, and it appears that most of the functions of this pathway are subsumed by the larger lateral corticospinal tract.

Tectospinal Tract

Remember that the tectum is the region of the posterior midbrain where the superior and inferior colliculi lie. The tectospinal tract arises from the colliculi and so receives information from visual and auditory systems. It influences movement of the neck, trunk, and shoulder muscles and is important in orienting the eyes and head to external stimuli (Figure 10–13).

Vestibulospinal Tract

The vestibulospinal tract involves the vestibular nuclei in the brainstem (described in Chapter 8) and provides input to muscles of the neck and upper back to aid in balancing the head (Figure 10–14). In addition, there are connections to the extensor muscles in the legs that aid in maintaining an upright, balanced posture.

Reticulospinal Tract

The reticulospinal tract, arising from the reticular formation in the pons and medulla, assists with upright posture. Like the vestibulospinal tract, there are connections to extensor leg muscles and to spinal reflexive circuits (Figure 10–15).

Motor Units and Muscle Innervation

The **neuromuscular junction**, as the name suggests, is where the nervous system connects with the muscular system. The description of neuron signaling in Chapter 3 and for sensory systems has focused primarily on neuron-to-neuron communication; however, at the neuromuscular junction, neurons synapse onto muscle fibers. This junction can specifically be broken down in terms of the motor unit, which consists of the LMN (cell body, axon, and axon terminal) and the muscle it innervates (Figure 10–16). The LMN axon terminal is called the motor end plate. Just as with the synapses described in Chapter 3, there is no physical connection between the axon terminal and the muscle fiber; rather, they are separated by a synaptic gap. The muscle fibers contain postsynaptic receptors that respond to the release of acetylcholine (ACh). Much is known about the motor unit and the specific tissues and structures within muscles that create muscle contraction. Here, we provide only a very broad description.

Acetylcholine is released from the LMN axon terminal and binds to receptors on the muscle fibers. This triggers a depolarization response in the muscle tissue that results in contraction (shortening) of the muscle. The more ACh released, the stronger the resulting muscle contraction.

Reflexes represent the most basic movements and provide a clear example of sensorimotor communication (Figure 10–17). In the patellar "stretch" reflex, the patellar tendon [extending from the kneecap (patella) to the tibia in the lower leg] is tapped with a reflex hammer, which causes

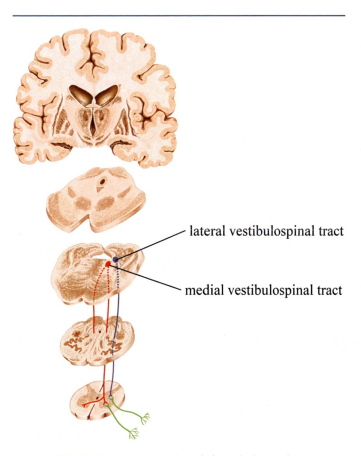

FIGURE 10–14. Lateral and medial vestibulospinal tracts.

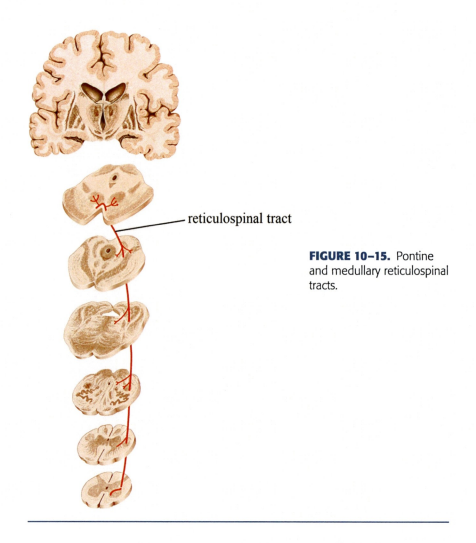

FIGURE 10–15. Pontine and medullary reticulospinal tracts.

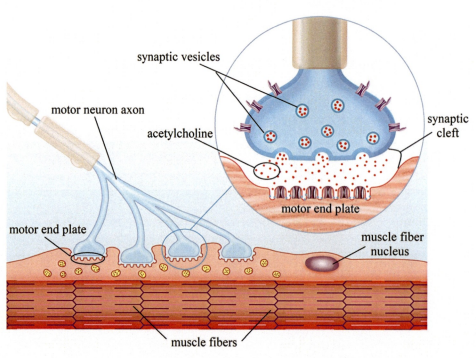

FIGURE 10–16. The neuromuscular junction.

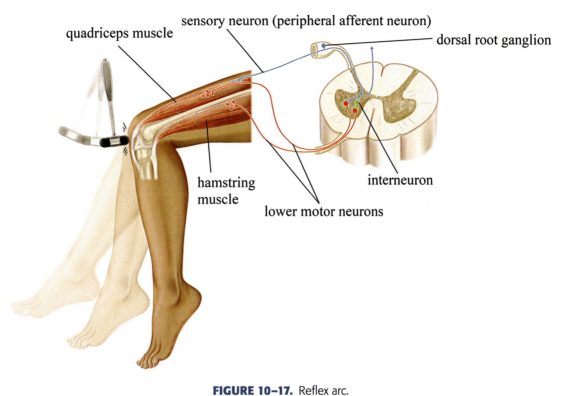

FIGURE 10–17. Reflex arc.

the tendon to stretch. Stretching momentarily lengthens the quadriceps muscle, activating a spindle afferent sensor. This stretching and subsequent activation of the spindle afferent causes depolarization of a somatosensory neuron (peripheral afferent neuron), resulting in an action potential sent through that neuron into the spinal cord. The axon of that sensory neuron has several collateral branches. One synapses onto an LMN in the ventral horn, causing an action potential to be sent down its axon to the quadriceps (anterior thigh) muscle, resulting in contraction of that muscle that extends the leg at the knee joint. A second collateral synapses onto an inhibitory interneuron within the spinal gray matter. The interneuron in turn synapses on an LMN that innervates the antagonistic or opposing muscle—in this case, the hamstring (posterior thigh). Because the interneuron is inhibitory, it essentially keeps the hamstring relaxed, which facilitates the extensor movement because the quadriceps muscle can contract unopposed. Thus, a signal from the patellar tendon results in excitation (contraction) of the target muscle and inhibition (relaxation) of the opposing muscle. This is called **reciprocal inhibition**. There is also a signal sent up the dorsal column–medial lemniscus tract to the primary sensory cortex, where the touch and resulting leg movement are consciously "felt." Although the reflex arc involves only the motor and sensory circuits between the spinal cord and effector muscles, cortical modulation (descending messages traveling from the brain toward the reflex circuit along UMNs) serves to dampen reflex responses in the absence of pathology or higher order control (i.e., anticipating reflexes can alter reflexes). The presence or absence of modulation is crucial in determining whether descending motor pathways are intact. Hyperactive reflexes are typically an indication of UMN damage, indicating damage to the descending motor pathway and a lack of cortical modulation. Conversely, hypoactive or absent reflexes are typically an indication of LMN damage because the signal to contract the muscle cannot reach the muscle.

Clinical Implications

Damage to the motor system causes a wide variety of disorders and impairments depending on which structure(s) or pathway(s) is affected.

For speech-language pathology, the key disorders resulting from motor system disruption are apraxia of speech, dysarthria, and dysphagia. **Apraxia of speech**

(Greek: *praxis = doing, action*) is caused by damage to the motor programming system and results in speech sound distortions and substitutions that are more prominent with longer words and increasing articulatory complexity. Alterations of speech rate and prosody are present along with articulatory "groping" as patients attempt to move the articulators into the correct position. **Dysarthria** (Greek: *arthron = joint, articulation*) is an umbrella term for a variety of speech disorders resulting from weakness or movement disorders such as incoordination of the articulators. The specific characteristics and type of dysarthria depend on the part of the motor system that is affected. **Dysphagia** (Greek: *phageon = to eat*), or swallowing dysfunction, is caused by weakness or incoordination of muscle groups (e.g., lips, tongue, palate, vocal folds) required for safe and efficient swallowing.

Good speech diagnosticians can aid neurologists in pinpointing the location of damage or disease within the nervous system based on a thorough oral mechanism examination and speech assessment from which to diagnose the type of dysarthria.

Motor Cortex

Damage to cortical areas involved in motor programming including the insula and regions around the inferior frontal gyrus can cause apraxia of speech. Damage to the primary motor cortex or the UMN axons in the corona radiata or internal capsule results in spasticity, characterized by hypertonia and resistance to stretching. Reflexes are brisk or hyperactive because there is a lack of cortical modulation and dampening of the reflex arc. UMN damage causes weakness or paralysis because of the increased tone and spasticity. Due to the decussation of the motor tracts, all signs will be present on the side of the body opposite the site of the lesion. A characteristic triple-flexion posturing with flexion of fingers, wrist, and elbow may be present (Figure 10–18).

UMN damage causes a **spastic dysarthria** characterized by a slow rate of speech and a strained, strangled vocal quality. If the damage is unilateral, the signs/symptoms are mild and often resolve spontaneously. Bilateral UMN damage, often due to traumatic brain injury or multiple sclerosis, results in more severe and often chronic spastic dysarthria.

Motor Pathways

Damage to both UMNs and LMNs results in weakness but for different reasons. There are other distinctive motor signs that aid in differentiating the source of weakness (Table 10–1). UMN damage, as noted previously, results

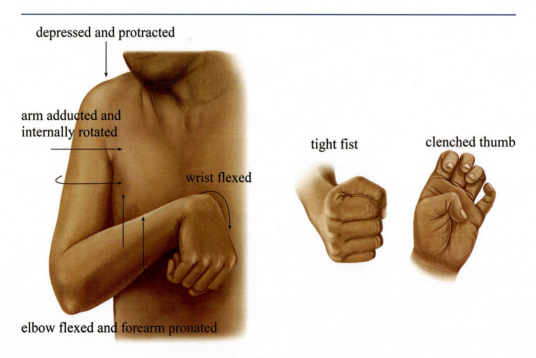

FIGURE 10–18. Triple-flexion posturing.

Table 10–1. Upper and Lower Motor Neuron Damage Characteristics

UMN Damage	LMN Damage
Weakness	Weakness
Hyperactive reflexes	Hypoactive reflexes
Increased tone	Decreased tone
No atrophy	Atrophy present
No fasciculations	Fasciculations present
Spasticity present	Flaccidity present

Note. LMN, lower motor neuron; UMN, upper motor neuron.

in spasticity and hypertonicity. Speech is characterized by spastic dysarthria, which is marked by strained, strangled quality and effortful articulation. LMN damage, in contrast, is characterized by hypoactive or absent reflexes, as the LMN innervation to muscle groups is either impaired or absent. As a result, muscle tone is also reduced. The reduction in tone, paired with hypoactive or absent reflexes, is referred to as **flaccidity**. Speech is characterized by **flaccid dysarthria**, with weak tongue movements and hypernasality (due to weakness of the velum) reducing intelligibility. The absence of signals from LMNs to muscle fibers results in **fasciculations**, which are involuntary twitches of small muscle groups (you could liken this to the flickering of a lightbulb that is about to burn out). **Fibrillations**, involuntary firing of individual muscle fibers, are not visible to the human eye but are also present for similar reasons. Both fasciculations and fibrillations can be detected through electromyography. Over time, muscles will atrophy as a result of LMN damage. This is the extreme case of "use it or lose it": The muscles deteriorate when they are not given signals to contract. UMN damage does not cause atrophy because LMNs can still carry signals to muscles, which results in the increased tone and hyperactive reflexes.

Diseases that impact axons or myelin cause characteristic positive and negative signs. Positive signs are added phenomena. These include **paresthesias**, or abnormal sensations such as tingling or pins and needles sensations that are caused by cross-talk across axons or hyperexcitability, which results in a sensory signal that is much more intense than the stimulus that caused it. Hyperexcitability can make a tap on the arm feel intensely painful. Negative signs are things that do not work anymore. Weakness, paralysis, and reduced reflexes are all negative signs. These and others can be caused by slowed or blocked conduction of action potentials or by an inability to sustain a high frequency of action potentials. Multiple sclerosis (see Chapter 3) causes both positive and negative signs due to the degeneration of myelin that disrupts the speed and timing of action potentials.

Amyotrophic lateral sclerosis (ALS; also called Lou Gehrig disease in the United States and motor neurone disease in the United Kingdom) causes degeneration of both UMNs and LMNs. The Latin translation means lack (a-) of muscle (myo-) growth (-trophic) accompanied by hardened scar tissue (sclerosis) in the lateral region of the spinal cord. The hardening is caused by astrocytes that migrate to the damaged areas. All muscle groups except the ocular (eye) muscles and voluntarily controlled bladder muscles are affected. Looking back at Table 10–1, you can expect to see mixed UMN and LMN signs/symptoms in patients with ALS. Most patients have bulbar-onset ALS, meaning that degeneration affects the cranial nerves first so that the early signs are related to speech and swallowing. The progression of ALS begins with mixed dysarthria becoming more predominantly flaccid and ultimately ends in a loss of speech production. Swallowing deteriorates progressively as well, leading to decisions about non-oral feeding, which is generally a necessity as the disease progresses. Patients with spinal-onset ALS, as you can guess, have initial signs in the limbs. Regardless of the location of the onset, as the disease progresses, both bulbar and spinal motor neurons will be affected. Two related disorders are **progressive bulbar palsy** and **spinal muscular atrophy**. Progressive bulbar palsy is caused by degeneration of only UMNs, whereas spinal muscular atrophy affects only LMNs. The latter is a developmental disorder seen primarily in infants.

Neuromuscular Junction

Disruptions to the synapse between the LMN and the muscle can occur for various reasons. There may be problems with the release of ACh from the LMN axon terminal, damage to the postsynaptic receptors on the muscle fiber, or the ACh may not be able to bind to the receptors. All of these will result in weakness or paralysis. Remember from Chapter 3 that certain toxins and drugs such as Botox, curare, and atropine cause weakness or paralysis by preventing the release or the binding of ACh.

Myasthenia gravis (MG), briefly described in Chapter 3, is an autoimmune disorder in which the postsynaptic ACh receptors are attacked and damaged by the immune system. The result is weakness because there are not enough intact receptors to create normal muscle contractions. Following rest, speech is often normal, but it declines rapidly, with loss of articulatory precision and hypernasality becoming more pronounced with continuous speech. A differential diagnostic characteristic of MG is a relatively rapid decline in strength and function during an activity with repeated muscle contraction and then recovery of strength after rest. During repeated contraction, ACh is released into the synapse, but once the ACh binds to the existing/functioning ACh receptors, there is no place for additional neurotransmitter to bind to increase the strength of the muscle contraction. A diagnostic test for MG is the injection of acetylcholinesterase (AChE) inhibitors such as prostigmine (also called neostigmine). Remember from Chapter 3 that AChEs are enzymes that destroy and remove ACh from the synapse. Inhibiting these enzymes will cause the ACh to remain in the synapse longer so that it can bind, release, and then rebind to the functioning receptors. Injection of these drugs results in a very rapid and quite astonishing return of strength. Check YouTube for videos of "tensilon tests" or "neostigmine tests" to see examples.

Box 10–5. Recognizing Signs of Myasthenia Gravis

Often, speech-language pathologists (SLPs) are the first professionals to recognize MG. Patients' concerns about troubles eating and speaking may seem subtle to primary care physicians and not necessarily recognized as symptoms of a neurological disorder. Placing direct demands on those structures through bedside assessments of speech and swallowing often exacerbates their impairments and allows detection. Although SLPs cannot make a diagnosis of MG, it is not uncommon for them to convey such suspicions to neurologists, who ultimately confirm the diagnosis through their testing. (See Case 16–12 in Chapter 16 for a clinical case of MG.)

Basal Ganglia

Because the basal ganglia are a set of structures, different presentations occur depending on the site of the damage or disease. Disorders can be generally classified into those with too much movement (**hyperkinetic**) and those with not enough movement (**hypokinetic**). **Parkinson disease (PD)**, resulting from degeneration of the substantia nigra and subsequent decrease in dopamine within basal ganglia circuits (see Chapter 3), is characterized primarily by reduced range of motion. This creates the "masked facies" or minimal facial expression, the poor articulation but rapid speech rate, and the shuffling gait. Movements are high velocity and low amplitude, resulting in soft phonation and rapid, mumbled bursts of speech. Together these are known as **hypokinetic dysarthria**. This affects multiple systems in the vocal tract: weak breathy voice due to failure to achieve tight adduction of the vocal folds, imprecise articulation caused by reduced extent of movement of articulators, and rapid rate of speech. It may initially seem counterintuitive that movements are both reduced and faster. Reduction in amplitude of movements accounts for the net reduced movement. However, if the articulators are not moving as far, they can move faster. Try saying "mama" quickly while opening your mouth as much as possible for each "a," then reduce the oral opening to only as much as needed to produce the sounds. Your rate is much faster when you use a smaller range of motion.

There is also a resting tremor associated with PD, which is an unwanted movement. This can include hand flapping and pill rolling tremors in the hands, but tremors are also common in the jaw, mouth, and tongue. These are resting tremors, meaning that they are present when the person is at rest, such as when they are sitting quietly, but they disappear when the person initiates movement. The tremors also cease with sleep. As described in Chapter 3, the contradictory presentations (not enough and too much movement) are due to the different dopamine receptors: Some create excitatory signals and others inhibitory.

Huntington disease (HD) is characterized by unwanted, uncontrollable movements. Degeneration of the caudate nucleus interrupts the balance between inhibition and excitation in the basal ganglia circuits, resulting in motor signals that should have been inhibited. Movements are characterized by low velocity and high amplitude qualities. In speech, this manifests as **hyperkinetic dysarthria** with jerky, inconsistent prosody, rate, and volume. Breathing and coordination of voicing are also disrupted. Note that "hyperkinetic" refers to too much or unwanted movement, and not movement that is too fast. In fact, individuals with HD often attempt to impose a rhythm to counteract the involuntary movements, which may result in slow, drawn-out speech. Often, adventitious (extra, unwanted) movements are present in the jaw and tongue.

Dystonias are another group of disorders characterized by too much or unwanted movements. Often, these appear as sustained contractions. Blepherospasm (eye twitching), torticollis (neck contractions), oromandibular dystonia (mouth and jaw), and spasmodic dysphonia (vocal folds) are all forms of focal dystonias. The precise mechanism of dystonias is not clear, but they are suspected to be related to basal ganglia function.

Cerebellum

Damage to the cerebellum results in disruptions to normal movements, but because it is not responsible for initiating movement, damage does not cause weakness or paralysis as does damage to the motor cortex or motor pathways. There are several motoric characteristics of cerebellar damage. First is **hypotonia** or reduced muscle tone. This can be accompanied by pendular reflexes; as the name suggests, the reflexive action continues back and forth like a clock pendulum because the damping process that typically stops the reflexive movement is disrupted. Second is a dual pattern of **atasia** and **abasia**. Atasia is the lack of coordination of limb and body postures across multiple joints. A person with atasia will have extreme difficulty walking because it requires close coordination of leg and trunk muscles. Abasia is the inability to maintain an upright posture against the force of gravity. Essentially, abasia is difficulty standing and atasia is difficulty walking.

The third is **ataxia** (Greek: -*taxis* = *order*) or uncoordinated movements. These are characterized by **dysmetria**, or abnormal targeting of movements, and **dysdiadochokinesis**, which is Greek for impairment of alternating movement. Related to speech production, dysdiadochokinesis affects the ability to repeat a consonant–vowel pair such as pa-pa-pa-pa. Control of voicing, intensity, and duration is affected. This can result in voicing substitutions (e.g., "pa" produced as "ba"), inconsistent volume across syllables, and inconsistent duration of successive syllables. These speech features together make up **ataxic dysarthria**. Ataxic speech shares the characteristics of drunken, intoxicated speech, marked by overshoots and undershoots, ultimately resulting in slurred quality with irregular timing.

Fourth is **action** or **intention tremor**, which occurs at the end of a movement. In normal movement, there is contraction of antagonistic muscles to stop the movement of the agonist muscles. Poor coordination of agonist and antagonist muscles results in tremors. In contrast to the resting tremor of PD, intention tremors are not present at rest but only appear during movement.

Box 10–6. Differential Effects of Tremors

The differential effects of resting and intention tremors can be seen by asking people to write their name. A person with PD may have significant resting tremor, but once they pick up a pen and begin to write, the tremors will disappear and their writing will be smooth. In contrast, a person with cerebellar degeneration with ataxia will have no tremors at rest, but once they begin writing, the tremors will appear, resulting in very shaky and possibly illegible writing.

Fifth is **nystagmus**. As described in Chapter 8, this beating movement of the eyes occurs when the semicircular canals are stimulated in the absence of head movement. Cerebellar damage that disrupts the vestibulocerebellar pathways may result in nystagmus.

Finally, many people with cerebellar damage report significant movement difficulties because they seem to have lost the ability for automatic or unconscious movements. Consider the last time you had to think about how your legs move when you walk. Maybe it was with a new pair of high-heeled shoes or walking along a slippery surface. Another example is walking through an unfamiliar space with obstacles on the ground, in complete darkness. The effort it takes to consciously attend to movements can be exhausting and limits the ability to do two things at once—like walking and chewing gum.

Summary

Multiple regions, structures, and pathways control bodily movement. Due to the precise, organized control and mapping of the motor system, damage or lesions to the motor system often can be predicted by careful evaluation of the motor deficits that appear (e.g., weakness, paralysis, incoordination, or too much movement).

Key Concepts

- The motor system consists of both direct (pyramidal) and indirect (extrapyramidal) systems. The pyramidal system produces and transmits gross motor signals to the body, and the extrapyramidal system is responsible for refining those signals.
- The lateral corticospinal tract innervates the arms and legs, crossing over at the caudal medulla and serving contralateral muscle groups.
- The anterior corticospinal tract innervates the trunk and crosses over in the spinal cord at the level it innervates.
- Damage to the pyramidal system results in weakness disorders, whereas damage to the extrapyramidal system results in movement disorders.
- There are four points of weakness to consider in differential diagnosis: UMN damage (cortical or in pathways), LMN damage (cranial and spinal nerves), dysfunction of the neuromuscular junction, or damage to the muscles themselves (e.g., sarcomas, trauma, or simply couch potato syndrome).
- Characteristics of reflexes can help distinguish UMN versus LMN weakness.
- Damage to the insula and regions around the inferior frontal gyrus can disrupt motor programming and cause apraxia of speech.
- Damage to the basal ganglia results in impairments to the coordination of movements, including too much or too little dampening (inhibition) of movements.
- Damage to the cerebellum results in problems with targeting and smooth tracking, such as dysmetria and tremor. Collectively, these movement impairments result in atasia, abasia, and ataxia. Changes to cognition also may accompany this damage.

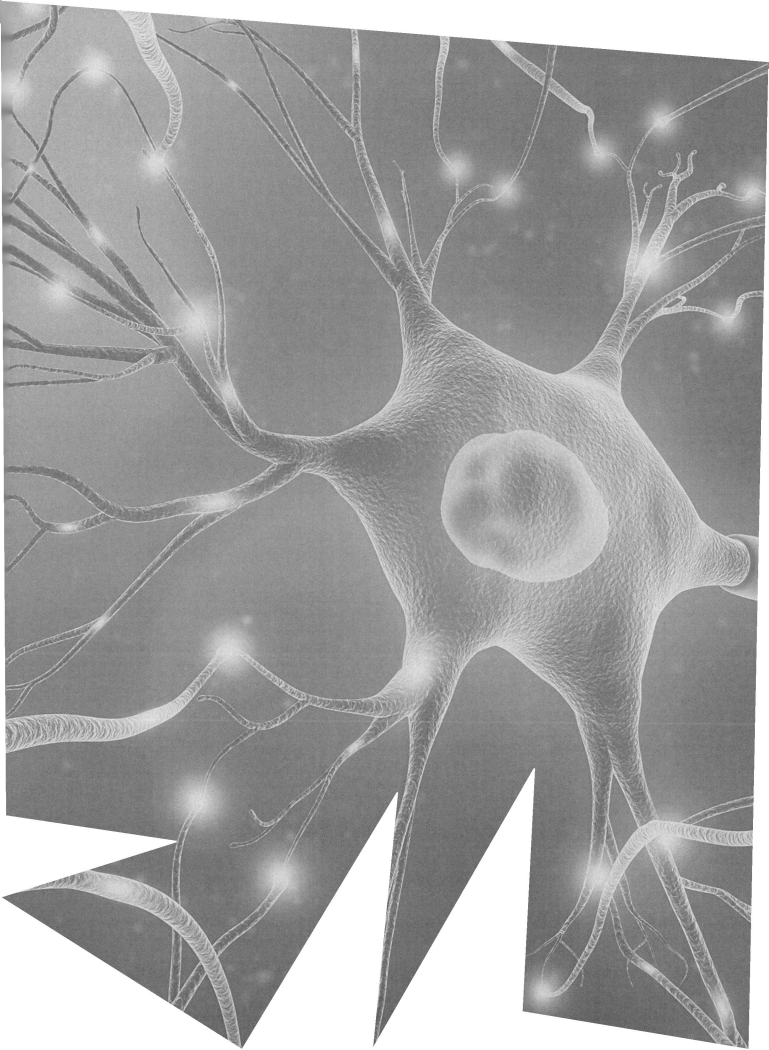

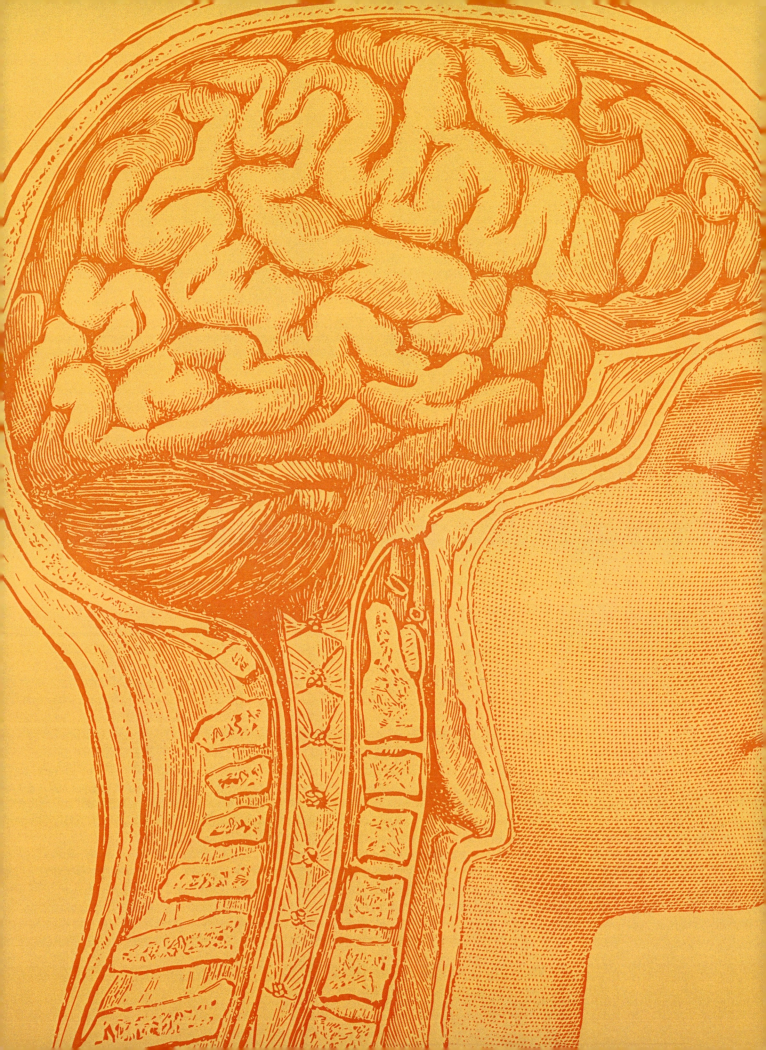

11

Cranial Nerves

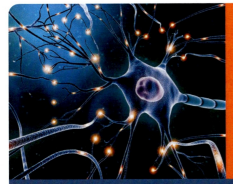

CHAPTER OUTLINE

Overview
   General Functions
Cranial Nerve Pathways
   Motor Pathways: Corticobulbar Tract
   Sensory Pathways
Cranial Nerves III, IV, and VI: Oculomotor, Trochlear, and Abducens
   Muscles of the Eye
   Oculomotor Nerve
   Trochlear Nerve
   Abducens Nerve
Cranial Nerve V: Trigeminal Nerve
Cranial Nerve VII: Facial Nerve
Cranial Nerve IX: Glossopharyngeal
Cranial Nerve X: Vagus Nerve
   Pharyngeal Branch of the Vagus
   Superior Laryngeal Nerve of the Vagus
   Recurrent Laryngeal Nerve of the Vagus
   Pharyngeal Plexus
Cranial Nerve XI: Spinal Accessory Nerve
Cranial Nerve XII: Hypoglossal Nerve
Integration of Cranial Nerve Functions
   Speech Production
   Swallowing
Clinical Implications: Examinations of Speech and Swallowing Mechanisms

Cranial Nerve/Oral Mechanism Examination
Smell and Taste
Vision
Extraocular Movements (CNs III, IV, and VI)
Jaw Movements and Mastication (CN V)
Facial Sensation (CN V)
Muscles of Facial Expression and Oral Preparation (CN VII)
Hearing (CN VIII)
Velar Functions—Motor and Sensory (CNs V, IX, and X)
Laryngeal Functions—Motor and Sensory (CN X)
Spinal Accessory (CN XI)
Lingual Motor Functions (CN XII with a Little Help from CN X)
Lingual Sensation (CNs V and IX)
Oral and Laryngeal Diadochokinetic Rate
Evidence for the Oral Mechanism Examination
Clinical Bedside Swallow Examination and Instrumental Assessment
Summary
Additional Resources

Overview

Cranial nerves are the nerves [part of the peripheral nervous system (PNS)] that exit from the brainstem and innervate structures and muscles of the head and neck. A thorough knowledge of cranial nerves is important for speech-language pathologists (SLPs) and audiologists (AuDs) because cranial nerves control all of the structures and muscles critical for speech and swallowing as well as the senses of hearing, taste, olfaction, and vision. A few of the cranial nerves were discussed in chapters on the special senses and are only touched upon here. It might be useful to review

173

head and neck anatomy (see Appendix) as a reminder of the muscles and structures innervated by the cranial nerves.

There are 12 pairs of cranial nerves, denoted by Roman numerals and numbered from superior to inferior based on where they enter/exit the brainstem. In this text, the abbreviation CN is used along with the appropriate Roman numeral to refer to the cranial nerves (e.g., the facial nerve is CN VII). Some cranial nerves, like spinal nerves, are made up of both sensory and motor axons. However, other cranial nerves are made up of only sensory or motor axons. The motor components of the cranial nerves make up the corticobulbar tracts (see Chapter 10 and Figure 11–1). The somatosensory components include pain, touch, temperature, and stretch from the muscles, joints, skin, and tissues of organs. These sensory pathways are similar to those covered in Chapter 6, including PNS ganglia for primary neuron cell bodies, a synapse in the thalamus, and the endpoint in the primary sensory strip in the postcentral gyrus. The sensory components for the special senses (smell, taste, vision, and hearing) have their own distinct pathways, as described in previous chapters. Cranial nerve nuclei are embedded in the brainstem (Figure 11–2) and are the location for synapses between upper motor neurons (UMNs) and lower motor neurons (LMNs) for the motor component and for incoming sensory information.

As shown in Table 11–1, there are a few traditional mnemonics to help remember the names, order, and general function of the cranial nerves. If none of these work for you, consider creating your own.

The olfactory, optic, and auditory–vestibular nerves were reviewed in detail in Chapters 9, 7, and 8, respectively. The remaining nine cranial nerves are described in detail here. In order to provide a more coherent review, they are grouped in regard to function instead of strictly by number.

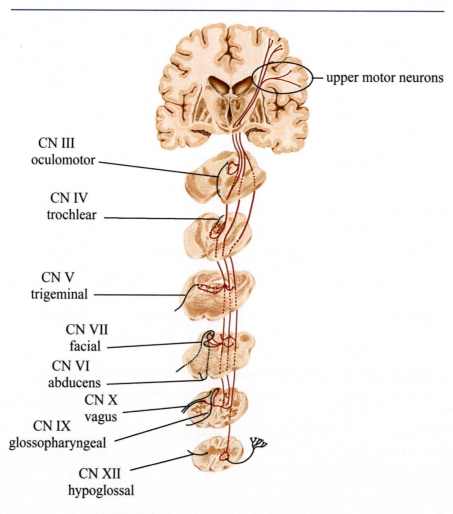

FIGURE 11–1. Corticobulbar pathways.

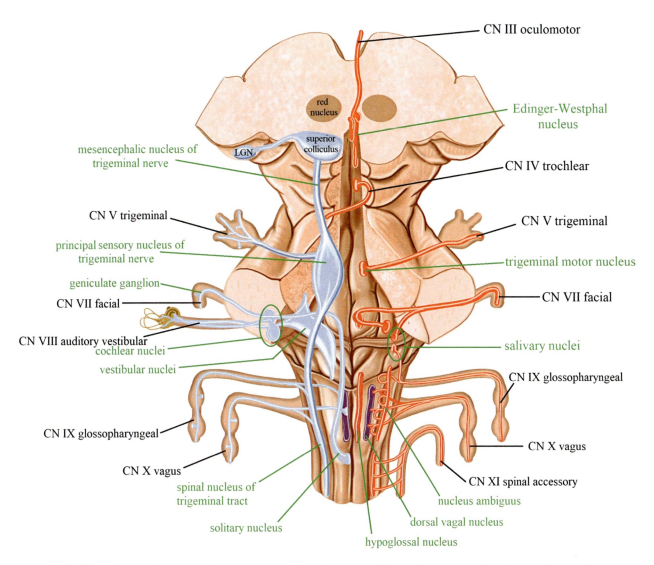

FIGURE 11–2. Cranial nerve nuclei for motor (*red*) and sensory (*blue*) pathways. LGN, lateral geniculate nucleus.

General Functions

Cranial nerve functions, as noted previously, can be motor (efferent), sensory (afferent), or both. The sensory and motor functions are further subdivided into those that impact somatic versus visceral systems. **Somatic** systems include the basic somatosensory components (pain, touch, temperature, and proprioception) and motor innervation of striated (skeletal and voluntary) muscles. **Visceral** systems include sensory signals from internal organs (Table 11–2). All of these seem pretty logical except the special efferent systems. These innervate the muscles of the face, neck, pharynx, and larynx. The reason why these are not classified as general efferent is that in embryonic development, they grew out of a segment called the brachial arch. Despite the different classification, their function is the same as that of general efferent for somatic muscles.

Motor inputs to the efferent components of cranial nerves arise from UMN cell bodies in the precentral gyrus and project along UMN axons. The UMN portion of the pathway can be referred to as the **supranuclear** region because it is superior to the cranial nerve nuclei. Damage to UMNs (i.e., supranuclear damage) in the corticobulbar tract results in contralateral weakness. Unilateral damage can be caused by strokes, tumors, or relatively focal traumatic injuries. Bilateral UMN damage is not uncommon after traumatic brain injuries. As described in Chapter 10, UMN damage results in spastic paresis or paralysis.

Table 11–1. Mnemonics for Cranial Nerves

Cranial Nerve	Name	Function	Name Mnemonic	Name Mnemonic	Function Mnemonic
I	Olfactory	Special sensory for smell	On	On	Some (sensory)
II	Optic	Special sensory for vision	Old	On	Saps
III	Oculomotor	Motor innervation of four of the six muscles of the eye	Olympus's	On	May (motor)
IV	Trochlear	Motor innervation of one of the six muscles of the eye	Towering	They	Marry
V	Trigeminal	Somatosensory for the face, dura, teeth, anterior tongue, mucous membranes of the mouth and nose Motor innervation of muscles of mastication and one velar muscle	Top	Traveled	But (both)
VI	Abducens	Motor innervation of one of the six muscles of the eye	A	And	My
VII	Facial	Special sensory for taste for the anterior tongue and anterior salivary glands Motor innervation of muscles of facial expression	Finn	Found	Brother
VIII	Auditory/vestibular	Special sensory for hearing and balance Motor innervation of auditory hair cells	And	Voldemort	Believes
IX	Glossopharyngeal	Somatosensory for pharynx (including nasopharynx), posterior tongue Special sensory for taste from posterior tongue Motor innervation of the stylopharyngeous muscle and posterior salivary glands	German	Guarding	Bad
X	Vagus	Somatosensory and motor for pharynx and larynx	Viewed	Very	Business
XI	Spinal accessory	Blends with vagus for motor innervation for velum, larynx; innervation of some neck muscles	Some	Ancient	Marriage
XII	Hypoglossal	Motor innervation of all intrinsic and three of four extrinsic tongue muscles	Hops	Horcruxes	Makes

Table 11–2. Cranial Nerve Functional Classifications

	General Afferent		General Efferent		Special Afferent		Special Efferent
	Somatic (GSA) Pain, temperature, and touch from striated muscle, skin, ligaments, and joints	Visceral (GVA) Pain, temperature, stretch, and pressure from organs	Somatic (GSE) Striated muscles of eyes and tongue	Visceral (GVE) Autonomic (parasympathetic) functions of smooth muscles and glands	Somatic (SSA) Specialized receptors for special senses	Visceral (SVA) Specialized receptors for chemical senses	Visceral (SVE) Muscles of face, neck, pharynx, and larynx
Cranial Nerve							
Olfactory						Smell	
Optic					Vision		
Oculomotor			Eye muscles	Pupil and lens			
Trochlear			Eye muscles				
Trigeminal	Face, oral cavity, meninges, ear canal						Muscles of mastication, velum
Abducens			Eye muscles				
Facial	External ear canal, scalp immediately posterior to pinna			Salivary and lacrimal glands		Taste	Muscles of facial expression
Auditory-vestibular				Outer hair cells in the cochlea*	Hearing, balance		
Glossopharyngeal	Tongue, palate, oropharynx, middle ear	Carotid artery		Mucosal glands		Taste	Pharyngeal muscle

continues

Table 11–2. continued

Cranial Nerve	General Afferent		General Efferent		Special Afferent		Special Efferent
	Somatic (GSA) Pain, temperature, and touch from striated muscle, skin, ligaments, and joints	Visceral (GVA) Pain, temperature, stretch, and pressure from organs	Somatic (GSE) Striated muscles of eyes and tongue	Visceral (GVE) Autonomic (parasympathetic) functions of smooth muscles and glands	Somatic (SSA) Specialized receptors for special senses	Visceral (SVA) Specialized receptors for chemical senses	Visceral (SVE) Muscles of face, neck, pharynx, and larynx
Vagus		Pharynx, larynx, thorax, abdomen		Trachea, esophagus, stomach, heart, blood vessels		Taste	Laryngeal and pharyngeal muscles
Spinal accessory							Neck muscles
Hypoglossal			Tongue muscles				

Note. GSA, general somatic afferent; GSE, general somatic efferent; GVA, general visceral afferent; SSA, special somatic afferent; SVA, special visceral afferent; SVE, special visceral efferent.
*There is limited evidence regarding the efferent portion of CN VIII, but some researchers have classified it as GVE (Ross & Jones, 1981).

Damage to cranial nerve LMNs will cause ipsilateral signs because the UMNs cross over prior to synapsing on LMN nuclei and sensory signals remain ipsilateral until after synapsing in the sensory nuclei. As discussed in Chapter 10, flaccid paresis or paralysis is a result of LMN damage. Cranial nerve damage can be caused by brainstem strokes or tumors that impact the LMN cell bodies in the CN nuclei or traumatic damage to the nerves themselves. It is rare to have bilateral damage to cranial nerves because the paired structures are located on opposite sides of the brainstem. A stroke or tumor large enough to affect both CN brainstem nuclei would likely have devastating effects and may be lethal given the autonomic functions controlled in the brainstem (see Chapter 1).

Cranial Nerve Pathways

Motor Pathways: Corticobulbar Tract

The motor components of the cranial nerves create the corticobulbar portion of the pyramidal tract. As described in Chapter 10, the corticobulbar tract is monosynaptic (one synapse between two neurons). Cell bodies of the UMNs are located in the inferior motor strip, where the head and neck are represented. The axons extend through the corona radiata and internal capsule down to the brainstem (Figure 11–1). At this point, the UMN axons will cross over immediately before synapsing onto LMN dendrites or cell bodies in the appropriate cranial nerve nucleus. For example, UMN axons innervating most of the muscles of the eye will decussate in the medulla prior to synapsing in the oculomotor nucleus. In contrast, the UMNs carrying signals that will innervate muscles of the tongue will remain ipsilateral through the majority of the brainstem before crossing over to synapse in the hypoglossal nucleus in the inferior medulla. LMN cell bodies are housed in the cranial nerve nuclei, and their axons extend out as cranial nerves to innervate the target muscles. Cranial nerve LMNs are entirely ipsilateral; damage to any cranial nerve will result in ipsilateral motor deficits.

Sensory Pathways

The sensory pathways for the general afferent components [general somatic afferent (GSA) and general visceral afferent (GVA)] have a three-neuron pathway similar to the spinal nerve somatosensory pathways. The first-order neuron lies primarily in the periphery with its cell body in a peripheral ganglion and an axon that extends into the brainstem, where it synapses onto the second-order neuron in the cranial nerve nucleus. The axon of the second-order neuron crosses the midline and extends up to the thalamus to synapse in the ventroposteromedial (VPM) nucleus. Remember from Chapter 5 that the ventroposterolateral nucleus of the thalamus is for the somatosensory pathways from the body and the VPM is for the somatosensory pathways from the head and neck. The third-order neurons' cell bodies are in the VPM, and their axons extend up to the inferior portion of the primary sensory strip (S1). The special afferent components [special somatic afferent and special visceral afferent (SVA)] each have their own unique pathways, which are described in detail in Chapters 7 (vision), 8 (auditory and vestibular), and 9 (olfaction and taste).

Cranial Nerves III, IV, and VI: Oculomotor, Trochlear, and Abducens

These three cranial nerves all innervate the muscles of the eyes. Each eyeball has six muscles that together can move the eye up, down, side to side, and everywhere in between. In addition, there are muscles that can constrict or dilate the pupils and adjust the lens for close versus distant vision. All three of these cranial nerves have extensive integration with nerves that innervate muscles of the neck and with the vestibular system to coordinate movement of the head and eyes.

Muscles of the Eye

The muscles of the eye include four that have a direct course from the orbit to the eyeball: the **medial rectus**, **lateral rectus**, **superior rectus**, and **inferior rectus** (Latin: *rectus = straight*). As the names suggest, these attach to the sides and the top and bottom of the eyeball. The remaining two muscles—the **superior oblique** and the **inferior oblique**—attach at an angle. The locations and functions of these muscles, and the cranial nerves that innervate them, are depicted in Figure 11–3 and Table 11–3.

Movement of the eye can be described in terms of adduction (medially, toward the nose), abduction (laterally, toward the temples), elevation (upward), depression (downward), intorsion (rotation down and toward the nose), and extorsion (rotation up and toward the nose).

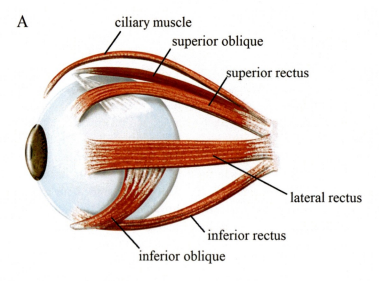
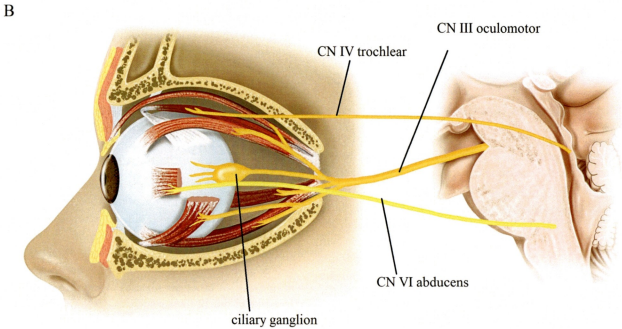

FIGURE 11-3. A. Muscles of the eye. **B.** Cranial nerves innervating muscles of the eye.

Table 11-3. Function and Innervation of Muscles of the Eye

Muscle	Function	Cranial Nerve Innervation
Medial rectus	Adduction	III: oculomotor
Lateral rectus	Abduction	VI: abducens
Superior rectus	Elevation	III: oculomotor
Inferior rectus	Depression	III: oculomotor
Superior oblique	Intorsion, depression, adduction	IV: trochlear
Inferior oblique	Extorsion, elevation, abduction	III: oculomotor

The function of the rectus muscles is straightforward: The lateral rectus will pull the lateral side of the eyeball, abducting the eye and causing you to look laterally; the inferior rectus will pull the eyeball downward, depressing the eye and causing you to look down. The oblique muscles also have a logical consequence if you track where they pull from. The superior oblique causes intorsion, rotating the eye down and medially as it pulls the top of the eyeball toward the nose. The inferior oblique causes extorsion, rotating the eye upward and medially.

Oculomotor Nerve

The oculomotor nerve, as the name suggests, is motor-only and innervates muscles of the eye. The LMN cell bodies lie either in the oculomotor or Edinger–Westphal nuclei in the caudal midbrain. As shown in Table 11–3 and Figure 11–3, this cranial nerve innervates four of the six muscles of the eye. It also innervates the levator palpebrae muscle, which elevates (opens) the eyelid. The oculomotor nerve also has special efferent (motor) functions [special visceral efferent (SVE)], as it innervates the constrictor muscles of the iris and is responsible for the pupillary light reflex in which the pupil constricts when a bright light is shone in the eye. This reflex is controlled through the Edinger–Westphal nucleus in the midbrain, which is connected to the parasympathetic nervous system.

Damage to the oculomotor nerve results in the following signs in the ipsilateral eye: lateral strabismus, reduced eye movement, ptosis, and mydriasis (Figure 11–4). Lateral **strabismus** (Greek: *strabos = squinting*) is the deviation of the eye to a lateral position. When looking straight ahead, the eye ipsilateral to the damage will deviate laterally. This is because the medial rectus is weak or paralyzed but the lateral rectus, innervated by the abducens nerve, is intact. Without the medial rectus to counteract the normal contraction of the lateral rectus, the eye is pulled laterally. The person will experience **diplopia** (double vision) because the two eyes are not focused on the same location. Adduction, elevation, depression, and extorsion of the eye all will be limited. **Ptosis** (Greek: *ptosis = to fall*) is drooping of the eyelid, caused by weakness of the levator palpebrae muscle. Finally, **mydriasis** is permanent dilation of the pupil. The pupil cannot constrict if the signals cannot reach the muscles in the iris.

Trochlear Nerve

The trochlear nerve innervates the superior oblique muscle. The Latin word *trochlear* means pulley and describes the connective tissue that creates a sling-like structure for the superior oblique muscle. The trochlear nucleus is in the caudal midbrain, and the nerve is the only cranial nerve to exit from the dorsal surface of the brainstem. Damage to the trochlear nerve will affect the introversion of the ipsilateral eye. When attempting to look down, a person will experience diplopia because the impaired side will not be able to track appropriately.

Abducens Nerve

Abducens is Latin for abducting or "drawing away," particularly from the midline. This bit of knowledge helps to remember the function of this nerve, which is to innervate

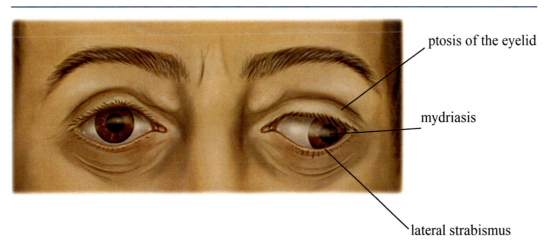

FIGURE 11–4. Signs of CN III damage.

the lateral rectus muscle—the muscle that abducts the eye. The abducens nucleus is in the posterior pons and the LMN axons extend out from the brainstem at the pontomedullary. Damage to the abducens will cause an ipsilateral medial strabismus in which the affected eye will be slightly adducted (deviated medially). This positioning, just like lateral strabismus, will result in diplopia.

Cranial Nerve V: Trigeminal Nerve

The trigeminal nerve is the largest cranial nerve. You can't miss it, extending out from the lateral pons as a large trunk that divides into three branches (Figure 11–5). These branches are the source of its name (Latin: *three twins*). The three sensory branches (ophthalmic, maxillary, and mandibular) convey somatosensory signals from the head, oral cavity, and meninges. The motor component innervates muscles of mastication—those that move the jaw for chewing (e.g., temporalis, masseter, and pterygoids; see full list in Table 11–4)—as well as the tensor veli palatini muscle that tenses the soft palate (velum) and the tensor tympani that dampens movement of the ossicles.

The three branches are named for the region they innervate. The **ophthalmic branch (V1)** is purely sensory and carries somatosensory signals from the superior face, eyes, sinuses, and the tentorium cerebelli. The **maxillary branch (V2)** innervates the midface, including the upper teeth and gums and the medial dura mater. The **mandibular branch (V3)** innervates the lower face and the lateral face up through to the scalp. This includes the anterior and middle meninges, the external auditory meatus, and the somatosensory (pain, touch, and temperature) from the anterior two-thirds of the tongue.

The trigeminal sensory pathways are a three-neuron system from the head to the cortex. The pseudounipolar first-order neurons have their dendrites in the periphery and cell bodies in the trigeminal ganglion just medial to the three trigeminal branches. The axons enter the brainstem through the pons and synapse onto second-order neurons in the trigeminal complex (Figure 11–6). This complex includes three distinct nuclei: the **mesencephalic nucleus** of the trigeminal nerve in the midbrain; the **principal sensory nucleus** in the superior–lateral pons; and the descending **spinal trigeminal nucleus**, which stretches down from the lateral pons into the medulla (Figure 11–2). Different sensory modalities are carried to different nuclei. First-order neurons responding to discriminative touch synapse in the principal sensory nucleus onto second-order neurons that extend up through the **trigeminothalamic tract** to the VPM nucleus of the thalamus, where they synapse onto third-order neurons. The third-order neuron axons

Table 11–4. Structures Innervated by Branches of the Trigeminal Nerve

Branch	Sensory Components	Motor Components
V1 ophthalmic	Upper face, eyeball, cornea, upper eyelid, lateral nose, sinuses Meninges: supratentorial dura, superior surface of the tentorium cerebelli	None
V2 maxillary	Midface (upper cheeks and lips, posterior nose), upper teeth and gums, soft palate, hard palate Meninges: anterior cranial fossa, anterior regions of the middle cranial fossa	None
V3 mandibular	Lower face, lower teeth and gums, lateral scalp, mucous membranes of the mouth, anterior two-thirds of the tongue, external auditory meatus Meninges: posterior regions of the middle cranial fossa	Muscles of mastication: masseter, temporalis, medial pterygoid, lateral pterygoid, mylohyoid, anterior belly of the digastric Tensor veli palatini Tensor tympani

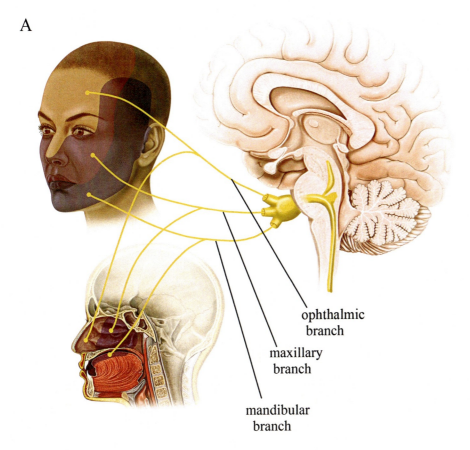

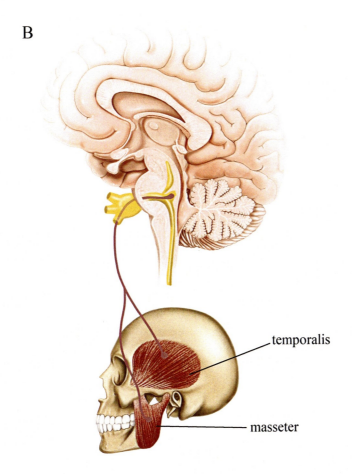

FIGURE 11–5. A. Sensory innervation of the branches of the trigeminal nerve. **B.** Motor innervation of the mandibular branch of the trigeminal nerve.

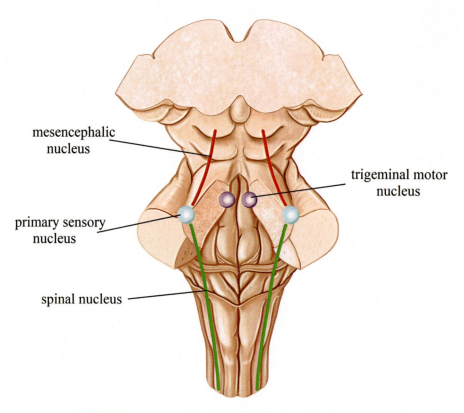

FIGURE 11-6. Cranial nerve nuclei for the trigeminal nerve.

extend to the inferior portion of the primary sensory area in the postcentral gyrus. First-order neurons responding to proprioceptive signals from muscles of mastication synapse in the mesencephalic nucleus onto second-order neurons that extend to the VPM. This pathway includes the reflexive bite reflex. Finally, sensory neurons carrying pain and temperature synapse in the descending spinal trigeminal tract. Here, signals are integrated with signals from several other cranial nerves, including the facial (CN VII), glossopharyngeal (IX), and vagus (X) nerves.

The motor component of the trigeminal nerve consists of UMNs with cell bodies in the facial region of the motor strip (M1) in the precentral gyrus (see Chapter 1, Figure 1–9). Axons from those UMNs extend down through the cortical bulbar pathway and cross over in the pons before synapsing onto LMN cell bodies in the trigeminal motor nucleus. Some UMN axons remain ipsilateral to provide bilateral innervation of muscles of mastication, which is important for voluntary control of jaw movement for chewing. The LMN axons extend out through the mandibular branch to innervate the muscles of mastication as well as the tensor veli palatini muscle, which tenses the soft palate, and the tensor tympani muscle, which can restrict movement of the ossicles and in turn the tympanic membrane (eardrum) to protect against cochlear damage due to loud noises. Both the tensor muscles (along with several others innervated by the vagus nerve) also play a role in opening the eustachian tube to equalize pressure in the middle ear.

LMN damage to the trigeminal nerve can result in ipsilateral **trigeminal neuralgia**, characterized by excruciating pain in the ophthalmic and mandibular branches. Weakness in muscles of mastication characterized by flaccidity also occurs ipsilaterally. A slight deviation of the jaw upon opening may be seen, but there will be minimal functional consequence. The muscles of the jaw are quite powerful, and the intact muscles on the contralateral side can make up for the unilateral weakness. Some people may find it difficult to chew crunchy or tough foods on the affected side, but that is easily compensated for by chewing on the unaffected side.

Unilateral UMN damage due to stroke or other focal injury will have limited effect on movement of the jaw due to both bilateral innervation and the strength of the masticator muscles. Extensive bilateral damage to UMNs can result in **masticator palsy**, or paralysis of the muscles of mastication. Because one of the functions of those muscles is to elevate the mandible, paralysis will lead to the jaw hanging open. As you can imagine, this has a dramatic effect on speech production because the shape of the oral cavity is changed, bilabials and labiodentals cannot be produced, and the tongue may not be able to approximate the hard and soft palates for production of the remaining speech sounds. Chewing and swallowing also are dramatically affected because the mouth hangs open, preventing chewing and causing problems keeping food or liquid within the oral cavity. As if all that weren't enough, social interaction may be affected by social biases in which people will assume intellectual deficits are associated with facial abnormalities and speech disorders.

Cranial Nerve VII: Facial Nerve

The facial nerve has both sensory and motor components. The nerve exits the pontomedullary region of the brainstem as two separate roots—a larger motor root and a smaller sensory root that fuse at the geniculate ganglion in the temporal bone and then split into branches to innervate the various regions of the face (Figure 11–7).

The facial nerve has only one small general somatic afferent from the external ear canal (external auditory meatus) and a small patch of the scalp just posterior to the outer ear (pinna). The SVA component carries taste from the anterior two-thirds of the tongue. Cell bodies for these first-order neurons are in the geniculate ganglion located in the temporal bone. The axons enter the brainstem and synapse in the superior (rostral) region of the **solitary nucleus** known as the gustatory nucleus. Second-order neurons extend bilaterally to the VPM of the thalamus, and third-order neurons extend to the insula as well as the primary sensory strip. As described in Chapter 9, there are other pathways to the hypothalamus and limbic system as well as connections to other nuclei in the brainstem that are involved in reflexive responses to taste.

The general visceral efferent (GVE) segment of the facial nerve innervates salivary and lacrimal glands. UMNs from the inferior motor strip in the precentral gyrus extend down to the pons, where the axons cross over before synapsing onto LMNs in the lacrimal or salivary nuclei. The sublingual and submandibular salivary glands in the mouth produce saliva. Lacrimal glands in the eyes produce tears. Interestingly, there are separate inputs for emotional and

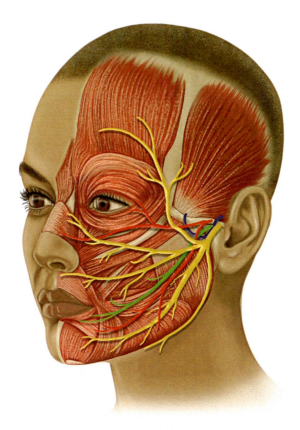

FIGURE 11–7. Branches of the facial nerve. *Yellow*, special visceral efferent (muscles of facial expression); *red*, general visceral efferent (glands); *green*, special visceral afferent (taste); *blue*, general somatic afferent (external ear canal).

non-emotional responses. Tears related to irritation of the eye are stimulated by the trigeminal inputs to the lacrimal nucleus—remember that the trigeminal nerve innervates pain and touch for the eyeballs. In contrast, emotional tears are stimulated by inputs from the hypothalamus to the lacrimal nucleus and carried through CN VII.

The SVE component of the facial nerve innervates muscles of facial expression, including the orbicularis oris that forms the lips, all of the muscles that elevate or depress the lips and the corners of the mouth, the orbicularis oculi around the eyes, and the frontalis muscle that elevates the eyebrows. The stapedius muscle in the middle ear also is innervated by CN VII. As with the GVE fibers, the UMN axons extend down to the pons, and most cross over before synapsing in the facial motor nucleus. The innervation of facial muscles is not strictly contralateral. The upper face including around the eyes and the frontalis muscle on the forehead receive bilateral innervation. Some UMNs targeting the upper face cross over in the pons and synapse contralaterally, whereas others remain ipsilateral. This provides bilateral innervation to the muscles in the upper face. LMNs to the lower face receive only contralateral innervation (Figure 11–8). This mixture of bilateral and unilateral innervation leads to specific patterns of weakness that aid in diagnosing the level of damage, as discussed later.

Several reflexes are mediated by the facial nerve, including the corneal, sucking, and stapedial reflex. The first two involve sensory signals carried through CN V (from the cornea and the lips, respectively), with synapses onto LMNs in the facial nuclei. The stapedial reflex is triggered by loud sounds that are carried through CN VIII to the LMNs of the facial nucleus to contract the stapedius muscle, which retracts the stapes from the oval window and limits the movement of the ossicles to protect the cochlea.

Unilateral UMN damage will result in contralateral lower facial weakness, with spared movement of the upper face (forehead). Essentially, the person will not be able to elevate/retract the lips on the contralateral side when asked to smile (lower face weakness) but will be able to raise both eyebrows (preserved upper face movement). This pattern is due to the bilateral innervation of the upper face: When UMNs from one side of the brain are damaged, the upper face still receives ipsilateral innervation (Figure 11–9). If damage occurs to the facial nerve unilaterally, the person

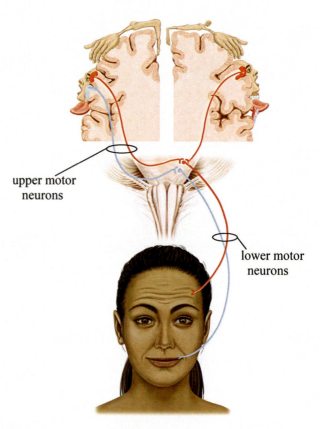

FIGURE 11–8. Innervation of facial muscles by the facial nerve.

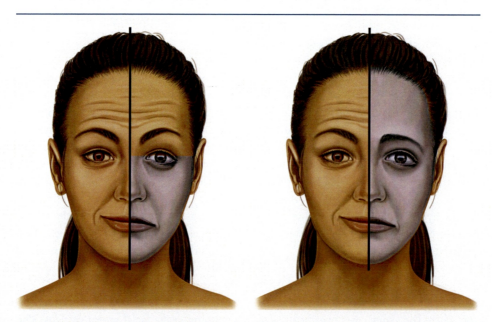

FIGURE 11–9. Supranuclear (UMN) versus LMN lesions to facial nerve. (*Left*) Damage to the UMN of the facial nerve will impair movement of the lower face (e.g., inability to retract lips for smile) contralateral to the lesion. (*Right*) Damage to the LMN of the facial nerve will impair movement of the entire face (e.g., inability to retract lips for smile and inability to raise eyebrow) ipsilateral to the lesion.

will exhibit weakness or paralysis to the entire ipsilateral face: They will not be able to elevate their lips in a smile or raise their eyebrow on the affected side. This is because the damage is to the LMN to the ipsilateral muscles of both the upper and lower face. Because of the clinical relevance of these movements, they are a common component of an oral mechanism exam (OME), as described later in this chapter.

Another characteristic of UMN damage is preservation of movement for emotional facial expression. Although weakness may be present contralaterally when the patient is asked to create different postures (e.g., smile, pucker lips), facial movement will be symmetrical when the expression is triggered by emotion (e.g., smiling due to happiness rather than on command). This phenomenon indicates that there are inputs to CN VII LMNs from structures (e.g., amygdala, limbic system) beyond the UMNs.

Cranial Nerve IX: Glossopharyngeal

The name of the glossopharyngeal nerve tells you that it innervates the tongue (glosso-) and the pharynx. It is a mixed nerve with both general and special components of the sensory and motor branches. Exiting from the medulla, there are multiple rootlets that fuse to form CN IX. As described later, some branches of the glossopharyngeal nerve blend with the vagus in a structure called the pharyngeal plexus.

The GSA component carries pain, touch, and temperature information from the posterior one-third of the tongue as well as the palate, oropharynx, and middle ear. Cell bodies of the first-order neurons are in the glossopharyngeal ganglion and synapse in the spinal nucleus of the trigeminal tract. From there, second-order neurons extend to the VPM of the thalamus, where they synapse onto third-order neurons that end in the primary sensory strip. The gag reflex is controlled by this component of CN IX.

Visceral (GVA) segments receive sensory signals from the carotid arteries in response to stretch receptors and chemoreceptors that monitor oxygen levels. Axons travel through the tractus solitarius to the nucleus solitarius with connections to the reticular formation and hypothalamus. This provides reflexive responses that control respiration, blood pressure, and heart rate.

The SVA branch carries taste information from the posterior one-third of the tongue. Axons synapse in the gustatory region of the nucleus solitarius along with those from the facial nerve, and they share the pathway from the brainstem through the VPM to the taste cortex in the insula (see Chapter 9, Figure 9–6 for the taste pathway).

The SVA motor components of the glossopharyngeal nerve innervate the parotid gland, which is the largest of the salivary glands. LMNs in the inferior salivatory nucleus receive input not only from UMNs but also from the olfactory cortex, which is responsible for salivation in response to the smell of food cooking, and the hypothalamus, which inhibits salivation in emotional situations, causing dry mouth in response to fear or other sympathetic responses (like taking your neuroanatomy exam, gulp!).

The SVE motor component consists of UMNs that bilaterally innervate LMNs in the rostral nucleus ambiguus. The LMNs extend out to innervate the stylopharyngeus muscle. This muscle, as the name indicates, originates on the styloid process and inserts into the pharynx. When contracted, it will elevate and retract the pharynx to aid in swallowing.

Cranial Nerve X: Vagus Nerve

Vagus is a Latin term for "wanderer" and is an apt name for this cranial nerve, which has multiple branches that extend throughout the neck, thorax, and abdomen, innervating a variety of quite disparate structures. The vagus nerve innervates several internal organs, including the stomach, liver, and small intestines, as well as the trachea and esophagus. Some branches innervate the cardiac muscles of the heart. The LMNs for these GVE branches originate in the dorsal nucleus of the vagus within the midregion of the medulla. These are beyond the scope of speech pathology and audiology, so they are not described further. The focus here is on just three branches of the vagus that innervate the pharynx and larynx and are critical for voicing, articulation, and swallowing. These are the pharyngeal, superior laryngeal, and recurrent laryngeal branches; the laryngeal branches are shown in Figure 11–10.

Pharyngeal Branch of the Vagus

The **pharyngeal branch** is motor only and includes both vagus and glossopharyngeal components. It innervates muscles of the velum, including the musculus uvula and levator veli palatini, and pharynx (salpingopharyngeus, palatopharyngeus, and pharyngeal constrictor muscles). It also innervates the palatoglossus, which can be classified as either a velar muscle or an extrinsic tongue muscle.

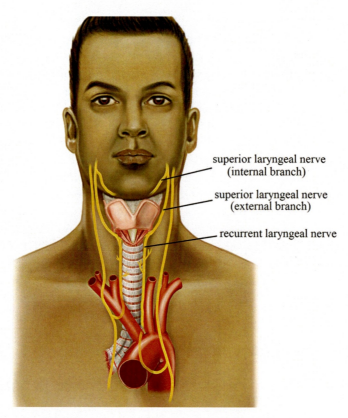

FIGURE 11–10. Laryngeal branches of the vagus nerve.

Damage to the pharyngeal branch will result in weakness of these muscles ipsilaterally. Weakness of the soft palate will cause hypernasality because the velum will be unable to completely close off the velopharyngeal port during production of non-nasal sounds. This also will impact swallowing with the potential for nasal regurgitation if the velopharyngeal port is not completely sealed as food/liquid is moved to the pharynx. The weakness of the pharyngeal constrictor muscles will impact the ability to move a bolus of food down through the pharynx to the esophagus. Food/liquid may pool in the piriform sinuses at the superior extent of the larynx, increasing the risk of penetration (food/liquid entering the larynx) and aspiration (food/liquid entering the trachea).

Superior Laryngeal Nerve of the Vagus

The **superior laryngeal nerve (SLN)** has two branches—the internal and external laryngeal nerves. The **internal laryngeal nerve** is purely sensory (GVA), carrying pain, touch, and temperature signals from the epiglottis and larynx above the vocal folds (i.e., sensation to the supraglottic mucosa). This branch also provides sense of taste from the epiglottis and esophagus. The **external laryngeal nerve** is purely motor (SVE). It innervates the cricothyroid muscle, which is responsible for lengthening the vocal folds. Along with the pharyngeal branch, it also innervates the inferior constrictor muscle.

Damage to the SLN will cause ipsilateral reduction of sensation in the superior aspect of the larynx. This increases the risk for penetration and aspiration because the person may not feel food or liquid entering the larynx and may have a reduction in the normal cough reflex that is designed to expel such "intruders." The damage also will reduce the ability to change vocal pitch because vocal fold lengthening is an important component of pitch manipulation.

Recurrent Laryngeal Nerve of the Vagus

The **recurrent laryngeal nerve (RLN)** has both motor and sensory components. The sensory fibers innervate the inferior region of the larynx, including the vocal folds and the conus elasticus tissue inferior to the folds, also known as the subglottal mucosa. The SVE motor component innervates all of the intrinsic muscles of the larynx (aside from the cricothyroid), including the transverse and oblique arytenoids, which adduct (close) the vocal folds by pulling the left and right folds closer to the midline; the posterior cricoarytenoid, which abducts (opens) the folds by moving them away from the midline; the lateral cricoarytenoid, which adducts and lengthens the vocal folds; and the thyroarytenoids (thyromuscularis and thyrovocalis segments), which tense and change the length of the folds.

Damage to the RLN will cause ipsilateral paresis or paralysis of the vocal folds. A paralyzed vocal fold will be in a paramedian position, meaning it is near the midline. In effect, it is halfway between full adduction and abduction. This will result in a breathy, hoarse vocal quality because the vocal folds will not be able to adduct completely. Coughing will be weak, and there will be an increased risk of penetration and aspiration because of the inability to completely adduct the vocal folds and close off the larynx during swallowing.

Over time, the muscles of the weakened vocal fold will atrophy, and the end result will be that the two vocal folds will no longer be the same thickness. Because of this, the right and left folds will vibrate at different speeds. The consequence of this is **diplophonia**, or two pitches. When asked to sustain a vowel (e.g., "ahhhhhh"), the person will produce two pitches at once—one from the vibration frequency of each of the vocal folds.

Pharyngeal Plexus

The **pharyngeal plexus** is a network of nerves created from branches of the glossopharyngeal and vagus nerves that innervate the pharynx and are critical for swallowing (Figure 11–11). From the vagus, the pharyngeal, superior laryngeal, and recurrent laryngeal nerves all contribute to the pharyngeal plexus. Through this plexus, branches of the pharyngeal and internal laryngeal branch of the vagus innervate all velar muscles except the tensor veli palatini and all pharyngeal muscles except the stylopharyngeus. The inferior constrictor muscle receives innervation from the plexus but also the external branch of the superior laryngeal nerve as well as the recurrent laryngeal nerve.

Cranial Nerve XI: Spinal Accessory Nerve

The spinal accessory nerve is motor only, with SVE innervation of several muscles of the neck (Figure 11–12). LMNs exit the brainstem from the lower medulla and innervate the sternocleidomastoid (SCM) muscle on the anterolateral neck and the trapezius muscle of the posterior neck and superior portion of the dorsal thorax (i.e., upper back). Other branches of the spinal accessory nerve blend with branches of the vagus nerve to innervate the velum and laryngeal muscles.

Damage to the spinal accessory nerve will impact movement of the head, including turning to the side (SCM muscle), moving the head toward the chest (SCM), and moving the head upward by pulling the occipital bone toward the back (trapezius). Vocalization and swallowing also may be affected due to damage to the branches that aid the vagus nerve functions.

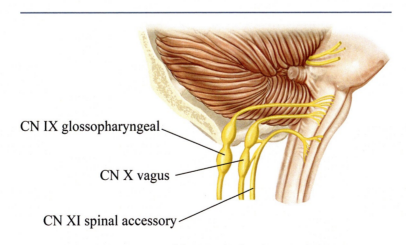

FIGURE 11–11. Cranial nerves in the pharyngeal plexus.

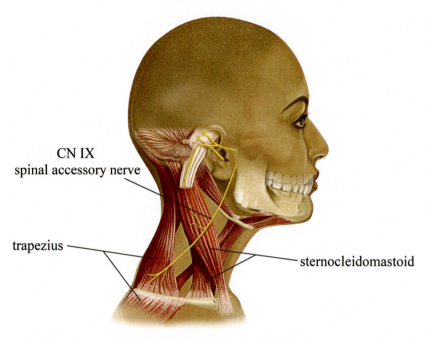

FIGURE 11–12. Spinal accessory nerve.

Cranial Nerve XII: Hypoglossal Nerve

The last cranial nerve is the hypoglossal. It is motor only. The LMN cell bodies are in the hypoglossal nucleus in the posterior and inferior medulla. They innervate all of the intrinsic muscles of the tongue and all but one of the extrinsic muscles (Figure 11–13). It helps to think about tongue muscles as "movers and shapers." Intrinsic muscles (the shapers), those that both originate and insert within the body of the tongue itself, change the shape of the tongue and can create fine movements such as elevating the tongue tip. These muscles can flatten or bunch up the tongue or curl it. They include the superior longitudinal, inferior longitudinal, transverse, and vertical muscles. Extrinsic tongue muscles (the movers) originate outside the tongue and insert into the body of the tongue. Their function is to create gross movements of the tongue—to pull it in or out of the mouth and to elevate the posterior part of the tongue to create velar sounds like /k/ and /g/.

Damage to the hypoglossal nerve will result in ipsilateral tongue weakness. This typically has only a slight effect on speech production because the tongue has much more strength than is needed for articulation of speech sounds and the intact side of the tongue can accomplish the movements and shape changes needed for intelligible articulation. Chewing may be difficult on the affected side because the tongue will be less able to move the food around onto the tooth surfaces for chewing. In addition, if food falls into the buccal cavity—the space between the teeth and the cheeks—it may be difficult to clear it out with the tongue.

Integration of Cranial Nerve Functions

Speech Production

Speech production requires the precise coordination of muscles and structures innervated by multiple cranial nerves (Table 11–5). Assuming that the respiratory system is functioning properly (the diaphragm and thoracic muscles are controlled by spinal nerves through input from the respiratory center in the medulla), voicing begins at the larynx where the RLN of the vagus innervates muscles to abduct and adduct the vocal folds. As the airstream travels superiorly through the pharynx, the velum, innervated by the pharyngeal branch of the vagus (combined with fibers from the spinal accessory nerve), may need to be elevated

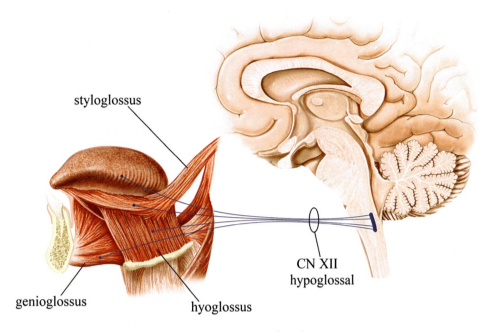

FIGURE 11–13. Hypoglossal nerve.

Table 11–5. Summary of Innervation of the Face and Mouth

Sensory	
Pain, touch, and temperature from the face and oral cavity	Trigeminal (V)
Pain, touch, and temperature from the anterior two-thirds of the tongue	Trigeminal (V)
Pain, touch, and temperature from the posterior one-third of the tongue	Glossopharyngeal (IX)
Taste from the anterior two-thirds of tongue	Facial (VII)
Taste from the posterior one-third of tongue	Glossopharyngeal (IX)
Motor	
Muscles of mastication	Trigeminal (V)
Muscles of facial expression	Facial (VII)
Tongue muscles	Hypoglossal (XII)
Velar muscles	Glossopharyngeal (IX) and vagus (X), pharyngeal branch

to close off the velopharyngeal port so that the air moves out through the mouth to create oral sounds. Articulation to shape the sound into phonemes requires movement of the tongue, controlled by the hypoglossal nerve, and movement of the lips, controlled by the facial nerve.

For example, production of a sustained /s/ requires abduction of the vocal folds (RLN of vagus), elevation of the velum/closure of the velopharyngeal port (pharyngeal branch of vagus, also trigeminal), elevation of the tongue tip (hypoglossal), elevation of the mandible (trigeminal), and small opening of the lips (facial). To move from just a sustained /s/ to the word "so," precise coordination is needed so that the vocal folds adduct at the same time that the tongue tip is lowered and the lips are rounded. The coordination is controlled by the motor system with sensory feedback from the articulators and the auditory system, which can confirm whether the articulatory movements achieved the desired phoneme combination.

Swallowing

Swallowing requires coordinated control of the lips (facial), tongue (hypoglossal), velum (trigeminal, pharyngeal branch of the vagus, and glossopharyngeal), pharynx (pharyngeal plexus including the pharyngeal branch of the vagus, glossopharyngeal, and cranial fibers of the spinal accessory), and larynx (superior laryngeal nerve, inferior laryngeal nerve, and recurrent laryngeal nerves of the vagus). Chewing is controlled by the mandible (trigeminal), whereas facial muscles (facial) help retrieve food from utensils and keep it positioned properly in the mouth.

Swallowing a sip of coffee, for example, begins with movement of the lips and other facial muscles (facial) to form a labial seal and suction—achieved in part through closure of the velopharyngeal port (trigeminal and pharyngeal plexus) and retraction of the tongue (hypoglossal). As the bolus (cohesive collection of liquid) of coffee enters the mouth, intrinsic tongue muscles (hypoglossal) help cup the tongue in order to collect the coffee, aided by buccal (cheek) muscles (facial) to keep the bolus on the tongue. Extrinsic tongue muscles (hypoglossal) begin to move the bolus posteriorly and elevate the tongue base toward the velum. As the base of the tongue passes between the faucial pillars (created by the palatoglossus and palatopharyngeus; pharyngeal plexus), the complex "patterned response" of the pharyngeal swallow is initiated. At this point, along with closure of the velopharyngeal port (trigeminal and pharyngeal plexus), pharyngeal constrictors contract in sequence from superior to middle to inferior (pharyngeal branch of vagus), and the larynx is elevated by suprahyoid muscles (pharyngeal plexus, trigeminal, facial, and hypoglossal)—inverting the epiglottis to deflect liquid away from the airway. The geniohyoid, thyrohyoid, and suprahyoid muscles are innervated by a branch of cervical nerve 1 (C1) from the cervical plexus, which courses with the hypoglossal nerve at the floor of the mouth. The laryngeal adductor reflex is also triggered (superior laryngeal branch of vagus), further preventing food from entering the airway. Once diverted to the esophagus, autonomic peristalsis is responsible for transfer to the gut (vagus also has a role in this parasympathetic and sympathetic process).

Secretion of saliva and mucus is triggered again through the pharyngeal plexus. Sensory signals carried by the plexus provide feedback regarding swallowing movements and trigger gag or coughing reflexes when food or liquid enters the larynx. Additional sensory information from the nasopharynx and velum is transmitted through the trigeminal nerve.

As with speech production, the muscles and structures must be precisely coordinated in order for swallowing to be safe and efficient. The following section provides clinical application through descriptions of oral motor and clinical bedside evaluations.

Clinical Implications: Examinations of Speech and Swallowing Mechanisms

Cranial Nerve/Oral Mechanism Examination

Now that you're familiar with the function of each of the cranial nerves, you are in a good position to make applications toward everyday practice. One of the most basic applications of cranial nerves to clinical practice is the OME. Although there is a heavy emphasis on components that relate to speech, hearing, and swallowing functions, most cranial nerves have a prominent role in the OME. Note that the following description does not include examination of oral structures such as teeth or gums because the focus is on the cranial nerve elements. A typical step for all sections is to examine the structures at rest for symmetry, atrophy, fasciculations, and tremor.

Smell and Taste

The olfactory nerve is rarely assessed in the OME by SLPs or AuDs, primarily because impaired sense of smell can be the result of numerous etiologies apart from direct damage to CN I (common cold, sinus infections, smoking, seasonal allergies, etc.). Furthermore, assessment of gustation (CNs I, VII, IX, and X) is also abbreviated, perhaps including only a question about sense of taste.

Vision

SLPs and AuDs may complete an informal or cursory examination of vision, which may be limited to a chart review or questions about changes to vision that could elicit information about visual field cuts. Questions about the need for glasses/contacts will provide information about visual acuity. Although acuity is most often related to peripheral functions rather than CN II functions, it will be important to know if patients can see well enough to perceive visual stimuli used in the OME.

Extraocular Movements (CNs III, IV, and VI)

Extraocular cranial nerve functions, if assessed at all, typically receive a fairly abbreviated examination by SLPs and AuDs. Those interested in alternative, nonverbal mechanisms for communication, such as eye gaze, tracking, or blinking, may complete a more comprehensive evaluation of CNs III, IV, and VI. Examine position of eyelids at rest and gaze direction. One way to assess extraocular movements is to have the client look in all directions without moving their head (up, down, right, left, down to left and right, up to left and right). You can facilitate this by having them follow (track) a finger/pen. Along with range of motion to each direction, examine whether tracking is smooth or tremulous. Also, ask questions about whether diplopia (double vision) occurs with any of the movements. It is not typical for SLPs or AuDs to examine pupil constriction and dilation, but this information may be gleaned from a chart review.

Jaw Movements and Mastication (CN V)

Mastication is an important function for swallowing (particularly oral preparation of chewable foods), making CN V assessment a staple of the OME. Most of this assessment addresses jaw range of motion and strength measures. For range of motion, instruct your client to open and close the jaw, as well as to move it from side to side (laterally) and protrude and retract the jaw. Strength assessment includes opening the jaw to resistance (achieved by holding a hand beneath the jaw to resist opening), closing to resistance (achieved by holding a finger/hand on the chin to resist closure), and bite strength (achieved by biting a tongue depressor and maintaining bite while the clinician attempts to pull the tongue depressor out anteriorly). Sometimes a jaw-jerk reflex is triggered by tapping on the tip of the chin with the client's jaw open slightly.

Facial Sensation (CN V)

Facial sensations are innervated by CN V. The trigeminal nerve carries sensation of pain, temperature, light and deep touch, proprioception, and vibration sense. Typically, CN V sensation is addressed through interview, although a cold metal object, such as a reflex hammer or tuning fork, can be used to check sensation of cold. A pin prick or the dull end of a clean paper clip can be used to assess sensation of deep touch. Light touch is typically examined by using a feather or lightly brushing the face with the back of one's hand/fingers. Begin by asking the client to close their eyes and distinguish whether the sensation is equal on both sides and/or asking them to raise a hand for the side touched. Be sure to check sensation in the ophthalmic (forehead), maxillary (upper cheeks), and mandibular (jaw) sections. Note that vibration sense is typically not tested.

Muscles of Facial Expression and Oral Preparation (CN VII)

Certainly, facial expressions have an important purpose in nonverbal communication. Furthermore, muscles of facial expression are responsible for oral preparation and lip movement for articulation of labial sounds. To distinguish between UMN and LMN facial nerve lesions, begin with examining forehead function. Simply ask the client to raise their eyebrows and/or wrinkle their forehead (brow) to examine whether forehead innervation is intact. You can assess strength by asking them to wrinkle their brow to resistance or resisting your attempts to pull wrinkles apart. Closing eyes tightly, with and without resistance (in the form of the examiner using two fingers to try to pry eyes open), is another useful assessment. Smiling is achieved by activating the zygomatic muscles, whereas drawing the corners of one's mouth back requires activation of the risorius muscles. Labial seal (an indication of activation of the orbicularis oris) can be examined by asking the client to purse their lips tightly. Asking the client to puff out their cheeks (cheek sufflating) can address integrity of the buccinators and requires some valving of the larynx, a velopharyngeal port seal, and a labial seal. Maintaining puffing to resistance (i.e., pushing the cheeks inward) helps examine strength.

As noted previously, unilateral weakness in the lower face affecting smiling and lip seal with preserved movement of the upper face (eyebrow raising) is an indicator of UMN damage with spared LMN function.

Hearing (CN VIII)

Knowledge about the integrity of hearing is relevant to both SLPs and AuDs. Note that each discipline will differ in how thoroughly it addresses this element of the OME. In the scope of a typical OME assessment, the hearing component may be fairly abbreviated. Similar to assessment of vision, auditory assessment in an OME provides some information about auditory acuity that may be related to peripheral or cochlear components rather than CN VIII function. The tasks likely include a subjective measure such as the clinician rubbing their fingers together near each of the client's ears and simply asking the client if they can hear it. It could include tapping a tuning fork and placing it at the mastoid process of each ear (Figure 11–14A) and then placing the still vibrating tuning fork 1 or 2 cm from the pinna (i.e., the Rinne test; Figure 11–14B). Another screener is the Weber test, whereby a vibrating tuning fork is placed at the top of the head (Figure 11–14C). Vestibular functions are typically not assessed by SLPs but can be gleaned from a chart review or interview questions.

Velar Functions—Motor and Sensory (CNs V, IX, and X)

Observation of the velum at rest allows you to determine symmetry and whether there may be unilateral weakness (indicated by one side of the velum drooping at rest). Asking the client to say "uh, uh, uh" examines activation of the tensor veli palatini (CN V), the levator veli palatini (CNs IX and X and pharyngeal plexus), and the uvula (CNs IX and X and pharyngeal plexus). Eliciting a sustained /ah/ allows you to examine the resonance quality, particularly whether there is hypernasality (an indication that the velum is not achieving effective closure of the velopharyngeal port). Eliciting a gag response is an accepted means to examine velar sensation. It is noteworthy, however, that approximately one-third of healthy adults have an absent gag. In addition to checking the gag response, velar sensitivity can be screened by lightly touching a tongue depressor to faucial pillars on each side, as well as the soft palate on each side.

Laryngeal Functions—Motor and Sensory (CN X)

In addition to the role CN X plays in velar function and sensation, it has central roles in pharyngeal and laryngeal functions. These are crucial to swallowing safety and phonation integrity. Strength of the pharyngeal swallow can be screened through laryngeal palpation of a dry swallow (or with a small sip of water, if necessary). This is accomplished by placing fingers on the thyroid cartilage and feeling for elevation. A number of potential measures can be used to examine laryngeal integrity. Typically, one or two measures are adequate. A sustained /ah/ can be used to subjectively evaluate voice quality (an indication of effective closure of the vocal folds). Vegetative functions such as throat clearing and a strong volitional cough can be used to further verify vocal fold closure and ability to clear potential aspirates (food or liquid that contacts vocal folds or enters lungs) or penetrants (food or liquid that enters the laryngeal vestibule or contacts vocal folds). A breath hold can be used to assess ability to achieve laryngeal valving, and counting can be used to examine endurance and breath support. Other potential measures include a glide up and down, along with examining s/z ratio (length of time producing the voiceless /s/ versus voiced /z/). Further details about laryngeal and pharyngeal function, including sensation, are elicited through interview questions.

Spinal Accessory (CN XI)

As the name implies, CN XI has an accessory role in phonation and swallowing functions. Integrity of this CN innervation is typically assessed through two tasks—the head turn and shoulder shrug. To elicit the head turn, the client is prompted to turn the head to look over the right and left shoulders, initially without resistance, followed by gentle resistance in each direction. Similarly, a shoulder shrug is first prompted without resistance and then with gentle resistance. This may be completed bilaterally, unless there is reason to believe one side is substantially weaker than the other, in which case you may wish to prompt shrugging of one shoulder at a time.

Lingual Motor Functions (CN XII with a Little Help from CN X)

CN XII has only motor functions, including gross and fine movements of the tongue. Recall that CN XII innervates all but one of the movers, responsible for protruding, elevat-

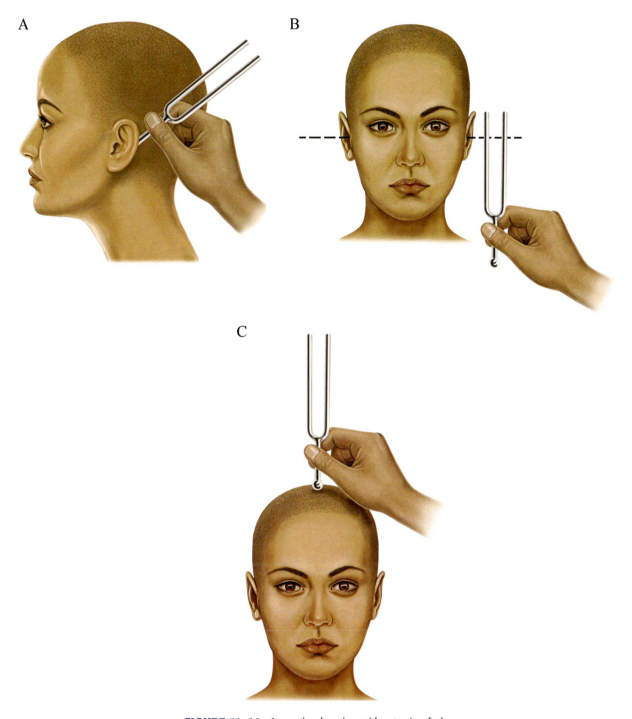

FIGURE 11–14. Assessing hearing with a tuning fork.

ing, retracting, and depressing the tongue. The exception is the palatoglossus (innervated by CN X). All of the fine (shaping) muscles are innervated by CN XII. Gross movement is the primary element assessed in the OME. This includes prompting tongue protrusion, lateral movement of the tongue (side to side), vertical movement (up and down), and drawing the tongue back along the surface of the palate. To assess strength, a tongue blade and/or gloved hand is then used to provide resistance. Ask the client to protrude the tongue against the tongue depressor, then protrude laterally to each side against the depressor, and finally protrude up and down against the depressor. Often, lateral strength is tested as well by having the client push the tongue against each cheek, with and without resistance.

Lingual Sensation (CNs V and IX)

Assessment of lingual sensation is subjective. A tongue depressor is used to apply gentle pressure to the anterior two-thirds (CN V) on each side and the posterior one-third (CN IX) on each side. The client is asked if they feel each touch and if it is equal from side to side and anterior to posterior.

Oral and Laryngeal Diadochokinetic Rate

Rapid alternating movements or speech alternating motion rates, also known as oral diadochokinetic (DDK) rates, are used to examine the agility and regularity of oral movements for speech. This is prompted by having the client repeat syllable productions such as /puh, puh, puh/, /tuh, tuh, tuh/, /kuh, kuh, kuh/. Sequential motion rates involve combining syllables /puh, tuh, kuh/ repeatedly over a short period of time. Similarly, laryngeal DDK can be conducted by prompting repetition of /huh, huh, huh/. The measure is used broadly to examine speed of repetitions, regularity-rhythm-coordination, and articulatory accuracy (or breakdowns in that accuracy). Disruptions to these variables can indicate impairments to strength, motor planning, coordination, and endurance.

Evidence for the Oral Mechanism Examination

There is evidence that the OME is a sensitive assessment when completed accurately and comprehensively. Most of the elements have good specificity on their own. Sensitivity to predicting risk for aspiration (food or liquid entering the lungs) or dysphagia (swallowing dysfunction) is strong collectively but not for individual measures. A great deal of evidence exists to validate the combined measures, including structural assessments and assessment of cranial nerve functions. We refer interested readers to the articles listed in Additional Resources.

Clinical Bedside Swallow Examination and Instrumental Assessment

The intent of this section is not to be a substitute for the breadth of diagnostic knowledge you will gain in dysphagia (swallowing disorders) courses. Rather, this is intended to serve as a snapshot that will aid you in understanding the functions of cranial nerves and the clinical Cases in Chapter 16.

The clinical bedside swallow examination (CBSE) has two main components:

1. The OME
2. Food trials
   a. These constitute a systematic, observational progression through liquid and solid consistencies, informed by your knowledge of OME outcomes and by clinical assessment of signs and symptoms of dysphagia. Symptoms may be seen at any of the stages of swallowing: oral preparatory phase (e.g., food falling out of the mouth anteriorly), oral phase (e.g., problems with anterior-to-posterior bolus transfer, characterized by food residuals after the swallow), pharyngeal phase (e.g., wet/gurgly voice, coughing, choking), or esophageal phase (e.g., complaints of reflux or food sticking in the "throat").
   b. Begin with small volumes and presentations controlled by the examiner (perhaps on a spoon or controlled sip). Progress through incrementally larger volumes and less control by the examiner and more independent feeding/drinking by the client.
   c. Move through various consistencies (viscosities) of liquids. Monitor for symptoms described previously.
   d. Move through various textures of solids. Monitor for symptoms described previously.
   e. Attempt trial therapies such as compensatory techniques or modified textures/viscosities. Monitor for symptom resolution or improvement.

Two primary techniques are used for instrumental assessment (although more exist):

1. The modified barium swallow (MBS) or fluoroscopic examination of swallowing uses a video x-ray to track foods/liquids mixed with radiopaque barium to examine speed/timing of processing across phases, effective clearance of boluses in each phase, and evidence of abnormalities (i.e., structural abnormalities or physiological abnormalities such as penetration or aspiration of liquids or solids). Like the CBSE, the MBS follows a systematic protocol for trials of various liquids and solids, along with opportunities to examine trial therapies (e.g., modified liquid/solids and/or compensatory strategies).

2. The flexible endoscopic evaluation of swallowing (FEES) uses an endoscope camera to observe swallowing in the moment. Placement of the endoscope through the nasal cavity to view the pharynx and larynx superiorly from the level just below the velum primarily limits assessment to the pharyngeal phase, although both oral and esophageal phases can be observed. Like the MBS, the FEES follows a similar systematic protocol for trials of liquids, solids, and trial therapies.

Summary

Cranial nerve function is essential for speech, swallowing, and communicating through nonverbal cues such as facial expressions. Knowledge of the cranial nerves and how to assess function is a critical skill for SLPs and AuDs. Differential diagnosis of motor speech disorders relies heavily on the proper implementation and interpretation of a thorough OME.

Key Concepts

- Cranial nerve functions are subdivided into general versus special, somatic versus visceral, and afferent versus efferent.
- Motor innervation via cranial nerves is through a monosynaptic pathway (UMN synapsing onto LMN extending out to muscles).
- Sensory innervation via cranial nerves includes cell bodies in presynaptic ganglia, synapses in the ventroposterolateral nucleus of the thalamus, and cortical synapses in the inferior postcentral gyrus.
- UMN or supranuclear damage typically results in contralateral signs/symptoms, whereas LMN or cranial nerve damage always causes ipsilateral signs/symptoms.
- For the facial nerve (CN VII), UMN damage will affect only the contralateral lower face, whereas LMN damage affects the entire ipsilateral face.
- Speech production and swallowing are accomplished by the precise timing and function of multiple cranial nerves.
- Oral mechanism exams are an efficient way to assess the function of cranial nerves involved in speech and swallowing.

Additional Resources

Festic, E., Soto, J. S., Pitre, L. A., Leveton, M., Ramsey, D. M., Freeman, W. D., . . . Lee, A. S. (2016). Novel bedside phonetic evaluation to identify dysphagia and aspiration risk. *Chest, 149*(3), 649–659.

Hara, K., Tohara, H., Wada, S., Iida, T., Ueda, K., & Ansai, T. (2014). Jaw-opening force test to screen for dysphagia: Preliminary results. *Archives of Physical Medicine and Rehabilitation, 95*(5), 867–874.

Knack, A. F. (2015). *Evaluating the relationship between diadochokinesis and severity of dysphagia as it relates to forced vital capacity in individuals with amyotrophic lateral sclerosis* [Unpublished doctoral dissertation]. Wayne State University.

Logemann, J. A., Veis, S., & Colangelo, L. (1999). A screening procedure for oropharyngeal dysphagia. *Dysphagia, 14*, 44–51.

Maccarini, A. R., Filippini, A., Padovani, D., Limarzi, M., Loffredo, M., & Casolino, D. (2007). Clinical non-instrumental evaluation of dysphagia. *Acta Otorhinolaryngologica Italica, 27*(6), 299–305.

Martino, R., Flowers, H. L., Shaw, S. M., & Diamant, N. E. (2013). A systematic review of current clinical and instrumental swallowing assessment methods. *Current Physical Medicine and Rehabilitation Reports, 1*(4), 267–279.

McCullough, G. H., & Martino, R. (2013). Clinical evaluation of patients with dysphagia: Importance of history taking and physical exam. In R. Shaker, C. Easterling, P. C. Belafsky, & G. N. Postma (Eds.), *Manual of diagnostic and therapeutic techniques for disorders of deglutition* (pp. 11–30). Springer.

McCullough, G. H., Rosenbek, J. C., Wertz, R. T., McCoy, S., Mann, G., & McCullough, K. (2005). Utility of clinical swallowing examination measures for detecting aspiration post-stroke. *Journal of Speech, Language, and Hearing Research, 48*(6), 1280–1293.

Perry, L., & Love, C. P. (2001). Screening for dysphagia and aspiration in acute stroke: A systematic review. *Dysphagia, 16*(1), 7–18.

Ramsey, D., Smithard, D., Donaldson, N., & Kalra, L. (2005). Is the gag reflex useful in the management of swallowing problems in acute stroke? *Dysphagia, 20*(2), 105–107.

Ross M. D., & Jones, H. R. (1981) The parasympathetic innervation of the inner ear and the problem of cochlear efferents: Enzyme and autoradiographic studies. In J. Syka & L. Aitkin (eds), *Neuronal mechanisms of hearing*. Springer. https://doi.org/10.1007/978-1-4684-3908-3_3

Terre, R., & Mearin, F. (2006). Oropharyngeal dysphagia after the acute phase of stroke: Predictors of aspiration. *Neurogastroenterology & Motility, 18*(3), 200–205.

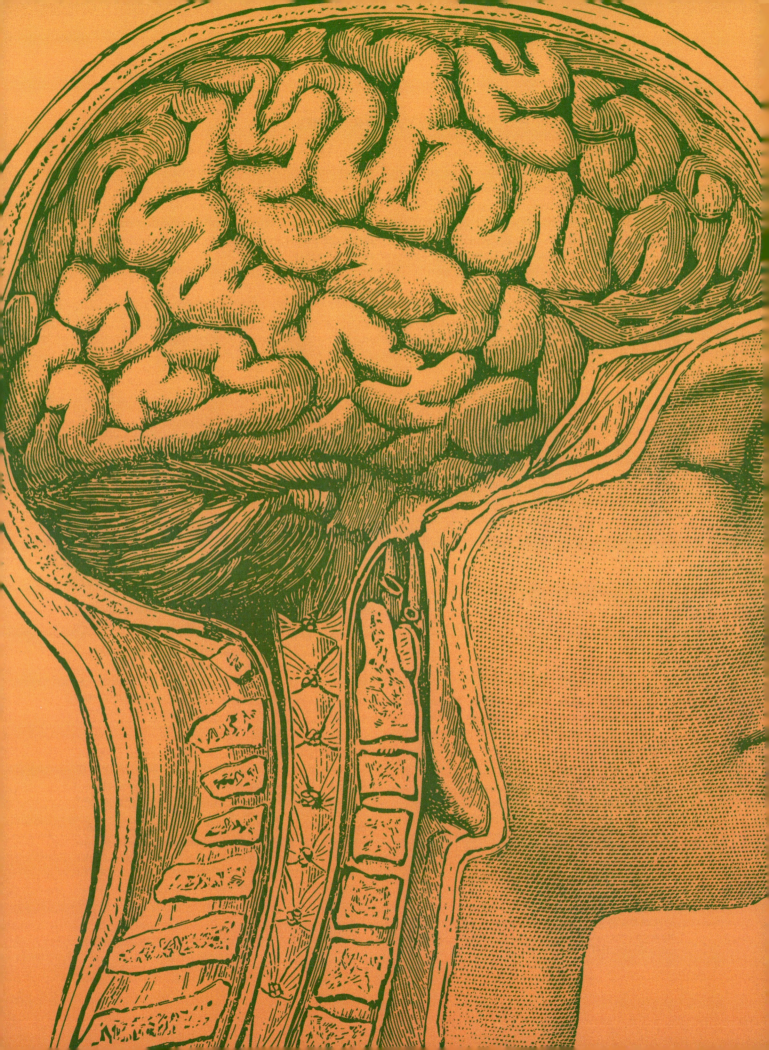

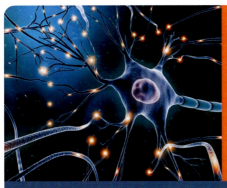

12
Limbic System and Reticular Formation

CHAPTER OUTLINE

Limbic System Structures and Functions
  Homeostasis
  Olfaction
  Memory
  Emotions

Integrating Limbic Information
Reticular Formation and Reticular Activating System
Summary
References and Additional Resources

Limbic System Structures and Functions

The limbic system and reticular formation fill a number of key roles relevant to speech-language pathology and audiology. The reticular formation regulates consciousness, alertness, and sleep functions. On a basic level, the reticular activating system (RAS) collaborates with the limbic system to process what we see, hear, and feel. The limbic system has four basic functions, eloquently captured by the mnemonic HOME: homeostasis, olfaction, memory, and emotion (Blumenfeld, 2010; see Box 12–1). These mechanisms are important for survival of the species (safety, nutrition, behaviors, and learning about experiences/the natural world). Furthermore, they have key roles in communication, cognition, and swallowing functions. Limbic cortices are heteromodal, meaning they have multiple modalities or functions. In fact, all components of the limbic system help carry out all limbic functions, even though key structures may be primary to certain functions. The limbic system is composed of the cingulate gyrus, hippocampus, parahippocampal gyrus, mammillary bodies, fornix, amygdala, hypothalamus, anterior thalamus, stria terminalis, and olfactory cortices (Figure 12–1).

 Box 12–1. Limbic HOME

H: *Homeostasis*—regulating drives (hunger, sexual, and thirst) and homeostatic mechanisms (temperature regulation, endocrine functions, stress responses, and other autonomic functions).

O: *Olfaction*—more than simply sense of smell or taste (gustation), the limbic system overlaps the entire rhinencephalon (piriform cortices, entorhinal cortices, periamygdaloid cortex, and amygdala) and has connections to emotions (amygdala) and memories (hippocampus/parahippocampal cortices).

M: *Memory*—including short-term, working memory, long-term memory, and explicit (declarative) and implicit (nondeclarative) types.

E: *Emotions*—this includes emotional regulation, emotional decision-making, and emotional memory. Many structures contribute to this function, but the amygdala is often thought about as a key structure.

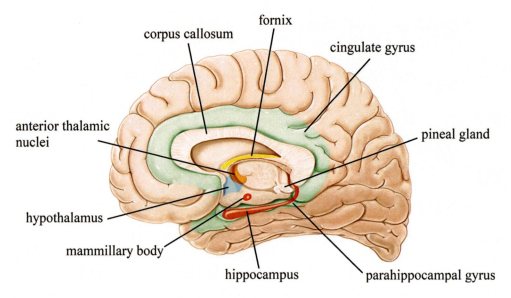

FIGURE 12–1. Limbic system structures.

Homeostasis

This is one of the key life-sustaining, survival mechanisms. Regulation of drives is a function of the **hypothalamus**, with some help from the rest of the limbic system/networks (Table 12–1). This includes autonomic, endocrine, and behavior regulation.

The lateral hypothalamus regulates the sense of hunger, whereas the ventromedial portion monitors the sense of satiety (see Box 12–2 for a clinical application). Orexin and leptin hormones help regulate appetite. Orexin is produced in the lateral hypothalamus, and along with stimulating appetite (cravings), it has a role in facilitating sleep. Conversely, leptin regulates satiety. Thirst is partially regulated by the hypothalamus but is primarily facilitated systemically given intra- and extracellular fluid composition. Specialized receptors in the hypothalamus, called osmoreceptors, are triggered by decreased intracellular water composition, stimulating thirst. Along with thirst, the pituitary gland releases antidiuretic hormone (also known as vasopressin) into the bloodstream systemically to conserve the body's fluid volume and help regulate blood pressure (see Box 12–3 for another clinical application). Note that thirst can be physiological (related to osmolarity) or behavioral (driven by habits or environmental cues). As a discipline that addresses swallowing and dysphagia, along with cognition and communication, recognizing these physiological and behavioral contributors to intake is crucial.

Sexual drives and responses include autonomic, endocrine, and behavioral components. Specifically, the hypothalamus triggers the **pituitary gland** to release sex hormones. The medial preoptic area of the hypothalamus has been implicated in the ability to engage in sexual behaviors. The preoptic region differs markedly for males versus females: In males, it is twice as large, which is a function of more testosterone and androstenedione in males. The amygdala is implicated in processing sexual arousal. Note that many of the body's reactions to sexual arousal parallel sympathetic reactions to a life-threatening experience, including increases in heart rate, blood pressure, respiratory rate, and pupillary dilation. The **nucleus accumbens** also has a crucial role because it is involved in experiences of pleasure sensation. Together, the **amygdala** and nucleus accumbens process motivation for sexual behaviors.

Regulation of temperature is controlled, in part, by the hypothalamus as well. Outputs of the hypothalamus for thermoregulation include the rostral ventromedial medulla, midbrain, and ventrolateral medulla (Morrison, 2016). These somatic and sympathetic premotor neurons stimulate sympathetic neurons in the spinal cord. Thermoreceptors within the viscera and skin receive information for cold and warm sensations. As described in Chapter 6, those thermoreceptors project to the dorsal root ganglia, ascending along a thermoreceptive-specific tract to trigeminal nuclei and the thalamus (Morrison, 2016). This facilitates perception, localization, and regulation of thermoregulation in viscera

Table 12–1. Inputs and Outputs of the Limbic System

Function	Key Structures	Inputs	Outputs
Homeostasis	Hypothalamus	Brainstem (via the dorsolongitudinal fasciculus) Median forebrain bundle Stria terminalis Amygdala (via the ventral amygdalofugal pathway) Hippocampus Septal nuclei Ventral striatum Orbitomedial PFC Retina Other cortical areas	Dorsolongitudinal (fasciculus to brainstem) Stria terminalis Amygdala (via ventral amygdalofugal pathway) Pituitary Anterior nuclei of thalamus via mammillothalamic tract Septal nuclei Widespread cortical areas
Olfaction	Rhinencephalon Piriform cortex Entorhinal cortex Periamygdaloid cortex Amygdala	Olfactory bulbs	Piriform cortices Amygdala Periamygdaloid cortices Parahippocampal gyrus Entorhinal cortices
Memory	Hippocampus	Entorhinal cortices Amygdala Contralateral hippocampus Cingulate gyrus Other cortical areas	Amygdala Orbitomedial PFC Septal nuclei Ventral striatum Hypothalamus Mammillary body Thalamus Cingulate gyrus Entorhinal cortices Other cortical areas
Emotion	Amygdala	Dorsomedial thalamus Orbitomedial PFC Ventromedial PFC Olfactory bulb and cortex Anterior cingulate Visual association cortex Hypothalamus Brainstem (periaqueductal gray, parabrachial nuclei) Septal nuclei (via stria terminalis)	Thalamus Orbitomedial PFC Ventromedial PFC Olfactory bulb and cortex Anterior cingulate Visual association cortex Primary visual cortex Hypothalamus Brainstem Septal nuclei (via stria terminalis) Hippocampus Ventral striatum

Note. Inputs and outputs of limbic structures/system provide insights into the interdependency and overlap in functions. As the table indicates, key structures have roles in the HOME functions, but you can see by looking at inputs and outputs that they carry out those functions with the help of other limbic structures and other areas of the brain. PFC, prefrontal cortex.

> **Box 12–2.** Alzheimer Disease and Declines in Homeostatic Mechanisms

Most people recognize that memory impairments are a prominent symptom of Alzheimer disease (AD). Atrophy to the anterior, medial temporal lobe accounts for those changes. Less well known are the changes to homeostasis. In AD, there is commonly atrophy to the hypothalamus, particularly laterally. This affects two homeostatic mechanisms fairly directly. There is a change in hunger drives that can result in less physical interest in food and failure to thrive, a phenomenon related to atrophy of the lateral hypothalamus. Furthermore, temperature regulation is impaired. In a memory care unit, it is common to see individuals wearing sweaters and wrapped in blankets, even on a hot summer day. Understanding the underlying mechanisms of these impairments in AD is crucial for being able to manage them effectively.

Incidentally, changes to the cytoarchitecture of structures is a two-way street. Just as physiological changes, such as atrophy in the lateral hypothalamus in AD results in decreased sense of hunger, structural changes can occur as a result of one's behavior as well. For instance, if you stop eating, atrophy is seen in the lateral hypothalamus. Likewise, damage to the medial hypothalamus is associated with overeating.

> **Box 12–3.** Syndrome of Inappropriate Antidiuretic Hormone

A common acute response to traumatic brain injury or intracranial hemorrhages is an alteration to the release of antidiuretic hormone (ADH). Brain swelling (increased intracranial pressure) compresses the pituitary gland, altering the regulation of ADH. Releasing too much ADH causes the body to retain too much water, which leads to hyponatremia, or low sodium in the bloodstream. This is exacerbated by the fact that extracellular fluid volume increases because regulation of kidney filtration is altered, adding more sodium to urine, causing diuresis (frequent urination) which causes more sodium to be flushed out with urine. Nausea, vomiting, headache, confusion, irritability, drowsiness/fatigue, muscle weakness/cramps, and seizures are all potential consequences of hyponatremia. Monitoring inputs and outputs of urine is essential for hospital staff. It is not uncommon for a patient with syndrome of inappropriate antidiuretic hormone (SIADH) to urinate numerous times in an hour. In the context of recovery from brain injury, it is important to distinguish between the physiological changes to blood serum affecting cognition/alertness and consequences of the brain injury. Clearly, very different treatments are indicated by metabolic dysregulation (medical treatment) and injury-related (speech-language therapy) cognitive disorders. For speech-language pathologists, sudden changes in participation and performance may indicate SIADH, so communication with nursing and physicians is crucial.

and skin. Damage to the hypothalamus results in impaired ability to regulate body temperature.

Note that the amygdala also has roles in homeostasis. Responses to environmental stimuli such as stress are mediated by the amygdala. The amygdala also helps regulate behaviors and motivation. The roles of the amygdala are expanded in the section on emotions.

Circadian rhythms regulate day–night cycles. The **suprachiasmic nucleus** (located superior to the optic chiasm) of the hypothalamus receives light inputs from the retina. Reciprocal connections to the reticular formation are also crucial in regulating sleep–wake cycles. This process is revisited in the section on the RAS.

Olfaction

Although the primary functions of olfaction are smell and taste (described in Chapter 9), it has a role in all four limbic functions (i.e., homeostasis, olfaction, memory, and emotions). The olfactory bulbs have direct projections to the piriform cortices, periamygdaloid cortices, and the amygdala (Figure 12–2). Projections from the piriform cortex to the anterior entorhinal cortex and reciprocal connections between the entorhinal cortex and the parahippocampal cortex may explain why odors can evoke memories (Figure 12–3). Likewise, outputs to the amygdala may account for emotions associated with odors and memories (see Box 12–4). See Table 12–1 for all inputs and outputs of the olfactory system. Note that although the olfactory bulbs and related cortices are the primary processors of olfaction and gustation, all limbic structures have a role in processing the relationship between olfaction, memory, emotional processing, and homeostasis (e.g., olfactory safety—smelling burning, noxious fumes, or gas).

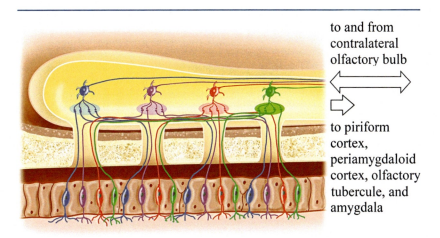

FIGURE 12–2. Olfactory bulb outputs.

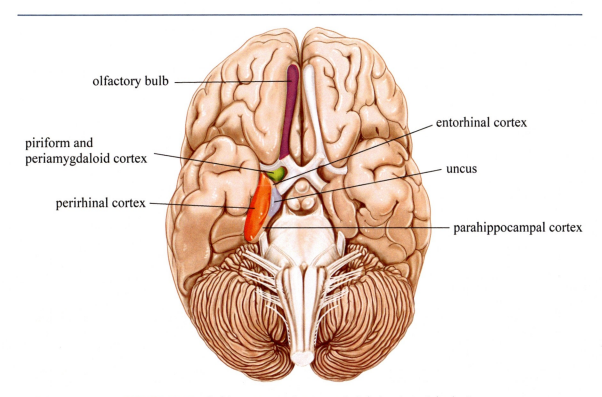

FIGURE 12–3. Limbic system regions seen in inferior view of the brain.

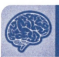

Box 12–4. Olfaction and Memories

Here is a personal connection from one of the authors. Waffle House is my favorite comfort food restaurant. There, I said it. It is not the friendly atmosphere or camaraderie that draws me in though. Growing up, I loved spending time at my grandmother's house. It was not an everyday occurrence, so I cherished those times. Per my memory (and this is important—in my memory, in my mind, not necessarily drawn 100% from historical fact or truth), every time we stayed overnight, we had waffles in the morning. In fact, I don't think my grandma ever had to wake us up in the morning; she simply opened the bedroom doors and let the aroma of waffles waft into our rooms. To this day, the smell of waffles and maple syrup brings me back to those moments. It is not just an olfactory moment, however. It is a multisensory experience. I can recall the smell of waffles on the waffle iron, bacon in the frying pan, and coffee on the stove range. This triggers vivid recall of the visual environment, including the avocado green appliances (slightly darker on the edges/corners than the body of the refrigerator and stove), avocado/golden linoleum in a scalloped diamond pattern with tanish-gold faux grout lines, cream/white Shaker cabinets that reached all the way up to the ceilings, a clock in the form of a sliced apple with seeds, and a door that led to the attic (where all of the good toys and cookies could be found). On the radio played polkas; I could sing to you the jingle and lead-in to "The Whoopee John Show!" (a local Minnesota polka band leader), even though that kitchen is the only place I heard that song. I was at a thrift store one day and found an old Whoopee John album for $1 and gave it serious consideration, even though I do not have a phonograph anymore. So many good memories flood my consciousness, all with a simple odor. Memories are generally strong either because they are activated often or because they are personally salient. I think you can guess why I gravitate to the Waffle House. Do you have any similar olfactory-related memories?

Memory

Memory is a very complex substrate, known to be a distributed process. Limbic memory structures are a critical component, but they do not account for all of the complex processes involved in memory. Although this section primarily addresses the limbic structures involved in memory, recall that the basal ganglia has roles in learning (skills, habits, and routines), the cerebellum is important for motor learning and procedural learning, and the prefrontal cortex has a role in working memory (see Chapter 14 for a broader discussion of memory processes). It is helpful to begin by considering three primary memory subsystems depicted in Figure 12–4.

The first subsystem, **working memory**, is involved in new learning and processing. Similar to other memory systems, it is not a focal system, but portions of the orbitomedial or ventromedial prefrontal cortex have an important role. Note the anatomical proximity between the orbitomedial/ventromedial prefrontal cortices and other key limbic structures involved in memory, such as the amygdala, hippocampus, and even olfactory bulbs/cortices. Working memory is a combination of our short-term memory and mental workspace. That mental workspace allows us to manipulate information. This is crucial for doing things such as making mental calculations; keeping track of characters in a story you read or hear; and simply retaining new information, such as directions, that allows you to complete a task. The information can be auditory or visual, allowing us to retain and use what we hear and see (including written information) in order to complete tasks. Working memory capacity varies across individuals and is frequently compromised by developmental and acquired brain changes. Furthermore, competing environmental or internal demands can cause working memory to decay more quickly.

The second subsystem, **declarative** or **explicit memory**, heavily involves limbic structures, such as those in the anterior, medial temporal lobe, and medial diencephalon. Declarative memory includes semantic and episodic memories. Semantic memory involves storage and subsequent recall of facts. This is the type of memory you use when you commit to memorizing definitions on flash cards. Episodic memory includes the ability to recall events and the timelines for those events. Remembering creating and studying those flash cards while being confined to your house during

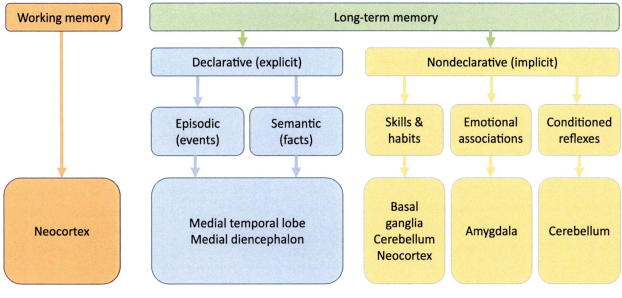

FIGURE 12–4. Memory systems and functions.

a winter storm is an episodic memory. The hippocampus is a key structure for declarative memory: It has roles in consolidation of new learning or working memory into long-term memory. The amygdala is a key structure for emotional memory, such as emotional episodic memories.

The third subsystem, **nondeclarative** or **implicit memory**, is facilitated by the amygdala, as well as basal ganglia, cerebellum, and other portions of the neocortex. Nondeclarative (implicit) memories are learned through doing or immersion in a context and can be described as knowing how to do things. We do not learn them explicitly, as we do with flash cards, but implicitly (without knowing). We often cannot describe these things in words yet can easily demonstrate them. (Think about trying to explain how to tie shoelaces compared to showing someone.) This includes the learning functions of routine or habit-based learning, procedural learning, and motor learning. See Figure 12–5 for a schematic of the memory systems that depicts which systems and anatomical structures carry out each type of memory process.

Nothing happens in isolation when it comes to the complex processes of memory because it is a distributed process. Recall that there is a major visual processing network (see Chapter 7) composed of two components, which communicate between the sensory and motor brain. The dorsal stream, also known as the "where" pathway, carries information about spatial information, movement, and orienting to space. The ventral stream, also known as the "what" pathway, carries information about shapes, colors, faces, and objects. The dorsal stream connects the parietal cortices to the hippocampus via the posterior cingulate gyrus. The posterior cingulate cortex receives inputs from the parietal cortices, receiving spatial information about actions. Furthermore, the posterior cingulate cortex has outputs to the hippocampus via the parahippocampal and entorhinal cortices (Rolls, 2019). The posterior cingulate cortex is a key pathway for transmitting visuospatial information to the hippocampus, where visual-object and reward-based information is combined to form episodic memories. Collectively, the posterior cingulate cortex and hippocampus have a role in action-outcome learning, essentially goal-oriented and causal learning (Rolls, 2019). Note that both the dorsal stream (the "where" pathway) and the ventral stream (the "what" pathway) converge in the hippocampus, allowing the formation of episodic memories of what happened where.

The anterior thalamus also has a role in memory and learning. Damage to anterior thalamic nuclei has been associated with anterograde amnesia (Dillingham et al., 2015), which disrupts the ability to form new memories. This is not surprising given dense, reciprocal connections to the hippocampus via the fornix. The mammillary bodies also provide inputs to anterior thalamic nuclei. Together, the mammillary bodies and anterior thalamus have several unique contributions to memory. These include mnemonic learning (Dillingham et al., 2015), spatial learning,

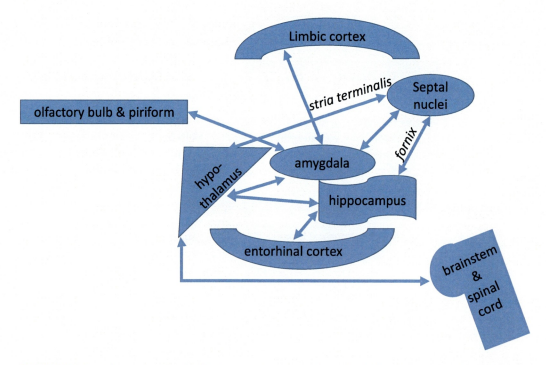

FIGURE 12–5. Schematic of key limbic inputs and outputs. Note the bidirectionality (reciprocal nature) of pathways.

spatial working memory, context-specific memory, and episodic memory.

Although it was previously noted that memory processes are distributed across many structures, the essential contributions of various structures are apparent in distinct deficits resulting from focal damage. For example, damage to the mammillary bodies and anterior thalamus results in anterograde amnesia with spared recognition memory. Similarly, contextualized fear conditioning is spared even though other context-specific memories are impaired. This dissociation is likely due to the amygdala's role in emotional memories.

Another structure with connections to the hippocampus and key roles in memory is the fornix. The fornix is a C-shaped white matter pathway that serves as an output pathway for the hippocampus (Figure 12–6). Damage to the fornix is also associated with anterograde amnesia. The left fornix carries verbal memory information, whereas the right fornix carries visuospatial memory information (Raslau et al., 2015). Furthermore, the medial aspect of the right fornix is important for object recognition and scene learning, whereas the lateral aspect of the right fornix has a role in emotional and motivational learning (Raslau et al., 2015).

Emotions

The amygdala carries out the emotional functions of the limbic system. This includes emotional regulation, emotional decisions, and emotional memory functions. As discussed previously, the olfactory bulb has direct inputs to the amygdala. Reciprocal connections between the amygdala and the prefrontal cortices, anterior–medial temporal lobe, insular cortex, and the thalamus facilitate communication between cognitive regions/substrates. These connections allow for learned responses to emotional stimuli, particularly anxiety and stress responses. Outputs to the septal nuclei, hypothalamus, and reticular formation help initiate behavior.

The orbitofrontal cortices and amygdala receive inputs from the ventral stream by way of the anterior cingulate gyrus. The cingulate gyrus, particularly the anterior portion, receives inputs from the orbitofrontal cortex and amygdala, which shares information about reward and nonreward outcomes (Rolls, 2019). Nonreward outcomes also include punishment, which is processed in the lateral orbitofrontal cortex. This network is implicated in learning the correct, goal-oriented actions to receive an award or avoid punishments, known as action–outcome learn-

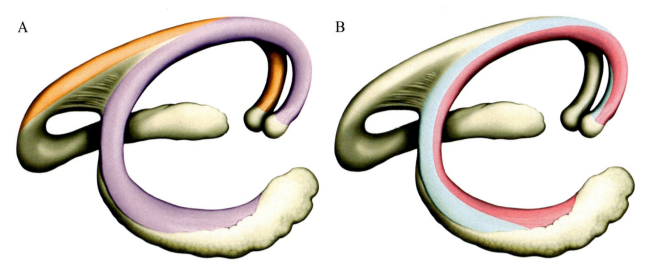

FIGURE 12-6 Functional organization of the fornix. *Orange*, left fornix (verbal memory); *purple*, right fornix (visuospatial memory); *seafoam*, medial right fornix (object recognition and scene learning); *magenta*, lateral right fornix (emotional and motivational learning). *Source*: Used with permission from the *American Journal of Neuroradiology*.

 Box 12-5. Treating Memory Disorders

Recall from Chapter 4 that explicit memory structures (i.e., anterior medial temporal lobe and prefrontal cortices) develop late and are susceptible to disease and trauma, whereas implicit memory structures (i.e., basal ganglia and cerebellum) develop earlier and are preserved later. This dichotomy is crucial for approaching clinical interventions. Interventions designed to utilize intact, implicit memory systems such as the basal ganglia and cerebellum pathways are typically more effective. Some examples of these are routine-based interventions in which a behavior or action is practiced repeatedly to create new habits or routines; errorless learning in which clients are asked to respond only if they are sure of the target response so that they do not guess and produce the wrong response; and spaced retrieval training in which clients are prompted to provide correct responses (using errorless learning) over a series of increasingly long delays. These treatments, because they do not rely on explicit memory systems affected by development, aging, or trauma, are typically effective for individuals with brain injury or even degenerative diseases such as dementias.

Consider how we acquire language functions. Nouns and verbs are sometimes learned more explicitly, but grammar and syntax are more likely learned implicitly. Learning a second language as an adult is difficult in part because we try to learn the language explicitly. Immersion programs are typically more effective because being surrounded by the context of that language is more likely to foster implicit learning.

ing. Linking reward and punishment elicits emotional responses to behaviors and actions. This may even influence autonomic responses to reward and punishment. Behaviors change, however, when the reward or punishment changes. In other words, altering the reward or punishment alters learning. This differs from implicit learning, such as stimulus-motor responses in the basal ganglia, whereby actions become habits after numerous incidents. In contrast to goal-, reward-directed learning, habits and routines are not sensitive to changes in goals/rewards.

The anterior cingulate cortex also has connections with the rostral superior temporal gyrus, the auditory superior temporal gyrus, and the superior temporal sulcus, sharing visual and auditory information regarding facial expression, gestures, and head movements. Again, the hippocampus receives this information via the parahippocampal gyrus and entorhinal cortex.

Box 12–6. That's Rewarding

The reward circuit includes the hippocampus, amygdala, prefrontal cortices, nucleus accumbens, ventral pallidum, and ventral tegmentum (Figure 12–7). The reward circuit has key functions in behaviors, as it coordinates connections between dopamine and serotonin pathways (Figure 12–8). Dopamine pathways have a key role in reward (motivation) and pleasure functions. Furthermore, compulsions and perseverations (getting stuck on an idea or repeating an action or statement) are a function of dopamine pathways. Serotonin pathways have roles in mood regulation, memory processing, sleep, and cognition.

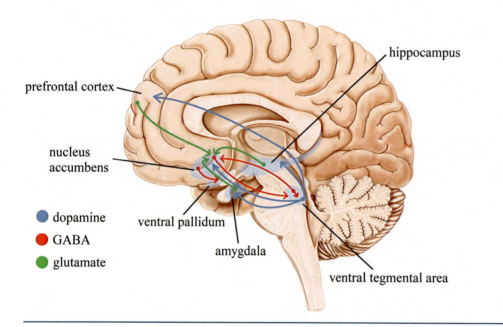

FIGURE 12–7. The reward circuit. GABA, γ-aminobutyric acid.

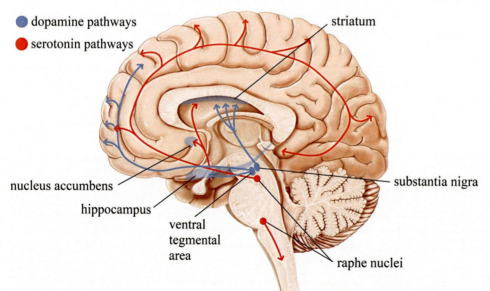

FIGURE 12–8. Dopamine versus serotonin pathways.

Box 12–7. Impacts of Disruption to Limbic Reward Circuits

Layla is a 19-year-old student who was recently suspended from her university for academic performance. Prior to this semester, Layla was a high achieving and interactive student. She was in the top 10% of her graduating high school class, had an ACT score of 35, and had a 3.89 grade point average for the first three semesters of her college career.

At the beginning of spring semester, Layla appeared to be off to her typical start. She engaged with small group discussions and regularly participated in whole class discussions for the first several weeks of the semester. She had received A's on her first several exams and completed her daily assignments. Somewhere around midterm, her professors started to notice a change. She continued to attend class but appeared sleepy, unkempt, and no longer engaged in small group discussions. Fellow students reached out to professors with genuine concern for Layla, as she was initially so interactive. They noted the hygiene concerns and that she mumbled to herself during small group time. Although she occasionally participated in whole class discussions, her questions and answers were frequently off the mark. Performance on exams began to falter from A's to B's and C's. Despite efforts to reach out to her, she avoided interactions with her professors, and subsequently, her attendance became more sporadic. When she did attend, she was not oriented to the content and was poorly groomed. She did not make eye contact with fellow students, teaching assistants, or professors. When confronted by a professor, as she left class one day, to set up a meeting to discuss how they may help her get back on track, she agreed to a meeting and quickly left that interaction. She did not follow through with that meeting and stopped attending classes completely. This ultimately resulted in academic suspension for one semester. She was encouraged to seek medical and counseling help.

She returned home and with the support of her parents was admitted to a stand-alone psychiatric facility for evaluation and treatment. She was having positive symptoms (auditory hallucinations and delusions of persecution from peers and emotional lability), cognitive symptoms [disorganized thinking, bradyphrenia (slowed thinking and processing), poor concentration, memory impairments, difficulty expressing thoughts, and difficulty regulating behaviors], and negative symptoms (inability to show emotions, apathy, and withdrawing from social relationships), which led to the diagnosis of schizophrenia. After regulating her medications, she returned home and eventually back to college after the one semester suspension. The university developed a support program to monitor her status. Grades in the first semester of returning began to rebound. Some inconsistency in performance continued, and with Layla's permission to share pertinent information, faculty were encouraged to collaboratively develop a proactive plan with Layla if they saw any of the warning signs, such as failure to make eye contact, poor hygiene, reductions in small group and/or whole class discussions, or substantial drops in performance on assignments or exams.

Note that positive symptoms are those that involve emergence of an aberrant behavior and negative symptoms involve a lack of typical responses, particularly affective and emotional responses. Along with dysfunction of limbic circuits, the reticular formation is also implicated in schizophrenia. Positive symptoms, including hallucinations, problems filtering out irrelevant sensory inputs, and sleep–wake disturbances, are caused by reticular dysfunction.

Integrating Limbic Information

Talk about well positioned and pulling all of the pieces together, the stria terminalis serves to communicate between limbic structures. Given its interconnectivity to limbic structures, it carries out all of the HOME processes. A portion of the stria terminalis, the bed nucleus, has an important role in regulating autonomic, neuroendocrine, and behavioral functions (Crestani et al., 2013). It has direct impacts on the functions of the amygdala and hypothalamus.

Reticular Formation and Reticular Activating System

The reticular formation is a set of nuclei in the brainstem beginning in the tegmentum gray matter in the midbrain and extending down to the medulla that help regulate sensory signals to the brain, control consciousness (arousal, alertness, circadian rhythm, and sleep–wake cycles), control motor functions (particularly muscle tone and posture), and regulate viscera (autonomic functions such as heartbeat and breathing). The ventral tegmentum of the reticular formation is connected to the limbic system (ventral striatum of the basal ganglia, hippocampus, and amygdala) via the **mesolimbic pathway** (Figure 12–9A). This dopamine pathway regulates reward and pleasure, with a role in learning. Excessive mesolimbic activity results in schizophrenia. The dopamine-regulated, **mesocortical**

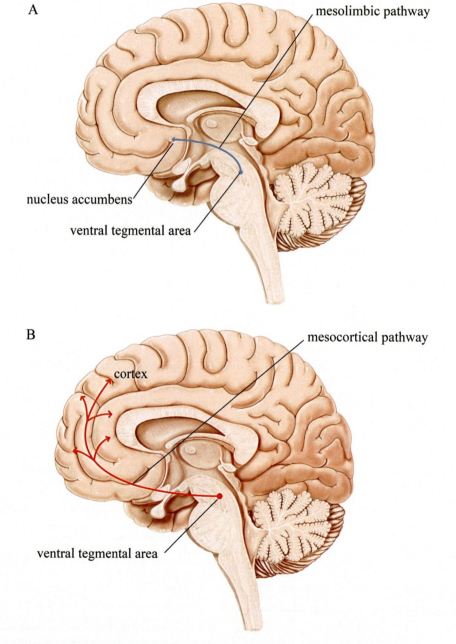

FIGURE 12–9. A and **B.** Dopamine pathways related to schizophrenia symptoms. *Note:* Overactivation of the mesolimbic pathway results in positive symptoms. Mesocortical pathway dysfunction results in negative and cognitive symptoms.

pathway (Figure 12–9B) connects the ventral tegmentum to the frontal lobes, anterior cingulate, and entorhinal cortices. It is believed to have an important role in motivation, executive functions, and emotional regulation.

The reticular formation is an important intermediary between the brain, body, and the outside world. While we sleep, the reticular formation is the gatekeeper, helping us ignore familiar sounds (a roommate's snore or even familiar sirens—depending on where you live) but respond to/awaken us with unfamiliar sounds (e.g., an unfamiliar commotion/noise of a roommate tripping on boots in the entryway). The reticular formation receives information from several ascending pathways in the spinal cord and auditory pathways. In turn, it sends information along ascending pathways toward the thalamus and cerebrum, along with descending pathways toward the body via the spinal cord. One of these, the **reticulospinal tract** (see Chapter 10), helps modulate tone, balance, posture, and coordination of body movement with inputs from visual–vestibular–proprioceptive systems. Damage to the reticulospinal tract, along with the **vestibulospinal tract**, can result in postural instability and ataxia. The reticular formation also has an active role in pain sensation and modulation. In order for pain to reach the somatosensory cortices, signals must pass through the reticular formation along an ascending tract. Descending pathways have a role in modulating pain by dampening pain in the PNS and blocking transmission back to the somatosensory cortices via the spinothalamic tract (see Chapter 6).

The **reticular activating system (RAS)** is a component of the reticular formation with extensive connections to both the brain and spinal cord (Figure 12–10). It regulates levels of arousal and rudimentary attention. The RAS also regulates autonomic functions, as well as working with the motor pathways to regulate reflexes and muscle tone. Among those autonomic functions are sympathetic fight-or-flight responses to environmental stimuli. Autonomic responses to environmental stimuli include motor/tone responses, such as a startle response, or more intentional motor responses (i.e., running away from danger). Caudal RAS projections run from mid pons to the spinal cord, activating the body.

The rostral portion extends from the rostral medulla and mid pons up to the thalamus, synapsing on the intralaminar nuclei of the thalamus and activating the cerebrum through diffuse connections. This increases attention and fosters conscious perception of sensory information (Figure 12–11). A second portion of the rostral projections

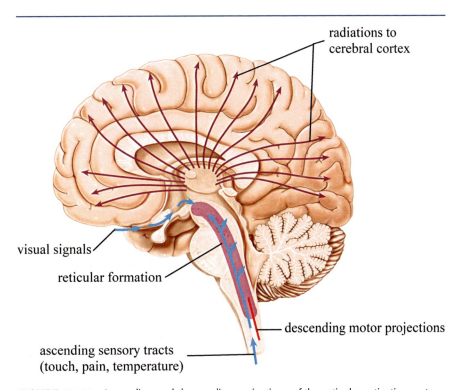

FIGURE 12–10. Ascending and descending projections of the reticular activating system.

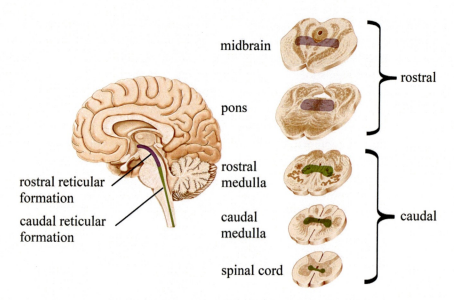

FIGURE 12–11. Rostral and caudal divisions of the reticular activating system.

extend to the hypothalamus to initiate regulation of behavior and coordination of sleep–wake cycles. The suprachiasmatic nucleus, found in the anterior hypothalamus, is the internal regulator of circadian rhythms—our internal day–night, wake–sleep generator. It inhibits external stimuli by reducing afferent (sensory) activity during sleep. Conversely, RAS neurons have a high rate of firing during wakefulness. Damage to the RAS has been associated with coma (see Box 12–8), sleep disorders (e.g., narcolepsy), chronic fatigue, and attention-deficit disorder. Conversely, overactivity of the RAS is associated with posttraumatic stress disorder.

> **Box 12–8.** Reticular Activating System in Altered States of Consciousness
>
> In cases of early coma emergence, the RAS is a key set of structures in clinical assessment and interventions. At the bedside, subtle stimuli such as "time to wake up" or even a gentle nudge to wake up are not likely to arouse an individual. In a sense, the RAS can be activated by activating the body. Sitting the person up in bed, shifting their weight from side to side, applying a wet/cool washcloth to the face, and moving arms to assist those actions can sometimes initiate arousal, allowing the person to more actively engage with the environment. The goal is to achieve differentiated responses to stimuli (i.e., responding directly to the stimuli, rather than indirect/undifferentiated responses such as agitation, irritability, or restlessness).

Box 12–9. Hypothalamic–Pituitary–Adrenal Axis

The hypothalamic–pituitary–adrenal (HPA) axis integrates neural network information and endocrine and immune responses to stress. The stress response is a normal and important part of maintaining homeostasis. Prolonged activation of this stress response results in disordered behaviors. HPA axis dysfunction plays an integral role in the symptoms of depression, disordered day–night rhythm, lack of reward feelings, disturbed eating, sex, and impaired cognitive functions. Disorders of this stress regulation system, such as major depressive disorders, are a consequence of susceptibility and environmental exposures (Lucassen et al., 2014). Several factors can influence susceptibility, including prenatal environmental stressors (e.g., placental insufficiency, inadequate nutrition, nicotine exposure via the mother); developmental stressors (e.g., early maternal separation, child abuse or neglect); and a host of stressors as an adult, including health and relationship stressors (Lucassen et al., 2014; Bao & Swaab, 2019). The HPA axis stimulates synthesis and release of cortisol. Chronically high levels of cortisol can lead to a host of psychological and physical impairments. Cortisol initiates negative feedback to the hypothalamus, pituitary gland, prefrontal cortices, and hippocampus. Along with being a culprit in mood disorders, it can affect regulation of endocrine functions systemically. Although not a direct clinical implication for speech-language pathologists and audiologists, understanding the developmental and adult environmental factors that contribute to susceptibility and HPA axis dysfunction has a great deal of relevance to our work. As a discipline, we encounter children with these developmental and environmental predispositions. Adults with acquired neurogenic disorders such as stroke and brain injury share these risk factors as well. Understanding these susceptibility factors is crucial for appropriate interdisciplinary management and prevention for such clients.

Summary

The limbic system plays some key functions in the work that speech-language pathologists and audiologists conduct. There's no place like HOME, and our limbic system carriers out those homeostatic, olfactory, memory, and emotional functions. The functions are interdependent and carried out by complex networks of limbic structures in concert with other cortical regions. Many of these structures are susceptible to disease, trauma, and developmental impairments, making them pertinent to our everyday work. The limbic system works in cooperation with the reticular formation and RAS. The reticular formation controls autonomic functions, such as heart rate and breathing. It also serves as an interface between brain and body by regulating sensory signals to the brain, controlling states of consciousness, regulating muscle tone and posture, and modulating visceral inputs such as pain. The RAS helps regulate our wake–sleep cycles and most rudimentary levels of attention. Several case examples involving the interplay between the limbic and reticular formation are included in this chapter, but further examples are present or expanded in Chapter 14 as well as Chapter 16.

Key Concepts

- Remember HOME. Homeostasis, olfaction, memory, and emotions are regulated by the limbic system. Although these functions are distributed throughout the system, each structure has unique contributions.
    - The hypothalamus is a primary structure for homeostasis.
    - The olfactory cortices, including the entorhinal and perirhinal cortices, are crucial for olfaction.
    - Although memory is a distributed function, the hippocampus is a key structure in memory functions.
    - The amygdala is a primary structure involved in emotional regulation, memory, and processing.

- Recall that several brain structures develop in the shape of a "C." This is true of the cingulate gyrus and fornix of the limbic system.
- The reticular formation controls autonomic functions such as heart rate and breathing. It also serves as an interface between brain and body, modulating sensory inputs to the brain, regulating consciousness, controlling tone and posture, and modulating visceral information including pain.
- The rostral RAS sends messages to the thalamus and cerebral cortex, enhancing alertness and attention to tasks.
- The caudal RAS sends messages to the body via the spinal cord. This helps regulate autonomic, sympathetic responses, including reflexes and muscle tone.
- Damage to the reticular formation has been implicated in schizophrenia, coma, posttraumatic stress disorder, and narcolepsy.

References and Additional Resources

Bao, A. M., & Swaab, D. F. (2019). The human hypothalamus in mood disorders: The HPA axis in the center. *IBRO Reports, 6*, 45–53.

Blumenfeld, H. (2010). *Neuroanatomy through clinical cases.* Sinauer.

Crestani, C. C., Alves, F. H., Gomes, F. V., Resstel, L., Correa, F., & Herman, J. P. (2013). Mechanisms in the bed nucleus of the stria terminalis involved in control of autonomic and neuroendocrine functions: A review. *Current Neuropharmacology, 11*(2), 141–159.

Dillingham, C. M., Frizzati, A., Nelson, A. J., & Vann, S. D. (2015). How do mammillary body inputs contribute to anterior thalamic function? *Neuroscience & Biobehavioral Reviews, 54*, 108–119.

Lucassen, P. J., Pruessner, J., Sousa, N., Almeida, O. F., Van Dam, A. M., Rajkowska, G., . . . Czéh, B. (2014). Neuropathology of stress. *Acta Neuropathologica, 127*(1), 109–135.

Morrison, S. F. (2016). Central neural control of thermoregulation and brown adipose tissue. *Autonomic Neuroscience, 196*, 14–24.

Raslau, F. D., Augustinack, J. C., Klein, A. P., Ulmer, J. L., Mathews, V. P., & Mark, L. P. (2015). Memory Part 3: The role of the fornix and clinical cases. *American Journal of Neuroradiology, 36*(9), 1604–1608. https://doi.org/10.3174/ajnr.A4371

Rolls, E. T. (2019). The cingulate cortex and limbic systems for emotion, action, and memory. *Brain Structure and Function, 224*, 3001–3018. https://doi.org/10.1007/s00429-019-01945-2

Shin, H., Lee, S. Y., Cho, H. U., Oh, Y., Kim, I. Y., Jang, D. P., & Min, H. K. (2019). Fornix stimulation induces metabolic activity and dopaminergic response in the nucleus accumbens. *Frontiers in Neuroscience, 13*, 1109.

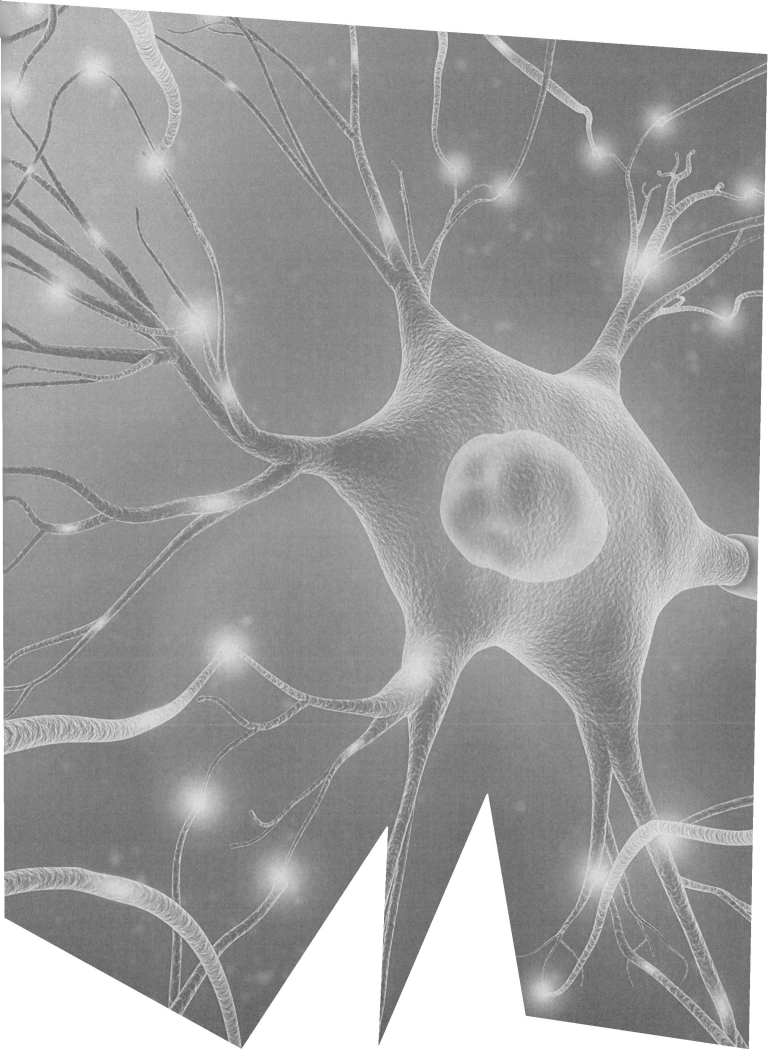

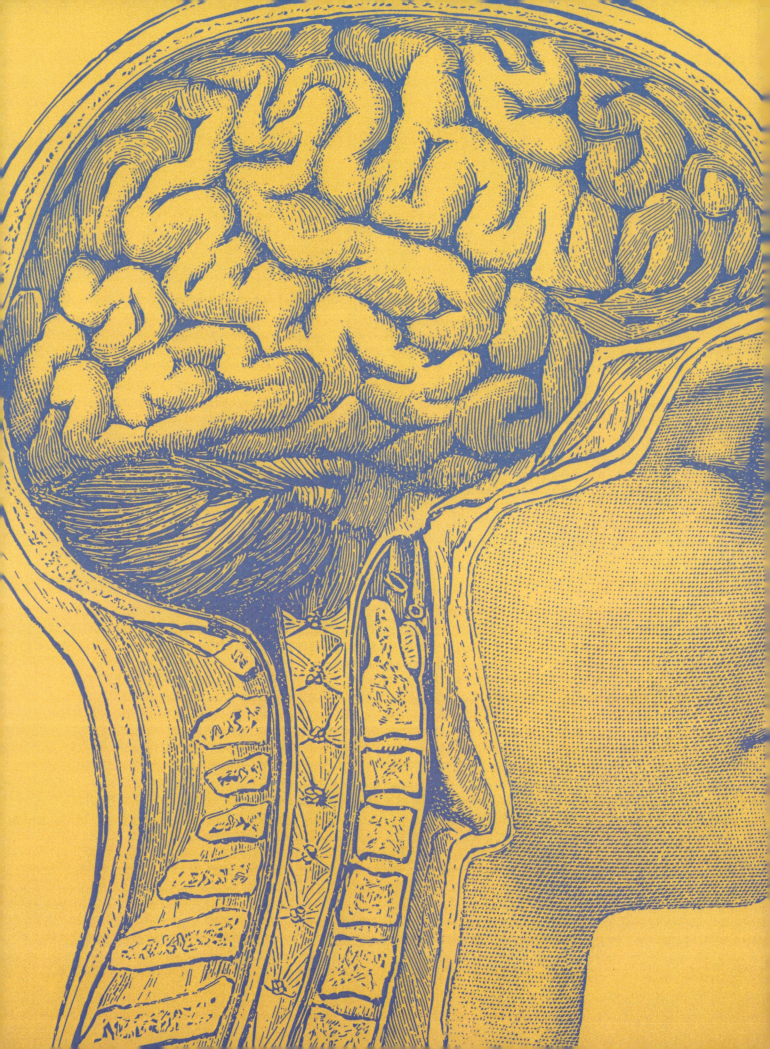

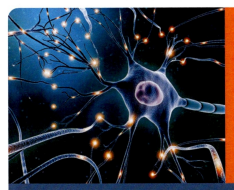

13
Cerebrovascular System

CHAPTER OUTLINE

Overview
Blood Supply and Functional Organization
Circle of Willis
Cerebral Blood Supply Distributions
Blood Supply to the Thalamus and Basal Ganglia
Blood Supply to the Cerebellum
Brainstem and Spinal Cord Distributions

Midbrain
Pons
Medulla
Spinal Cord
Blood–Brain Barrier
Disruptions to Blood Supply
Summary
References and Additional Resources

Overview

The overlap between cerebrovascular distributions and functional organization of the brain makes understanding this system particularly relevant to speech-language pathologists and audiologists. Neural tissue requires a constant supply of oxygenated blood to carry out its roles. Thus, restrictions to blood flow result in changes or impairments to brain functions. As described in Chapter 3, neurons cannot store their own oxygen and thus are dependent on the vascular system to provide it. The bloodstream also carries nutrients to the neurons and glial cells to support their normal functions. Due to a protective structure called the blood–brain barrier, not everything that is in the bloodstream can get to the neural tissue.

Interruption to the blood supply will starve neurons of oxygen and impair their normal function. Learning the pattern of arteries and which arteries supply what areas of the brain is critical for understanding relationships between localization of damage and subsequent patterns of impairments.

Blood Supply and Functional Organization

The relationship between cerebral blood supply and **functional organization** of cerebral structures is a key concept, particularly in clinical applications. As discussed in Chapter 1, basic sensory and motor functions can be precisely mapped within the cortex, whereas more complex functions such as language, communication, and cognition involve collaboration of multiple regions. Nevertheless, understanding the overlap between basic functional organization (e.g., Brodmann areas) and blood supply distributions does help predict functions/impairments when a blood supply is restricted (Figure 13–1). For instance, structures such as the motor strip, somatosensory strip, premotor area, Broca area, and Wernicke area all fall within the **middle cerebral artery (MCA)** distribution. We would predict that restrictions to MCA **perfusion** (the delivery of blood to tissues) would affect functions of these structures. Likewise, if we identified behavioral impairments related to these structures (e.g., aphasia, unilateral paralysis), we

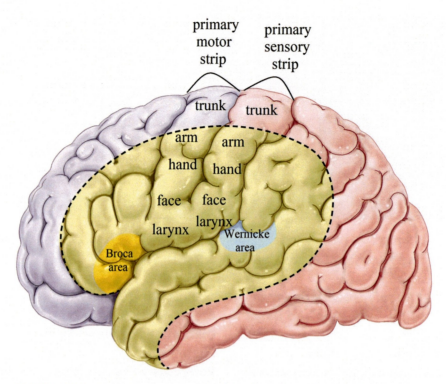

FIGURE 13–1. Overlap between cerebral blood supply and topographical organization. The *yellow*, center region is the middle cerebral artery distribution; the *blue*, anterior/dorsal region is the anterior cerebral artery distribution; and the *pink*, posterior/inferior region is the posterior cerebral artery distribution.

could predict that MCA blood supply may have been disrupted (acknowledging that not all etiologies are vascular in nature). To understand this concept more deeply, it is helpful to understand the source and tributaries of the cerebrovascular system.

The blood supply to the brain consists of two pairs of major arteries that carry blood from the heart, up the neck, and into the cranium. On the inferior surface of the cerebrum, they join with other arteries to form the **circle of Willis**, from which branches extend out to supply the entire brain.

In order to get a clear understanding of the system, begin with the source—the heart. Fresh, oxygenated blood begins in the heart and respiratory system. The aorta distributes that blood, branching off into the left and right subclavian and **common carotid arteries**. The subclavian arteries branch off into the left and right **vertebral arteries**, which merge near the inferior pons to form the **basilar artery**. The basilar artery serves the posterior portion of the circle of Willis and supplies blood to the posterior and inferior regions of the brain. The common carotids give rise to the **internal** and **external carotid arteries**. The left and right internal carotids supply the anterior portions of the circle of Willis and, by extension, the brain (Figures 13–2 through 13–4). Note that we have provided several images because perspective is crucial to understanding where these vessels are situated in the neck and head.

Circle of Willis

The circle of Willis is a crucial distributor system in the cerebrum (see Figures 13–2 through 13–5). The internal carotid and basilar arteries bring oxygenated blood into the circle of Willis, and that blood is distributed to the brain through **cerebral arteries.** The circle itself is created by these major arteries and anastomoses called **communicating arteries. Anastomoses** are small-diameter, connecting

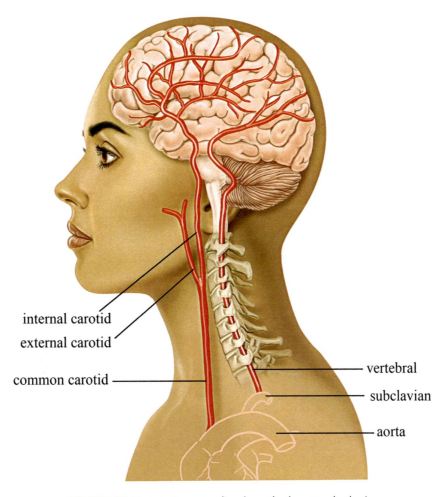

FIGURE 13-2. Arteries extending from the heart to the brain.

blood vessels that span between two larger vessels. In the case of the circle of Willis, anastomoses connect the main arteries, allowing for collateral circulation—a protective mechanism that may provide perfusion to major blood supply territories given a short-term obstruction. The **basilar artery** serves the **posterior cerebral artery** (PCA) distribution and is joined to the anterior distribution through the **posterior communicating artery** (PCoA or PComA; the posterior anastomosis). The **internal carotid** serves both the **middle cerebral artery** (MCA) and the **anterior cerebral artery** (ACA) distributions. Those distributions are joined through the **anterior communicating artery** (ACoA or AComA; the anterior anastomosis). It is worth noting that there are variations across individuals; some individuals have larger or smaller diameter anastomosis lumens connecting major arteries, and in up to 50% of people, the circle is incomplete, such as when the ACoA that connects left and right ACA distributions is absent.

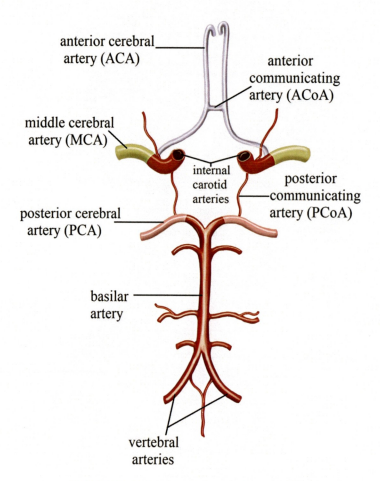

FIGURE 13–3. Arteries within the circle of Willis.

 Box 13–1. Arteries of the Circle of Willis

The arteries leading into the circle of Willis are the bilateral internal carotids and the single basilar (created by merging of the bilateral vertebrals). The arteries leading out of the circle of Willis to the brain are the bilateral anterior, middle, and posterior cerebral arteries. A single anterior communicating artery connects the right and left anterior cerebral arteries, and the paired posterior communicating arteries connect the middle to the posterior cerebral arteries.

Chapter 13 – Cerebrovascular System   221

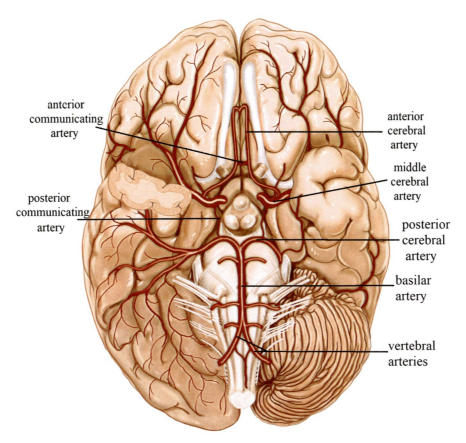

FIGURE 13–4. Circle of Willis in the context of the inferior surface of the brain.

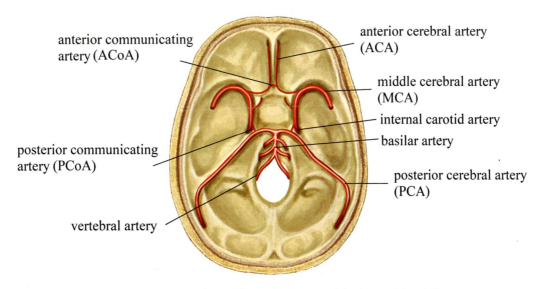

FIGURE 13–5. Circle of Willis in the context of the base of the skull.

Cerebral Blood Supply Distributions

Three main paired vessels account for the majority of cerebral blood supply: the ACA, MCA, and PCA (Figures 13–6 and 13–7). The anterior choroidal artery, a small branch off of the MCA, accounts for a small distribution. Arising out of the internal carotid, the ACA and MCA supply much of the lateral surfaces of the cerebrum. Although only accounting for a small portion of the lateral surface, the ACA supplies most of the anterior half of the medial

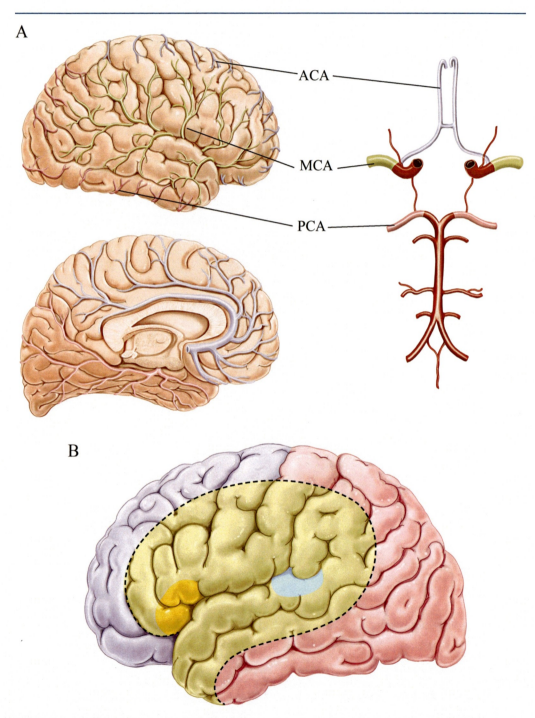

FIGURE 13–6. A. Cerebral artery branches on the lateral, medial, and inferior surfaces of the brain. **B.** Blood supply distributions on the lateral surface of the left hemisphere. *continues*

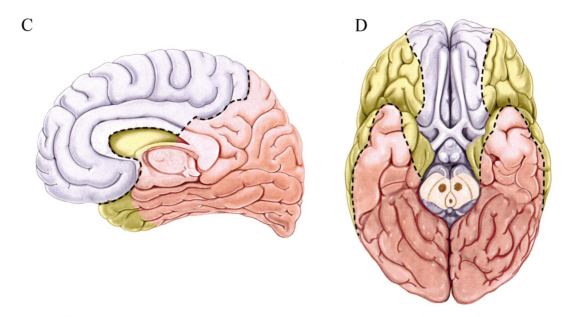

FIGURE 13–6. *continued* **C.** Blood supply distributions on the medial surface. ACA, anterior cerebral artery (*blue*); MCA, middle cerebral artery (*yellow*); PCA, posterior cerebral artery (*pink*).

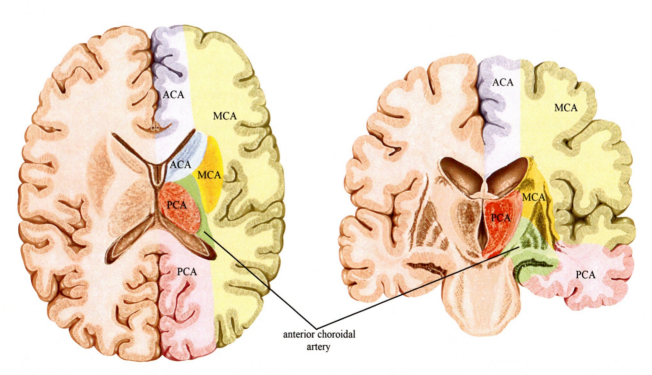

FIGURE 13–7. Blood supply distributions shown in horizontal and coronal slices. Distributions from deep branches of the cerebral arteries are shown in darker colors. The anterior choroidal artery is shown in *green*. ACA, anterior cerebral artery (*blue*); MCA, middle cerebral artery (*yellow*); PCA, posterior cerebral artery (*pink*).

surface. Likewise, the PCA supplies most of the posterior half of the medial surface, along with the perimeter of the lateral surface. It also supplies the inferior region of the temporal lobe. Cross-referencing the perspectives shown in the figures, you can see that the MCA distribution covers a substantial portion of the blood supply to the cerebrum.

> **Box 13–2.** Middle Versus Medial, Not Potay-Toe Versus Potah-Toe!
>
> This is one of those instances in which using anatomical terminology is critical. In everyday usage, middle means "between two things." The middle of the brain could be the center (along the midline), or it could be halfway between the front (anterior) and back (posterior). In anatomical naming, middle is always used in reference to other things that will clarify the location. The middle cerebral artery is located between the anterior and posterior cerebral arteries. This provides the context for you to know that middle is the region between the front and back of the brain. Remember that medial means "toward the midline" (another meaning of middle). The MCA does not supply blood to the midline; that's the job of the ACA.

The MCA distribution serves the middle portion of the lateral surface of the cerebrum, including parts of the frontal, temporal, and parietal lobes. Anterior to the central sulcus and superior to the lateral sulcus is the superior branch of the MCA, which supplies portions of the motor strip/precentral gyrus (gross motor innervation to the hands, arms, and face); the premotor area (motor planning); and, in the left hemisphere, Broca area (language production). Posterior to the central sulcus and inferior to the lateral sulcus is the inferior MCA branch, which supplies the postcentral gyrus/primary somatosensory cortices (Brodmann areas 3, 1, and 2); somatosensory association cortices; Heschl gyrus (primary auditory cortex); and, in the left hemisphere, Wernicke area (language comprehension). Deep branches of the MCA serve the putamen and globus pallidus. The anterior choroidal artery serves the posterior limb of the internal capsule.

The PCA distribution serves the perimeter of the posterolateral cerebral surface, along with the majority of the posterior half of the medial surface. This includes the visual cortices (Brodmann areas 17–19) in the occipital lobes, superior and medial parietal lobes, and temporal lobes. It also supplies the inferior surface of the temporal lobe. Deep branches of the PCA serve the thalamus.

Watershed regions exist between each of the main cerebral blood supply distributions (Figure 13–8). A watershed region is an area of overlap between distributions, in which the brain tissue receives blood supply from both distributions through the final, smallest diameter branches of each artery. The anatomy provides both benefits and short-

The ACA distribution includes the lateral and medial surfaces of the prefrontal cortices, which house executive functions and working memory processes. It also supplies the anterior portion of the cingulate gyrus, lateral and medial portions of the supplementary motor area (motor planning), and lateral and medial portions of the motor strip/precentral gyrus (gross motor innervation to trunk, legs, and feet). Deep branches of the ACA serve the anterior limb of the internal capsule, the head of the caudate, and the hippocampal formation.

> **Box 13–3.** Left Superior Branch of MCA Cerebrovascular Accident With tPA Therapy
>
> Darius was a 63-year-old male who experienced acute onset of right-sided weakness, confusion, and global aphasia (see Chapter 14) following a suspected left cerebrovascular accident (CVA). Imaging revealed a large ischemic stroke affecting the left superior branch of the MCA. Etiology was determined to be cardioembolic, secondary to atrial fibrillation. A "clot-busting" drug called tPA was administered. Darius' condition improved over the course of the initial 48 hours of hospitalization. Aphasia began to resolve toward a mild to moderate, nonfluent aphasia. Right hemiparesis persisted with upper extremity weakness worse than lower extremity weakness. Darius was transferred to inpatient rehabilitation, where he stayed for 2 weeks for physical, occupational, and speech therapy services. At discharge, he could walk independently with a four-point cane for household ambulation. He was able to dress himself with adaptive equipment from occupational therapy. Mild, nonfluent aphasia persisted at discharge. Atrial fibrillation was managed with an anticoagulant and calcium channel blocker post CVA. The arrhythmia resolved. (See Case 16–5 in Chapter 16 for an expanded version of this case.)

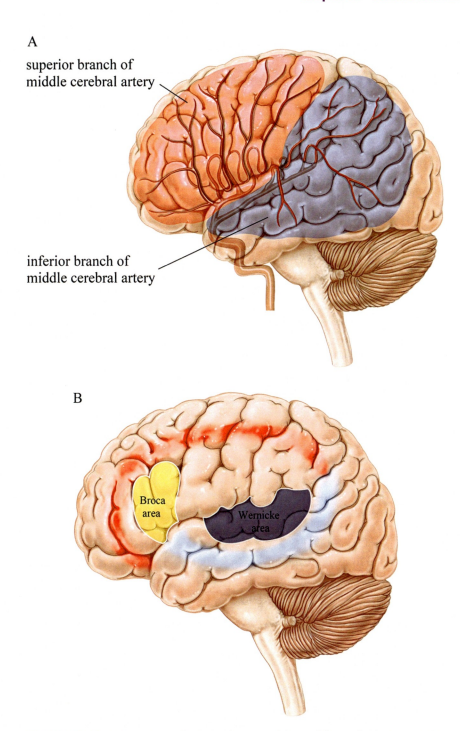

FIGURE 13–8. A. Superior and inferior divisions of the middle cerebral artery (MCA). **B.** Watershed areas between divisions of the MCA and anterior cerebral artery (*red*) and posterior cerebral artery (*blue*).

comings. An obvious benefit is double coverage, meaning that if one of the blood vessel distributions is interrupted, these areas are still served by the adjacent vessels. A shortcoming is that these narrow lumen vessels are more susceptible to atherosclerosis (deposits of plaque or fatty material on walls of vessels) and small vessel disease.

Box 13–4. Small Vessel Disease, Vascular Dementia

Harold was an 86-year-old male who presented with severe, bilateral carotid stenosis (narrowing of the lumen of the arteries) caused by buildup of fatty plaques on the walls of the arteries. His carotid arteries were 80% occluded on the right side and 90% the left side. Given his age and medical history, it was determined he was not a good candidate for a carotid endarterectomy, a procedure in which the plaques are cleared out. Harold experienced insidious (gradual) onset of aphasia and confusion. Along with difficulties with word retrieval, comprehension was impaired for conversation-level exchanges. The family noted gradual changes in memory and decision-making as well. This prompted his family to move Harold from an assisted living setting to a skilled nursing facility. Suspected diagnosis of small vessel ischemic disease was confirmed with magnetic resonance imaging MRI with diffusion-weighted MRI and magnetic resonance angiography (MRA). Microemboli were suspected. Harold received physical, occupational, and speech therapy services for several weeks, noting improvements in communication, memory, decision-making, and activities of daily living in the short term. He remained in the skilled nursing facility following discharge from rehabilitation therapies. (See Case 16–6 in Chapter 16 for an expanded version of this case.)

Blood Supply to the Thalamus and Basal Ganglia

Blood supply to the thalamus and basal ganglia was briefly covered in the discussion of cerebral blood supply distributions, but it may be helpful to map those distributions directly to those structures (Figures 13–9 and 13–10, Table 13–1). As discussed in Chapter 5, the thalamus is a major gatekeeper for all portions of the brain because it is a point of synapse for most brain-to-body and body-to-brain messages, as well as many cortex-to-cortex communications. It is also a foundational structure for global attention and awareness. The thalamus receives blood supply from the PCA. The basal ganglia, key components of the motor system and cognition (see Chapter 10), are served by the ACA, MCA, and anterior choroidal arteries.

Blood Supply to the Cerebellum

The cerebellum is supplied by three arteries: the **posterior inferior cerebellar artery (PICA)**, **anterior inferior cerebellar artery (AICA)**, and the **superior cerebellar artery (SCA)** (Figure 13–11). Note that the blood supply distri-

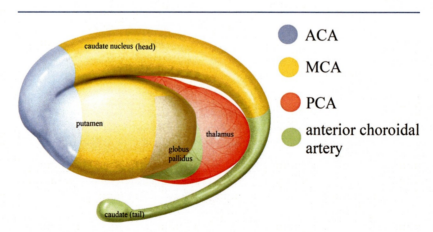

FIGURE 13–9. Blood supply to basal ganglia and thalamus. ACA, anterior cerebral artery; MCA, middle cerebral artery; PCA, posterior cerebral artery.

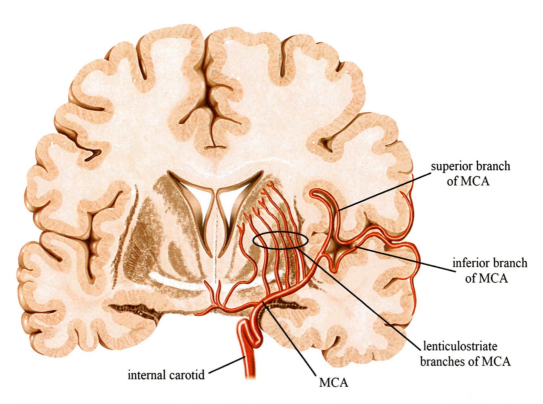

FIGURE 13–10. Blood supply to internal capsule and globus pallidus. MCA, middle cerebral artery.

Table 13–1. Blood Supply to the Thalamus and Basal Ganglia

Structure	Blood Supply
Thalamus	PCA
Basal ganglia	
Putamen	ACA and MCA
Head of caudate	ACA and MCA
Tail of caudate	Anterior choroidal artery
Globus pallidus	MCA and anterior choroidal artery

Note. ACA, anterior cerebral artery; MCA, middle cerebral artery; PCA, posterior cerebral artery.

butions are organized perpendicular to the functional organization regions: Blood supply regions run horizontally, stacked on top of each other whereas functional areas run vertically and are divided into columns. The most medial portion of the cerebellum, the vermis, is partially covered by each of the three arteries, as are the intermediate and lateral portions. Therefore, it is unusual to experience loss of discrete functions after cerebellar strokes. Instead, vascular lesions result in mixed impairments (i.e., ocular, trunkal, limb, and speech ataxia). However, it is helpful to consider distributions and typical consequences associated with each.

The SCA serves the superior cerebellar hemispheres, vermis, and parts of the midbrain. Ipsilateral limb ataxia, nystagmus, vertigo, ataxic dysarthria, and gait ataxia are the predominant symptoms for SCA infarcts. The distribution and size of the PICA differ across individuals and vary proportionately to the AICA (i.e., the larger the PICA, the smaller the AICA and vice versa). The PICA distribution typically includes the inferior posterior surface and inferior vermis. Infarcts to the PICA distribution result predominantly in more trunkal ataxia and are often concomitant with symptoms of Wallenberg syndrome/lateral medullary syndrome (see the section on the medulla and Case 16–10 in Chapter 16 for a description of this syndrome). Severe headache and neck pain are also common given rapid effects of swelling associated with cerebellar infarcts. The AICA distribution serves the mid-anterior portion of the cerebellum. AICA infarcts are rarer and include more severe vertigo and hearing dysfunction, facial sensation

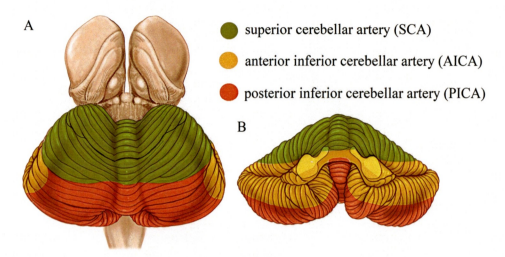

FIGURE 13–11. Cerebellar vascular distributions.

> **Box 13–5.** Cerebellar Cerebrovascular Accident
>
> Devin was a 52-year-old non-binary person who initially presented with "slurred," confused speech and clumsy, "drunken" gait. Radiologic findings identified a cerebellar, ischemic stroke in the anterior lobe. Devin was somewhat obtunded (reduced alertness and slow responses to stimuli) and confused initially but became oriented to person and place by the second day of hospitalization. Speech was characterized by ataxic dysarthria, marked by imprecise and irregular articulation qualities. Similar to characteristics of their gait, Devin's speech shared features of "drunken" speech, including overshooting and undershooting targets, irregular rate, and timing problems. Their gait was unsteady and marked by similar overshoots, such as swinging the right leg across the left leg as they attempted to walk a straight line. Devin's eye movements were also disrupted, including the presence of nystagmus (the eyes make rapid twitching movement—either side to side or, in this case, up and down). Cognition improved markedly over the first few days, but speech and gait impairments remained persistent upon discharge. (See Case 16–9 in Chapter 16 for an expanded version of this case.)

and motor impairments, and Horner syndrome (decreased pupil size, ptosis, and decreased sweating on the affected side of face). Across distributions, ataxias are ipsilateral to the side of lesions.

Brainstem and Spinal Cord Distributions

Blood supply for the brainstem and spinal cord also arises from the **vertebral** and **basilar** arteries (Figure 13–12 and Table 13–2). The pathophysiology of strokes (interruption of blood supply to the brain) is covered later, but for each of these sections the impairments caused by interruption of blood supply is included to highlight the functions affected.

Midbrain

The PCA, created from the bifurcation of the basilar artery, serves the posterior two-thirds of the midbrain, whereas the basilar artery supplies the anteromedial one-third. Lesions to the inferior midbrain are difficult to localize but typically result in dizziness; vertigo; hearing loss; speech, appendicular trunk, and gait ataxia; limb weakness; and pseudobulbar affect syndrome (disproportionate and contextually inappropriate emotional behaviors). Visual impairments and extraocular palsies caused by damage to cranial nerves (CNs)

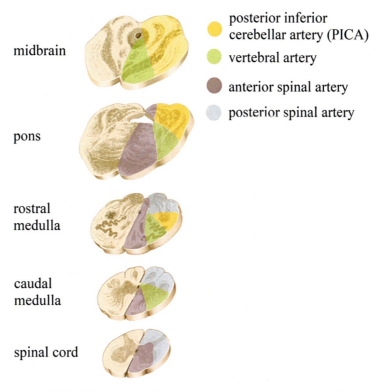

FIGURE 13–12. Blood supply to brainstem and spinal cord.

III, IV, or VI are also common. Superior midbrain lesions tend to involve the thalamus as well, with serious impairments to consciousness. The higher the lesion, the greater the likelihood of coma.

Pons

The posterior one-third of the pons is served by the AICA, whereas the anterior–medial two-thirds is covered by the basilar artery. Infarcts within the AICA distribution (lateral pontine syndrome) are characterized by ipsilateral facial weakness, limb and gait ataxia, vertigo, and unilateral ipsilateral deafness from labyrinthine artery ischemia (insufficient oxygenated blood to inner ear). Infarcts within the inferior medial pontine, basilar artery distribution (Foville syndrome) are characterized by contralateral arm and leg weakness, ipsilateral face weakness (lower motor facial weakness of the entire face due to damage to CN VII), and lateral gaze weakness (related to CN VI).

Medulla

The posterolateral portion of the rostral medulla is served by the PICA, whereas the vertebral artery serves the posterior–medial portion and the anterior spinal artery serves the anterior–medial one-third. The posterior one-third of the caudal medulla is served by the posterior spinal artery and PICA, the medial one-third is served by the vertebral artery, and the anterior one-third is served by the anterior spinal artery. Infarcts to the PICA distribution result in lateral medullary syndrome (Wallenberg syndrome), characterized by vertigo, dizziness, nystagmus, ataxia, nausea and vomiting, severe dysphagia, and hiccups. Infarcts involving the vertebral arteries result in damage to the medial medulla and are characterized by dizziness, vertigo, diplopia, numbness around the mouth, blurred vision, tinnitus, ataxia, and orthostatic hypotension (rapid drops in blood pressure when going from sitting to standing that can result in syncope/fainting). Lesions to the anterior spinal artery result in similar impairments.

Spinal Cord

The posterior spinal artery serves the posterior and lateral spinal cord, whereas the anterior spinal artery serves the anterior–medial portion. For more information regarding the functions of the ascending and descending tracts that make up the spinal cord white matter, see Chapters 6 and 10.

Table 13–2. Blood Supply to the Brainstem and Spinal Cord

Structure	Blood Supply
Midbrain	
Posterior two-thirds (includes the vestibular nuclei, solitary nuclei/tract, spinotrigeminal nuclei/tract, and spinothalamic tract)	PCA
Anterior one-third (includes the corticospinal tract fibers, medial lemniscus, and inferior olivary complex)	Basilar artery
Pons	
Posterior one-third	AICA
Anterior–medial two-thirds	Basilar artery
Medulla	
Rostral portion	
Posterior–lateral	PICA
Posterior–medial	Vertebral
Anterior–medial	Anterior spinal artery
Caudal portion	
Posterior one-third (includes the spinal trigeminal tract/nucleus, medullary portions of fasciculus gracilis, and fasciculus cuneatus)	Posterior spinal artery and PICA
Medial one-third (includes the posterior spinocerebellar tract and spinothalamic tract)	Vertebral artery
Anterior one-third (includes the pyramidal decussation and spinothalamic tract)	Anterior spinal artery
Spinal cord	
Posterior–lateral portion (includes the posterior cerebellar tract, fasciculus gracilis, and fasiculus cuneatus)	Posterior spinal artery
Anterior–medial portion (includes the lateral corticospinal tract, rubrospinal tract, and spinothalamic tract)	Anterior spinal artery

Note. AICA, anterior inferior cerebellar artery; PCA, posterior cerebral artery; PICA, posterior inferior cerebellar artery.

Blood–Brain Barrier

The blood–brain barrier (BBB) is a morphological (structural) difference in the composition of blood vessels within the brain compared to the rest of the body. In the body, there are open junctions between endothelial cells that compose the walls of blood vessels. This allows for efficient and easy transport of nutrients (e.g., glucose) and oxygen from the bloodstream to structures. It also allows for the transport of pathogens and viruses (usually fairly large in relative terms) from the bloodstream to the body. The BBB is a protective mechanism that prevents larger pathogens and viruses from entering the brain. It was first discovered in the 1800s. Dye injected into peripheral vessels stained organs outside of the vessels, whereas the brain did not change color, reflecting the tight junctions present

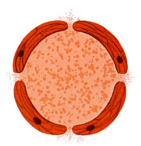
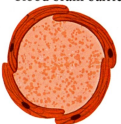

FIGURE 13–13. Vessel morphology throughout the body versus the blood–brain barrier.

with the BBB (Figure 13–13). Because the junctions in brain blood vessels are tight or stacked (overlapping), only small molecules can pass. For instance, alcohol is a small compound, so it enters quite easily. Many pathogens and viruses that affect the body are too big to pass (e.g., the common cold). Some sneaky pathogens do, which makes them particularly nasty. For instance, syphilis, the AIDS virus, and prion-based pathogens can pass, either because of size or because of composition. Prions are small protein particles when they enter the body (rod-like structures) but expand into crystalline projections once in the brain. If you can imagine a crystal in the brain, it causes some damage. The generic disorder manifestation is called spongiform encephalopathy because of the spongy holes that it creates in brain tissue. Most spongiform encephalopathies have a dormant period when the disease does not progress. Examples include Creutzfeldt–Jakob disease (CJD) and kuru, but there are a number of variants (some transmissible to humans and others not). Note that diseases such as CJD produce swift and profound damage to the brain and thus neurological function once they reach their active phase.

In addition to restricting some viruses and pathogens, the BBB also protects the brain from some drugs. Generally, this is a good thing, but in some cases it makes pharmaceutical treatments more complicated. Parkinson disease (PD) is a result of too little dopamine in the central nervous system (CNS; see Chapters 3 and 10). Ideally, patients with PD could simply take dopamine pills or injections. However, dopamine molecules cannot cross the BBB. This led to the use of levodopa or L-dopa, which is an amino acid and a precursor to dopamine. The amino acid component is the "ticket" to cross the BBB. Once in the CNS, L-dopa is converted into dopamine.

Disruptions to Blood Supply

Blockages or restrictions to blood flow perfusion interrupt the distribution of nutrients and oxygenation to tissues served by specific blood supply distributions. In the brain, such interruptions are called **cerebrovascular accidents** or, more commonly, **strokes**. Such an interruption in blood flow causes **ischemia** or inadequate blood perfusion to the tissues that a particular blood vessel serves. Furthermore, an interruption in perfusion causes **hypoxia** (inadequate oxygenation) or **anoxia** (no oxygenation) of those tissues. It is possible to have hypoxia without ischemia, meaning that blood flow reached the tissues but it was inadequately oxygenated. Conversely, it is not possible to have ischemia without hypoxia because restricted blood flow always results in restricted oxygenation. If blood supply

Box 13–6. Factors That Escalate Ischemia to Infarction

- 10 seconds of brain ischemia leads to a loss of consciousness.
- 20 seconds of brain ischemia leads to ceasing of electrical activity (action potentials).
- Blood flow >20 ml/100 g/min is insufficient for electrical signaling (55 ml/100 g of CNS tissue/min is the typical level).
- Blood flow <10 ml/100 g/min for more than a few minutes, or a few minutes of total ischemia = irreversible brain damage (infarction).

is not restored, the result is an **infarct**, a region of dead, nonfunctioning brain tissue.

Several mechanisms can result in ischemia, including local or distal blockages, edema, or hemorrhages. A **thrombus** (plural: thrombi) is a local blockage. Atherosclerosis or plaque accumulation can also narrow or obstruct vessels within the brain. Conversely, an **embolus** (plural: emboli) develops in some other part of the body (e.g., the heart, lungs, or femoral arteries), breaks off, and travels through the vascular system toward the brain. Emboli may be composed of air, adipose (fat), or clotted blood. Cardiac arrhythmias, such as atrial fibrillation, can result in shower emboli—that is, multiple small emboli that affect multiple blood supply distributions. Communication disorders can result from shower emboli caused by atrial fibrillation because emboli may affect multiple vascular territories, including the left or right MCA distributions that supply critical areas for communication (right hemisphere) or language (left hemisphere). Right-sided emboli are more common in individuals with atrial fibrillation—approximately a 60:40 right:left ratio (Park et al., 2014). Some inhalants or toxins can produce ischemia without a true blockage. Likewise, **vasospasm** (literally *vessel spasm*) can constrict blood vessels, causing ischemic damage.

A secondary mechanism of damage, edema (swelling), can compress surrounding tissues and vessels, further constricting perfusion. The edematous area surrounding that primary lesion (infarcted area) is referred to as the **penumbra** (Figure 13–14). Tissues in the penumbra are hypoperfused but can recover with appropriate medical and pharmacological management. Restoration of blood flow to the penumbra can reduce secondary damage. Conversely, poor medical management can result in extension of the primary lesion. Ischemia can be identified through a variety of radio imaging tests, including computed tomography (CT), MRI, and cerebral angiography (or CT angiography or MRA).

Hemorrhagic strokes occur when blood leaks out of the vessels into surrounding brain tissue. These account for approximately 20% of strokes. Like ischemic events, hemorrhagic etiologies result in both primary and secondary consequences. Primary consequences include direct damage to brain tissues as blood comes into contact with the brain tissues and reduction in perfusion to brain tissues served by that vessel. Secondary damage includes the effects of edema and cytotoxic damage to surrounding tissues. Individuals with ruptured aneurysms are monitored closely for onset of vasospasm because risk increases following intracranial hemorrhage.

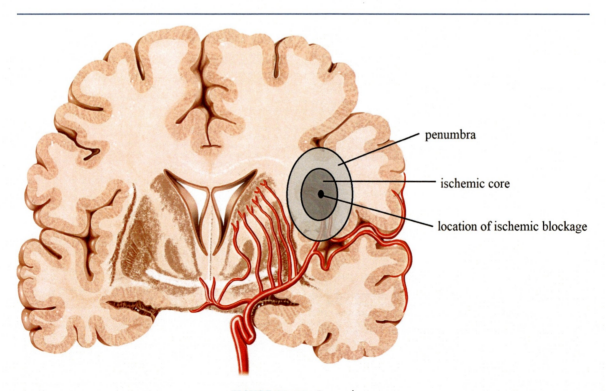

FIGURE 13–14. Penumbra.

Box 13–7. Right MCA Cerebrovascular Accident

Anton was a 62-year-old male who initially presented with lethargy and inattention. His partner brought him to a local hospital after noticing his difficulty focusing or even responding to simple questions. He was diagnosed with a large, inferior branch, ischemic stroke of the right MCA. For the first few days, he had a strong gaze preference to the right/left inattention along with very limited endurance and difficulty maintaining attention to task. When he was alert, he was impulsive when eating, taking large bites and consuming food/liquids at a rapid rate. He needed support to get the spoon to the center of his mouth and tended to miss to the left side without that hand-over-hand support. After a few minutes of self-feeding, he was exhausted and leaned heavily to the right. At this point, he required maximal assistance to eat, including physical cues/efforts to turn his head toward midline. A few days later, his endurance improved markedly and his gaze preference was equal (left/right), with the exception of more complex tasks such as walking and navigating the hospital (right gaze preference/left inattention returned during tasks that required a lot of attention). He required moderate assistance to maintain safety when ambulating, even though his balance and gait were fairly functional. For instance, he would collide with doorways with his left shoulder and lost balance/feel to the right when inattentive or when asked to engage in a task while standing. Anton's speech was characterized by mild, spastic dysarthria, and his communication was marked by rambling and egocentrism (a pervasive tendency to focus on himself). (See Case 16–8 in Chapter 16 for an expanded version of this case.)

Hemorrhagic strokes can result from several etiologies. Weaknesses in vessel walls can result in a ballooning effect called an **aneurysm**. Aneurysms may result from prolonged hypertension, genetic predisposition, or environmental exposures including smoking and a variety of medications.

There are three main types of aneurysms: saccular/berry (a sac-like outpouching attached to one side of an artery), fusiform (ballooning on all sides of an artery), and mycotic (caused by an infection that weakens artery walls). Some aneurysms are present in key vascular locations, such as the

Box 13–8. Ruptured Aneurysm and Vasospasm

Marjorie was a 45-year-old female smoker who was otherwise healthy before experiencing acute onset of confusion, severe attention impairments, and language impairments. She had two daughters who were in their early teens at the time of this event. She was admitted to the hospital with an intracranial hemorrhage due to a large (25-mm) saccular (berry) aneurysm on the circle of Willis, near the junction of the left internal carotid and MCA/ACA branches. The hemorrhage caused her cognitive status to deteriorate rapidly upon admission, resulting in a somnolent (sleepy) status as she was taken to surgery. A neurosurgeon evacuated the intracranial hemorrhage and placed a clip on the aneurysm. Initial response to the neurosurgical intervention was good. Marjorie awoke with anomia, somewhat agrammatic spoken language expression, impaired comprehension of spoken language, attention impairments, executive dysfunction, and confusion (including disorientation to place, time, and situation). Over the course of 4 or 5 days, her condition began to stabilize further, and cognitive communication functions began to improve substantially. At that point, her communication was characterized by anomia, mild nonspecific language impairments, poor attentional control and endurance, and executive dysfunction (characterized by poor inhibition and self-regulation). She remained disoriented, although overall cognitive communication status was improving. Seven or eight days after initial admission, she was oriented to person, place, time, and situation. Latent onset of diffuse cerebrovascular vasospasm resulted in severe declines in cognitive status. (See Case 16–7 in Chapter 16 for an expanded version of this case.)

circle of Willis. **Arteriovenous malformations (AVMs)** are an aberrant tangle of arteries and veins that alter blood flow, resulting in ischemia and hypoxia. Aneurysms and AVMs can be identified through a variety of radio imaging tests, including CT, MRI, and cerebral angiography (or CT angiography or MRA).

Traumatic or spontaneous dissections of arteries can result in intracranial hemorrhages as well. These occur when there is a tear in the inner layer of the wall of the artery and blood flows into this false opening, creating a pouch. The dissection weakens the walls of the artery, and the altered blood flow can create blood clots that then flow to the brain and cause a stroke. Clotting disorders or anticlotting (antithrombotic—either anticoagulants or antiplatelet classes) medications can increase the likelihood of spontaneous or traumatic hemorrhages as well. Finally, some metastatic tumors (e.g., renal tumors that metastasize to the brain) have a propensity for bleeding.

Ischemia and hemorrhages elsewhere in the body are labeled and described differently. For instance, cardiac ischemia is known as a myocardial infarction or heart attack. Although speech-language pathologists and audiologists may not deal directly with ischemic events outside of the brain, understanding the potential for concomitant impairments throughout the body is important because susceptibility for vascular impairments is sometimes systemic and not limited to cerebral structures (e.g., a person with a myocardial infarction may also have atrial fibrillation, which places them at risk for shower emboli and cerebral ischemic events/CVA).

Summary

The cerebrovascular system is responsible for the distribution of oxygenated and nutrient-rich blood to brain and spinal structures and thus is essential to the function of those structures. Understanding the source, flow, and distribution of blood supply underlies the understanding of disruptions to that blood supply. Furthermore, understanding functional organization of brain regions aids in identifying probable consequences when blood supply to a particular vascular territory or distribution is disrupted.

Key Concepts

- The vascular system serves the entire body, but the brain is one of the first structures to receive oxygen-rich blood from the heart by way of the aorta and its branches.
- Like branches on a tree, each subsequent vessel within the cerebrovascular system is incrementally smaller than the segment that feeds it. Therefore, final tips and branches of a given vascular territory are small in diameter.
- Terminal branches of blood vessels in the brain overlap with adjacent vascular territories, creating watershed areas.
- Blood supply distributions or vascular territories overlap with functionally organized brain regions, so disruption to a particular distribution or territory results in disruptions to functions of that area.
- Ischemic events, hemorrhages, trauma, and tumors can all disrupt blood supply and perfusion to critical brain tissues.
- Secondary damage includes edema, which can further restrict perfusion.
- The blood–brain barrier is a protective mechanism found within the walls of blood vessels in the brain. It has stacked endothelial cell junctions, which prevent passage of larger molecules and viruses from passing from the bloodstream into the brain.

References and Additional Resources

Blumenfeld, H. (2010). *Neuroanatomy through clinical cases* (pp. 230–237). Sinauer.

Kandell, E., Schwartz, J., & Jessell, T. (2000). *Principles of neural science* (4th ed.). McGraw-Hill.

Nolte, J. (2002). *The human brain: An introduction to its functional neuroanatomy* (pp. 570–573). Mosby.

Park, K. Y., Kim, Y. B., Chung, P. W., Moon, H. S., Suh, B. C., Yoon, K. J., & Lee, Y. T. (2014). Right-side propensity of cardiogenic emboli in acute ischemic stroke with atrial fibrillation. *Scandinavian Cardiovascular Journal, 48*(6), 335–338.

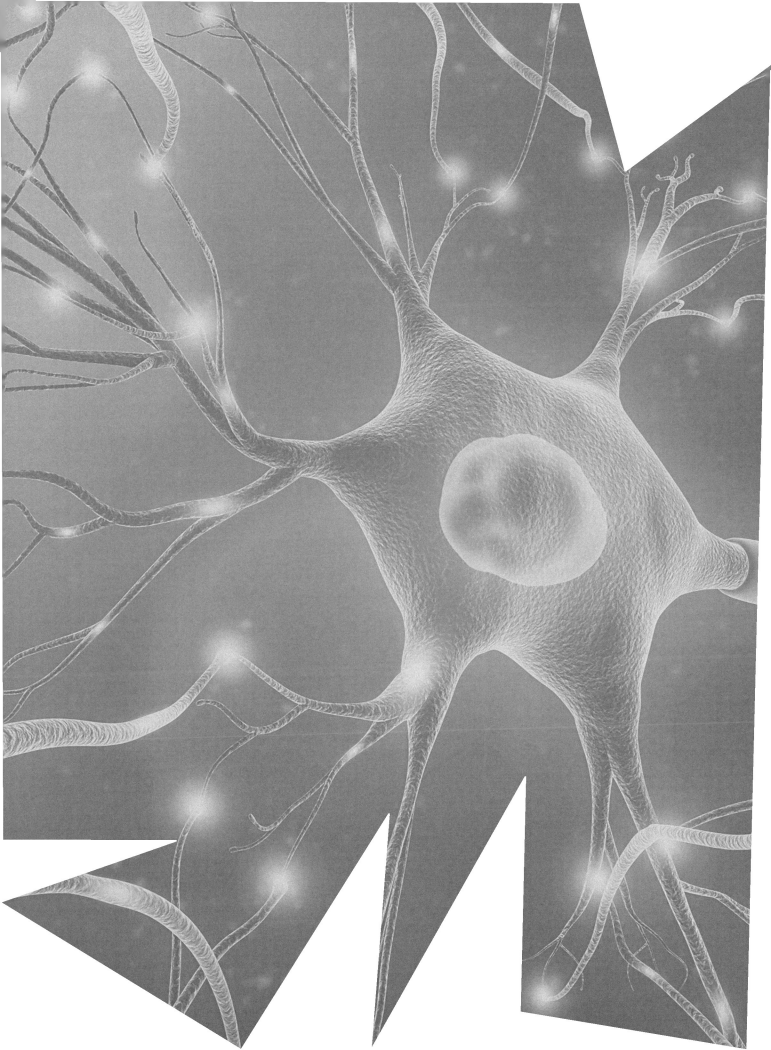

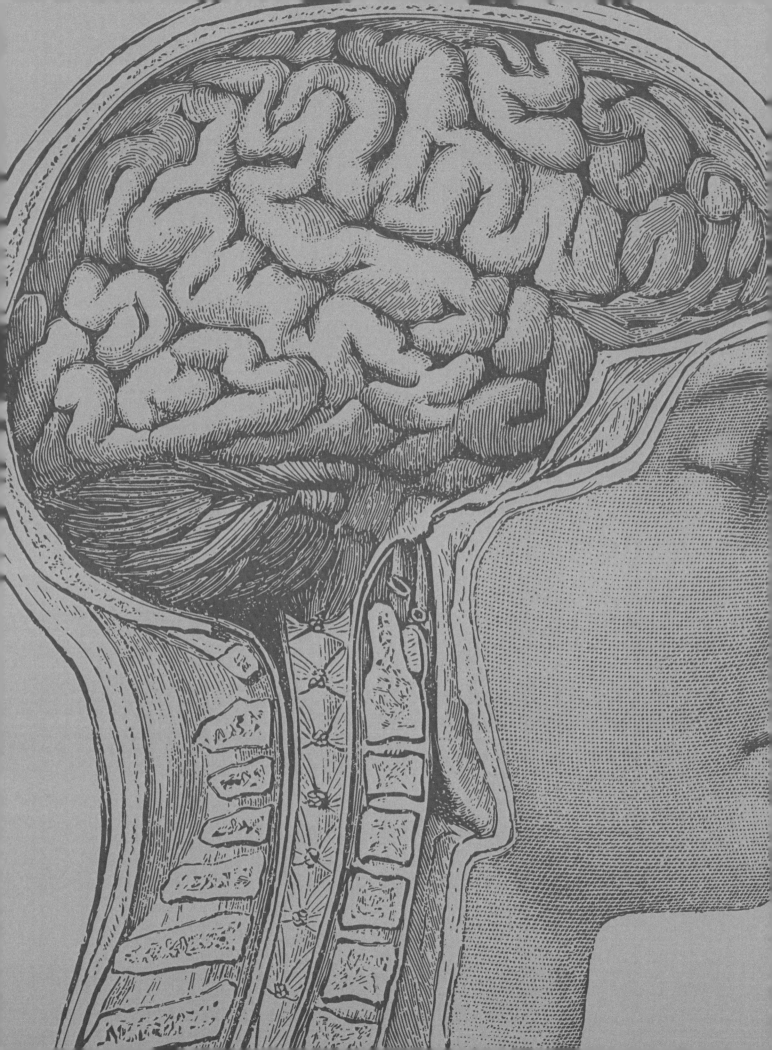

14

Communication and Cognition

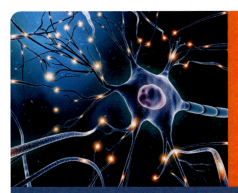

CHAPTER OUTLINE

Overview
Common Developmental Disruptions
   Developmental Language Disorders
   Autism Spectrum Disorder
   Down Syndrome
   Fragile X Syndrome
Common Neurologic Insults and Diseases
   Traumatic Brain Injury
   Degenerative Diseases and Tumors
Communication
   Language
     Networks
     Development
     Lesions and Disorders
   Pragmatics and Social Cognition
     Networks
     Development
     Lesions and Disorders
Cognition
   Executive Functions
     Networks
     Development
     Lesions and Disorders
   Memory
     Networks
     Development
     Lesions and Disorders
   Attention
     Networks
     Development
     Lesions and Disorders
Summary
References and Additional Resources

Overview

The professions of speech-language pathology and audiology focus on assessment and treatment of communication and cognition. A solid grasp of the neurologic underpinnings of development and the impact of neurologic damage on communication and cognition is an important part of understanding the disorders that we diagnose and treat. It is easy to fall into the trap of thinking that neuroanatomy and neurophysiology are important only for acquired disorders you see in adults in medical settings. Understanding development and disruptions to normal development is equally important for providing appropriate services for children because developmental disorders that impact communication rarely affect isolated areas of the nervous system. In addition, children can have acquired neurologic injuries, such as traumatic brain injuries and even strokes. Knowing the timeline of neurodevelopment will provide information about which skills might be affected by neurological damage and which may have been fully developed prior to the injury.

However, there are no clear, one-to-one relationships between complex social, cognitive, and communicative behavior, development, and brain structures (Kilford et al., 2016). Researchers use knowledge of the adult systems to evaluate the functions of developing nervous systems, but with the complexity of social and cognitive networks it is not possible to pinpoint specific structures or connections that explain multifaceted behaviors or developmental processes. In addition, development may be a process of interactive specialization, in which experiences and learning interact with brain maturation (Johnson, 2011), which adds even more complexity. The endpoint of this interactive development is smaller and/or more efficient networks or regions controlling specific functions (Happe & Frith, 2014).

Box 14–1. Kids Have Brains Too

Infants and children through age 4 years have the highest incidence of traumatic brain injuries (TBIs), yet most speech-language pathologists (SLPs) think of adolescents and adults when they hear "TBI." Often in our fields, there is a clear distinction between adult/medical and pediatric/school topics in academic classes and clinical education offerings. But as Ciccia and colleagues (2021) note, this is a false dichotomy and instead there should be a smooth continuum of care between medical SLPs and school SLPs to support children with acquired brain injuries (including not only TBI but also tumors or other neurologic disorders that impact children and teens) so that services can be conducted in a relevant environment: the schools.

The purpose of this chapter is to provide foundational content about networks controlling cognitive and communicative functions, including development of those networks, impacts of common developmental disorders, and the impact of acquired damage. Damage to motor systems affecting voice and speech production resulting in dysarthrias was covered in Chapters 10 and 11, so this chapter focuses on language and cognitive–communication processes.

As has been described in the previous chapters, the location of neurological damage or disruption plays a key role in the resulting disorders or impairments. These are most clearly delineated in the motor system, in which damage to different components or pathways causes different forms of dysarthria (see Chapter 10). Communication and cognition are not so precisely organized, in part because they are more complex processes and rely on inputs from many different regions and systems. Despite this, there are regions of the brain that are more important or have a primary role. The general functions ascribed to the lobes of the brain in Chapter 1 provide a basis for predicting deficits based on location of lesion or disruption.

Common Developmental Disruptions

Developmental neurologic disorders can be divided broadly into prenatal (before birth) and postnatal (after birth) onset. They may interfere with meeting typical developmental timelines or compromise development altogether. Some disorders are inherited, carried within the genetic code of their parents (e.g., Down syndrome, epilepsy, Friedreich ataxia, muscular dystrophy, phenylketonuria, Tay–Sachs disease, and Wilson disease), whereas others (e.g., cerebral palsy, prenatal stroke, and fetal alcohol syndrome) are caused by exposure to environmental conditions or external forces that cause structural damage or disrupt developmental processes. Environmental conditions can include inadequate nutrition, specific nutritional deficiencies (e.g., folic acid), or the presence of drugs or alcohol. A few common developmental syndromes are covered here to provide illustrations of how disruption to neurodevelopment can affect communication and cognitive function.

Developmental Language Disorders

Developmental language disorders (DLDs; previously known as specific language impairment) occur in the absence of other genetic syndromes and cognitive impairments. DLDs were once thought to be the product of environmental factors, including the quality of parental care, subtle brain damage at birth, or hearing impairments (Bishop, 2006). It is now known that they are multifactorial in etiology, and ties to anatomical underpinnings are somewhat more evident. Neural imaging studies have discovered abnormalities in the caudate nuclei, cerebellum, and Broca area (Vargha-Khadem et al., 2005). Children with DLDs also may have greater proportions of white matter compared to typically developing children (Herbert et al., 2004). In most cases, greater volumes of white matter correspond to greater preservation of redundant or less efficient pathways and less selective pruning. That results in breakdowns in efficiency and quality of signaling within language systems that require complex, coordinated signals. Currently, it is not possible to demonstrate a one-to-one correspondence between structural evidence and language impairments.

Autism Spectrum Disorder

Autism spectrum disorder (ASD) is characterized by deficits in social cognition and communication, repetitive behaviors, and restricted areas of interest. It has a strong genetic component. During the first year of life, children who are later diagnosed with ASD undergo a phase of rapid brain growth, resulting in brains that are larger than those of their typically developing peers (Shen & Piven, 2017). This enlarged size is due to increased amounts of white matter, particularly in association tracts within each hemisphere, and greater surface area of gray matter (Herbert et al., 2004). In addition, there is an excessive amount of cerebrospinal fluid (CSF) in the subarachnoid space. The characteristics of neurologic development are associated with behavioral symptoms. The excess CSF occurs at the time that motor deficits are often identified; the increase in cortical surface area in regions associated with somatosensory and attention processing corresponds to emergence of sensory and attention deficits; and the expansion of white matter tracts has been linked to the onset of deficits in social cognition and communication. Studies of ASD also show unexpected patterns of hemispheric asymmetry in some brain areas. In the general population, some areas tend to be larger in the right hemisphere (RH) compared to the left hemisphere (LH) and vice versa. In ASD, many of these areas show reduced amounts of asymmetry so that they are more symmetrical than expected either because they are thinner or because they have less surface area. These include smaller RH fusiform gyrus, superior temporal lobe, and medial orbitofrontal regions and smaller LH isthmus of the cingulate, medial orbitofrontal region, rostral anterior cingulate, rostral middle frontal gyrus, superior frontal lobe, and lateral orbitofrontal gyrus. In contrast, the left putamen showed greater asymmetry, meaning that it was even larger than expected in the ASD groups compared to the right putamen. Although many of these areas are associated with social cognition and communication, because those functions are complex, it is not possible to directly link an asymmetry to a behavior. Nonetheless, these results indicate that the brains of people with ASD do not develop in the same pattern, and the interaction between the two hemispheres may function differently (Postema et al., 2019).

Down Syndrome

Down syndrome (DS) is the result of an extra 21st chromosome (called trisomy 21). Most individuals have some level of intellectual disability, although visuoperceptual skills and visual memory tend to be relatively good (Lott & Diersson, 2010; Martin et al., 2009). Language expression is affected more than comprehension, with impairments primarily in morphosyntax. Phonological development may be slow, and speech production can be affected both by language processing disruptions and by structural differences such as a small oral cavity, enlarged tongue, and altered development of some facial muscles and reduced muscle tone. Pragmatics and social skills tend to be areas of strength.

Brains of people with DS are small, particularly in frontal and temporal lobes, with reduction of the hippocampal volume (Lott, 2012). The cerebellum is also notably small. Despite these reductions, subcortical gray matter, such as the basal ganglia, tends to be within expected limits. At the cellular level, DS is characterized by fewer neurons overall, fewer synapses, and less dendritic branching. The total number of neurons is a result of both reduced neurogenesis and increased neuronal death or pruning. People with DS show neurologic characteristics of Alzheimer disease at approximately age 40 years. Due to the widespread effects of trisomy 21 on neural development and the complexity of cognition and communication, it is not possible to directly tie specific symptoms to isolated neurodevelopmental disruptions.

Fragile X Syndrome

Fragile X syndrome has clearly ascribed genetic underpinnings related to the *FMR1* gene. It is the most common inherited intellectual disability and is known to significantly limit language development (Crawford et al., 2001; Finestack et al., 2009). The reduction of a specific protein (FMRP) leads to disruption of multiple additional proteins that are critical for development of synaptic connections (**synaptogenesis**) and synaptic plasticity (Salcedo-Arellano et al., 2020). It may also play a role in axon guidance (the process of sending out axons to the correct targets) during early neural development. FMRP is found not only in neurons but also in astrocytes, Schwann cells, and oligodendrocytes. It has also been suggested that fragile X affects γ-aminobutyric acid-ergic and glutamanergic synapses, resulting in an imbalance of inhibitory and excitatory signals within the central nervous system. The disruption of FMRP and the consequent effects on the variety of areas it impacts result in intellectual disability and other characteristic features of fragile X. In addition, structural differences can be seen in several regions of the brain. The caudate nucleus and ventricles are enlarged and the vermis of the cerebellum is smaller than typical. The volume of gray matter tends to be decreased in frontal and temporal lobes but increased posteriorly in parietal and occipital lobes.

Fragile X commonly co-occurs with autism and DS. For most children, it is not detected until age 3 or 4 years, when signs of delay in language become prominent. It can be detected through prenatal genetic testing. Although gaps in language ability are small early on, the gaps continue to grow as individuals approach adulthood. This speaks to the severity of language impairments and other cognitive impairments. Cognitive impairments include problems with sequential processing, working memory, and attention. Psychopathology and challenging behaviors are also common, including hyperarousal, hyperactivity, and anxiety (Abbeduto et al., 2005).

Common Neurologic Insults and Diseases

Acquired neurologic disorders can be divided into those with sudden or traumatic onset (stroke, traumatic brain injury) and degenerative diseases with a slow onset and progressive deterioration (Parkinson disease, dementias). As described in Chapter 13, strokes occur suddenly as a result of interruption of blood flow to the brain. The impact of neurologic diseases and disorders on communication and cognition is directly related to the location of the damage.

Traumatic Brain Injury

Traumatic brain injuries are a result of a blow to the head or rapid movement of the head that results in movement of the brain within the skull. The meninges and the CSF within the meningeal layers are designed to prevent the brain from moving within the skull (see Chapter 2). However, in the case of violent movements of the head, the brain can move with enough force to displace the CSF and hit the inner surface of the cranium. The two forms of damage that occur are **contusions** (bruises) or lesions that occur due to impact of the brain against the inner surface of the skull and **diffuse axonal injury** (DAI; also called traumatic axonal injury) caused by tearing or shearing of axons. A secondary mechanism of damage is edema (swelling). As described in Chapter 3, swelling around the directly damaged area causes compression of adjacent tissues, reducing blood flow and the ability of neurons to carry out normal neurophysiological processes, including regulation and restoration of cell membrane potentials before and after discharge.

Linear movement, such as front-to-back or side-to-side, often occurs in motor vehicle accidents or when the head is hit by or against a solid object. These commonly result in contusions both at the point of impact (called a coup injury) and opposite the impact (contrecoup injury) that occur when the brain "rebounds" within the skull and bounces back to impact with the skull a second time. Imagine a car accident in which the driver's head hits the steering wheel. The coup injury in the frontal lobe, where the impact occurred, would be accompanied by a contrecoup injury in the occipital lobe that resulted from the brain rebounding and moving posteriorly after the rapid anterior movement.

Rotational injuries, as the name suggests, occur when the impact causes the head and brain to rotate. The most common result of this head movement is DAI. When the brain rotates, axons are stretched and torn. This leads to degeneration of axons (see Chapter 3). In severe TBIs, damage occurs to axons spread throughout the brain, which is why it is labeled a "diffuse" injury.

Another cause of diffuse brain injury is **hypoxia** (reduced oxygen) or **anoxia** (absence of oxygen) when the supply of oxygen to the brain is severely reduced or cut off for a period of time (see Chapter 13). Remember from Chapter 3 that neurons cannot store oxygen, so they are dependent on the vascular system to provide a continuous supply of oxygen. Hypoxia can be caused by stopping or reducing the blood supply to the brain as occurs in a heart attack. It also occurs with carbon monoxide poisoning, when carbon monoxide attaches to blood cells instead of oxygen, or from reduced oxygenation of the blood that can occur with emphysema or at high altitudes with low environmental oxygen levels.

Degenerative Diseases and Tumors

Degenerative neurologic diseases most commonly are a result of interruption of neuronal function in specific regions. As described in Chapters 3 and 10, diseases can affect the myelin (multiple sclerosis), neurotransmitter systems (Parkinson disease), synaptic function (myasthenia gravis), or the neurons themselves (amyotrophic lateral sclerosis, Alzheimer and other dementias). Another form of degenerative disease is vascular dementia, which is the result of multiple small strokes. Symptoms may not be apparent initially because the region of damage is quite small. Over time, however, the amount of brain tissue that is no longer functional adds up and symptoms become apparent. Tumors also generally have a progressive course: As a tumor grows and impacts neuronal function either by interrupting normal functions or creating pressure on neural tissue, cognitive and communication functions will progressively deteriorate. Onset of degenerative diseases and tumors is typically insidious (gradual), with subtle changes initially leading to more debilitating effects over time. Recognition of early signs and symptoms by SLPs and audiologists can lead to more effective management of these disorders.

To understand how neural structures are affected by dementia, it is necessary to delineate classifications of dementia. Classifications are based on the type of pathology: **proteinopathies** (i.e., the presence of abnormal protein aggregates found in neurons, glial cells, and extracellular fluid) versus **vascular dementia** etiologies and **mixed dementias** (Elahi & Miller, 2017). Each proteinopathy is associated with vulnerability to damage in particular parts of the brain. There are four types of proteinopathies: prion-related dementia, Alzheimer dementias, frontotemporal dementias, and Lewy body dementia. Note that proteinopathies can be primarily cortical or subcortical in distribution or both. Dementias such as Alzheimer dementia and frontotemporal dementia, once thought to be fairly homogeneous, are now recognized as quite heterogeneous. Table 14–1 presents the types and pathology distributions.

Vascular dementias affect the patency of vessels of all diameters (large and small vessels), resulting in hemorrhages, infarcts, and white matter damage (i.e., demyelination, axonal damage, and astrocytosis). There are three main vascular subtypes: cerebral atherosclerosis, small vessel disease (SVD), and cerebral amyloid angiopathy (Grinberg & Thal, 2010). All subtypes can lead to ischemic infarcts and hemorrhages. Atherosclerosis involves large- to medium-diameter arteries, frequently including vessels of the circle of Willis. Involvement of small vessels is commonly seen as well with co-occurring SVD. Chronic cerebral SVD is caused by a problem with blood–brain barrier dysfunction that can cause cortical and subcortical microinfarcts, white matter disease, and hippocampal atrophy. Watershed regions are particularly susceptible to SVD. Cerebral amyloid angiopathy is characterized by deposits of amyloid β-protein in cerebral and leptomeningeal vessels (including arteries, veins, and capillaries). These deposits can result in ischemia, hemorrhage, and angiitis (swelling of the vessel walls). Although these three subtypes are distinct, they correlate/co-occur with each other and with Alzheimer dementia.

Mixed dementias include more than one type. The most common co-occurrence is Alzheimer and vascular dementias.

Communication

Human communication involves not only *what* we say (the sounds, words, and sentences) but also *how* we say it (the intonation or prosody and the accompanying body language and facial expression) and the way that the "what" and the "how" are interpreted by another person. This interpretation may take into consideration *where* and *when* it was said (in what context or setting and in response to what) and *why* it was said (what the person meant or wanted to communicate), determined in part by the speaker's knowledge, beliefs, and perspectives.

All of the components are interconnected and rely on extensive networks within the brain. However, different domains of communication can be roughly localized to different areas of the brain. The LH is primarily in charge of what we say. **Phonology** (sounds), **morphology** (minimal units of meaning), and **syntax** (rules for combining words into sentences) are controlled almost exclusively by the LH in most humans. The LH is the primary site of **semantics** (word meanings), although the RH also plays a role. The RH is predominantly in charge of the "how" of communication. This is the domain of **pragmatics**, or the use and interpretation of language and communication within context. Pragmatics, as described later in this chapter, includes not only words and sentences but also prosody and nonverbal cues. The interpretation of communication is part of **social cognition**, which is controlled by a bilateral network situated primarily in the frontal lobes with extensions to temporal and parietal lobes. The right/left distinction for communication is true for approximately 90% of the population. In the remainder, some people have more equal distribution across the two hemispheres or even a reversal of roles.

The LH's role in basic language functions is the reason it is often called the "dominant hemisphere." This label is misleading and inaccurate unless used very narrowly to refer to basic language control. The RH has a substantial role in communication, and both hemispheres share sensorimotor control of the body. Indeed, the RH plays a dominant role in visuoperception and some forms of attention. Human communication and cognition are a result of intricate and continuous connections between the hemispheres.

Table 14–1. Types and Pathologies of Proteinopathic Dementias

Classification	Subtypes	Cortical	Subcortical	Brain Regions Affected
Prion	Creutzfeld–Jakob disease (CJD)	✓	✓	Cortex, basal ganglia, thalamus, cerebellum (potentially throughout the central nervous system—primarily gray matter)
	Fatal familial insomnia (FFI)			
	Gerstmann–Sträussler–Scheinker disease (GSS)			
Alzheimer	Amnestic	✓		Medial temporal lobe, entorhinal cortex
	Behavioral and dysexecutive	✓		Prefrontal cortices, entorhinal cortex
	Logopenic primary progressive aphasia (PPA)	✓		Left middle posterior temporal gyrus, angular gyrus, precuneus, hippocampus, left inferior parietal
	Visuoperceptive	✓		Right inferior parietal, posterior temporal
	Posterior cortical atrophy	✓		Parietal, occipital and occipitotemporal cortices
Frontotemporal	Behavioral	✓		Orbitomedial prefrontal cortices and anterior temporal lobes
	Nonfluent primary progressive aphasia (PPA)	✓		Left inferior frontal gyrus, supplementary motor area, motor strip, insula
	Semantic primary progressive aphasia (PPA)	✓		Anterior temporal lobe bilaterally (left > right)
	Frontotemporal dementia with motor neuron disease (FTD-MND)	✓		Frontal and temporal lobes, hypoglossal nucleus motor neurons, spinal motor neurons
	Corticobasal degeneration (CBD)	✓	✓	Superior frontoparietal regions, primary motor and somatosensory cortices, anterior corpus callosum, putamen, median substantia nigra
	Progressive supranuclear palsy (PSP)		✓	Subthalamic nucleus, globus pallidus, striatum, red nucleus, substantia nigra, pontine tegmentum, oculomotor nucleus, medulla, dentate nucleus
Lewy body	Lewy body dementia (LBD)		✓	Basal ganglia, subthalamic nucleus, substantia nigra, globus pallidus, brainstem
	Parkinson dementia			

Language

Networks

Language is a complex process, carried out by networks of neurons in a distributed process. Most of these are within the **peri-sylvian region** of the LH. In discussing language areas of the brain, it is important to begin with the caveat that although those discrete brain regions are involved in language production and comprehension, language cannot be isolated to those areas (Figure 14–1). Separating speech (motoric production of sounds) from language (set of symbols to convey meaning) with regard to anatomical substrates is difficult, given their interconnectedness. Current models of LH language processing suggest that language is processed through two crucial pathways—the dorsal and ventral streams (Figure 14–2). In this dual-stream model, the **dorsal stream** consists of the arcuate fasciculus (AF)/superior longitudinal fasciculus (SLF), which carries information about **phonological processing** from the posterosuperior temporal to the inferior frontal cortices (Chang et al., 2015). The dorsal stream connects the frontal, parietal, and temporal lobes in order to convert voices to phonemes, retrieve words, repeat words, and articulate words. This pathway carries information about the motor aspects of speech, including the mapping of phonological processes to articulation. A second component of this pathway is involved in learning new vocabulary. Converting sounds into phonemes occurs in the superior temporal gyrus (STG), which is adjacent to the Heschl gyrus (Fujii et al., 2016). The STG also has a role in auditory short-term memory. The posterior STG is connected to the supramarginal gyrus via the AF/SLF. Phonological processing occurs in association with the precentral gyrus, AF/SLF, and Broca area (Fujii et al., 2016). The left middle–inferior precentral gyrus and subcortical fibers have a key role in articulation.

Semantic processing is carried through the **ventral stream** through the inferior fronto-occipital fasciculus (IFOF) and intratemporal networks (Chang et al., 2015). The middle temporal gyrus (MTG) has a role in assigning meaning to the word and lexical access. Specifically, the posterior MTG accesses the lexicon through connections to comprehension and expression via the AF, including word selection and phonemic processing for production (Fujii et al., 2016). The anterior MTG is involved in semantic processing and word selection. Integration of phonological and semantic word processing is carried out by the intratemporal network, which includes the middle longitudinal fasciculus, inferior longitudinal fasciculus, IFOF, and other short association fibers.

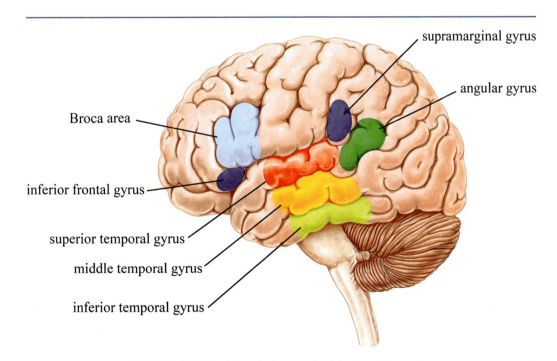

FIGURE 14–1. Left hemisphere peri-sylvian language areas.

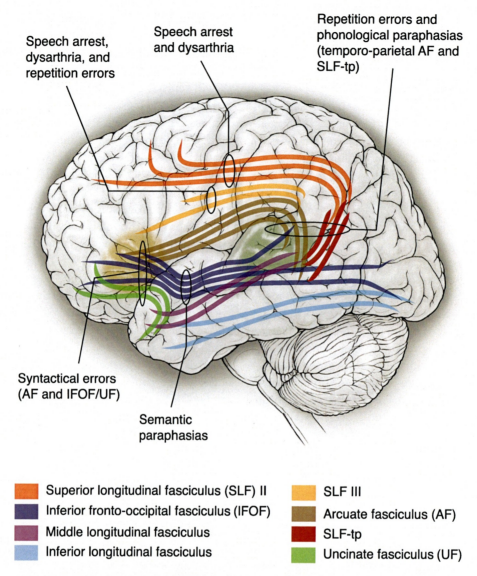

FIGURE 14–2. Model of left hemisphere language networks. *Source:* Reused with permission. Copyright 2015 Dr. Edward Chang. Chang, E. F., Raygor, K. P., & Berger, M. S. (2015). Contemporary model of language organization: An overview for neurosurgeons. *Journal of Neurosurgery, 122*(2), 250–261.

Lexical processing is not isolated to the temporal lobe, particularly in more complex contexts, such as sentences and discourse. The inferior parietal lobule and inferior frontal gyrus have a role in processing syntax, contextual semantics, and word selection in association with semantic memory. This suggests that language comprehension and expression are integrated. Indeed, the IFOF is an important structure for this integration. Another crucial tract, the frontal aslant tract (FAT), connects the supplementary motor area to Broca area, playing an important role in initiating speech and speech spontaneity. The intrafrontal network or FAT connects the medial aspect of the frontal lobes, the inferior frontal gyrus, and the middle–inferior portion of the precentral gyrus. Hickok and Poeppel (2007) argue that speech perception and comprehension are processed bilaterally, based on evidence from stroke studies, Wada tests, and functional imaging. As described later, lesion-based and functional imaging studies have identified the RH as having a role in interpreting prosodic features, particularly emotional tone (Chang et al., 2015).

Box 14–2. Dorsal and Ventral Streams in Multiple Modalities

There are at least four different systems that involve dual pathways, one more dorsal and one more ventral. In the visual system (see Chapter 7), the dorsal pathway is the "where" pathway, situating visual images within space, whereas the ventral pathway is the "what" pathway, responsible for recognition and identification of visual images. Language processing is also processed through two pathways: The dorsal stream predominantly controls the motor aspects of speech, word learning, and retrieval of words, whereas the ventral stream is important for semantics or word meanings. There are also dorsal and ventral streams for processing emotional prosody in the RH. Similar to the LH language areas, the dorsal stream and anterior regions process production of emotional prosody and the ventral stream and posterior areas process emotional prosody recognition and comprehension. Finally, attention functions are controlled through the dorsal attentional network responsible for sustained attention, whereas the ventral attention network responds to unexpected or salient stimuli.

Development

Describing anatomical underpinnings of language from a developmental standpoint is challenging. Much of our knowledge of language function comes from adults, and much of that information is based on lesion studies. Most positron emission tomography studies in children are conducted with clinical populations, so it is questionable whether these findings apply to typically developing children. Functional magnetic resonance imaging has been identified as a safe tool for examining language development in typically developing children and will continue to provide important evidence about the neural underpinnings of language development.

Our understanding of development of language areas in the brain is still fairly limited, but evidence suggests that in infants and small children, neural activity during language tasks occurs in both LH peri-sylvian language areas and the RH homologs of those areas. Synaptic density peaks at 3 months in the auditory cortex and at 15 months in the middle frontal gyrus (Huttenlocher & Dabholkar, 1997). Synaptogenesis and pruning occur during the critical period for language development (Thompson & Nelson, 2001), along with myelination (Figure 14–3). Together, these processes improve the speed and efficiency of neuronal connections.

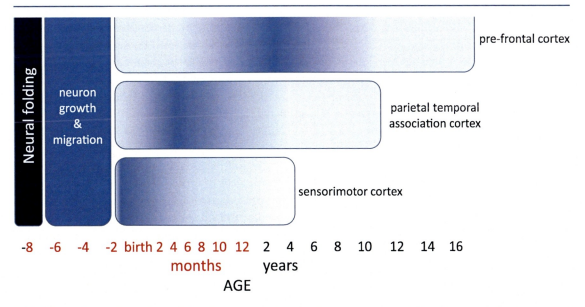

FIGURE 14–3. Timeline of neural development. Darker shading represents peak time frames of development of different systems.

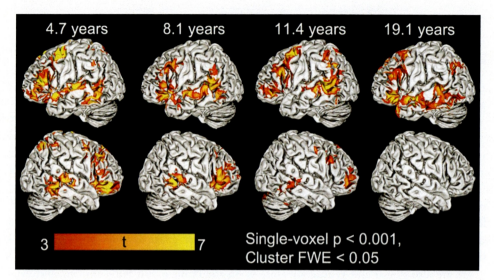

FIGURE 14–4. Left and right hemisphere language activation over time. Language activation maps from different age groups show right hemisphere activation is strong in young children but decreases over time, with little activation in adults. *Source*: Olulade et al. (2020).

Over time, language processing becomes more lateralized to the LH (Figure 14–4) so that by adulthood, there is limited, if any, activation of the RH during imaging studies of basic language processing (Basser, 1962; Lenneberg, 1967; Olulade et al., 2020). This is particularly true for areas traditionally associated with language, such as the frontal regions (e.g., Broca area) and posterior temporal areas (e.g., Wernicke area and the angular gyrus). Lesions to either the RH or LH in prelingual children (aged 18–24 months) are equally likely to cause language impairments, suggesting that lateralization continues to progress through early childhood. In addition, LH activation becomes more focused in peri-sylvian areas, which has been interpreted as increasing efficiency of the language networks (Szaflarski et al., 2006).

Lesions and Disorders

Aphasia is a language disorder associated with damage to the left cerebral hemisphere. It is characterized by impairments in naming (e.g., finding the right word), repetition, fluency of language production, and comprehension of language. Types of aphasia are defined by patterns of strengths and weaknesses across these areas of impairment (Table 14–2). The location of damage within the language networks is related to the pattern of deficit. This chapter is not designed to prepare you for differential diagnosis of types of aphasia but, rather, to link neurologic function with language abilities. Figure 14–5 shows approximate lesion locations that result in different forms of aphasia. Importantly, aphasia types cannot be isolated discretely into the cortical regions shown in the figure. Damage to other areas not shown in the figure, such as the thalamus, basal ganglia, and cerebellum, can also result in aphasia. For those who are interested in learning more about aphasias, see References and Additional Resources.

As described previously, the peri-sylvian language areas are highly interconnected, but there are regions that are more responsible for certain language functions. Damage to the dorsal language stream network causes sound-based word errors (called phonemic paraphasias) and impairments of repetition and auditory short-term memory.

Lesions to motor areas that are part of the language network, such as middle and inferior precentral gyrus, anterior precentral gyrus (Brodmann area 4), and premotor areas (Brodmann area 6), impact speech and language production, including motor programming for speech (a disorder called apraxia of speech), the inability to initiate speech (anarthria), disruptions to expressive linguistic prosody, and distortions of phonemes (Fujii et al., 2016).

Disruptions to the ventral pathway result in errors related to lexical concepts, syntax, morphosyntax, and speech recognition. Although damage to these regions accounts for most disruptions to naming, damage to both the temporal and parietal areas has been associated with naming dysfunction (Chang et al., 2015).

Table 14–2. Types of Aphasia and Language Characteristics

	Fluent?	Good Comprehension?	Good Repetition?
Global aphasia	No	No	No
Mixed transcortical	No	No	Yes
Broca aphasia	No	Yes	No
Transcortical motor	No	Yes	Yes
Wernicke aphasia	Yes	No	No
Transcortical sensory	Yes	No	Yes
Conduction	Yes	Yes	No
Anomic	Yes	Yes	Yes

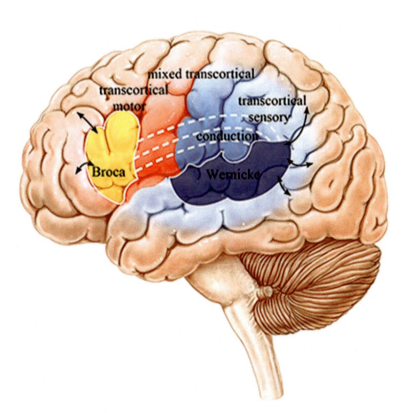

FIGURE 14–5. Location of damage and aphasia type based on language impairments.

Pragmatics and Social Cognition

Pragmatics is one of the five domains of language (along with phonology, morphology, syntax, and semantics). It involves "conveying meaning or intent within a specific context through **linguistic** (word and syntactic selection), **paralinguistic** (vocal manipulation), and **extralinguistic** (posture, facial expression, gestures, eye contact) components" (Minga et al., 2021). The linguistic aspect has to do with the choice of words and syntactic construction based on the social situation. Use of syntactic slang or profane language with friends but not co-workers is one example. Telling your friend she looks "glowing" versus "sweaty" in order not to offend her is another example. Paralinguistics is the use of intonation or prosody. This includes grammatical prosody used to differentiate homophonic nouns from verbs (*con*flict versus con*flict*), mark clause or sentence boundaries, or differentiate questions from statements or commands; pragmatic prosody that includes signaling turn-taking or emphatic stress to highlight new or important information; and emotional prosody. Finally, extralinguistics are the nonverbal cues that convey meaning, such as body language, gestures, eye contact, and facial expressions.

Pragmatics goes hand in hand with social cognition, which, as defined by Cornwell et al. (2021), is

> a set of cognitive processes that allow us to attend to, recognize, and interpret the broad contexts in which communication occurs. It includes recognition and interpretation of emotional/affective cues, theory of mind, and social inferential reasoning to integrate all of the components into a gestalt.

With good social cognition, we can correctly interpret people's intended meaning by integrating what they say with how and when and where they say it. One component of social cognition is **theory of mind**, which is the ability to understand that other people think and feel differently than you do. With good **cognitive theory of mind**, you are aware that other people have thoughts, ideas, perspectives, and knowledge that might differ from your own. Good **affective theory of mind** allows you to be aware that other people have feelings and emotions that might differ from your own.

Networks

Several fairly extensive, bilateral networks have been described that control pragmatics, social cognition, and emotion. As you might suspect from the similar nature and integrated functions of these processes, their neural networks physically overlap to some extent.

Pragmatic networks connect multiple lobes across both hemispheres. The **mentalizing network**, responsible for theory of mind processing, extends throughout the frontal, temporal, and parietal lobes (Figure 14–6). The more ventral regions, including the inferior frontal gyrus, ventromedial prefrontal cortex, and orbitofrontal cortex, are important for affective (emotional) processing, whereas the more dorsal regions (dorsomedial and dorsolateral prefrontal, dorsal anterior cingulate, superior temporal sulcus, and temporoparietal junction) have been linked to cognitive theory of mind.

The **empathy network** overlaps the social cognition networks and includes the dorsal and anterior cingulate gyrus, insula, and supplementary motor areas. The RH component appears to be more important for emotional empathy (sharing another person's feelings or emotions) and the LH component for cognitive empathy (understanding another person's feelings or emotions).

Emotional processing was one of the earliest functions attributed to the RH. The right frontal (inferior frontal gyrus, frontal operculum, orbitofrontal, and dorsolateral frontal cortex), temporal, and anterior insula cortices are important for emotional processing. Subcortical structures including the amygdala and portions of the basal ganglia and thalamus also are part of the emotional networks. Left hemisphere regions including the pars orbitalis segment of the inferior frontal gyrus, anterior insula, and amygdala also are involved in emotional processing. These may be associated with different stages of processing.

Right hemisphere networks for production and comprehension of emotional prosody (Figure 14–7) roughly follow the dual-stream pattern of language processing networks (Zezinka Durfee et al., 2021; Schirmer & Kotz, 2006). Emotional prosody production is controlled by a dorsal stream that involves the orbitofrontal cortex, supramarginal gyrus, and the underlying white matter including the superior longitudinal fasciculus. In contrast, emotional prosody comprehension is processed in a ventral stream that involves the posterior superior temporal lobe. The ventral white matter tracts, the inferior fronto-occipital fasciculus, and the uncinate fasciculus appear to be involved in both comprehension and production, similar to their function in language processing in the LH. Again, similar to the LH, anterior peri-sylvian lesions in the RH often result in expressive deficits, whereas more posterior lesions affect comprehension.

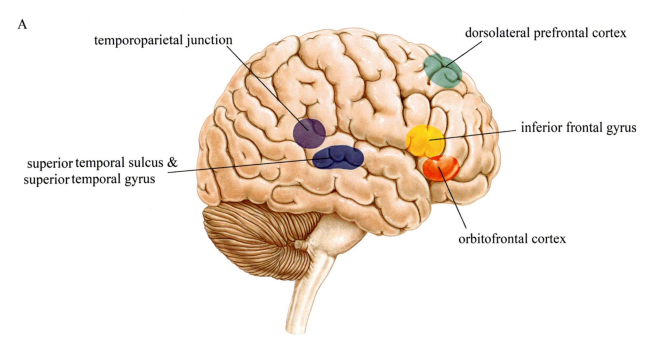
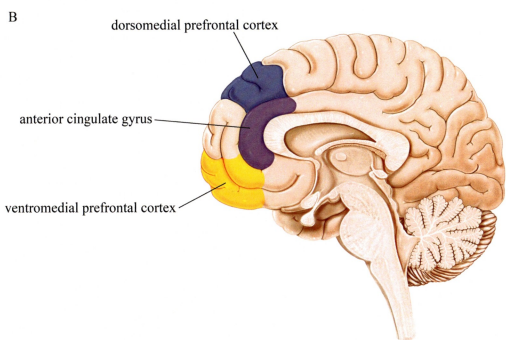

FIGURE 14–6. Right hemisphere areas involved in cognitive (*cool colors*, more dorsal regions) and affective (*warm colors*, more ventral regions) theory of mind.

Development

Differences in the structure and function of the RH and LH occur early in development. Growth of the cerebral hemispheres, in terms of volume and gray matter density, is not linear but, rather, there are multiple spurts of development of lobes as well as hemispheres (Chiron et al., 1997; Remer et al., 2017). Hemispheric development may occur in a cyclical manner (Thatcher, 1997), with alternating growth spurts in the RH and LH. Some studies suggest

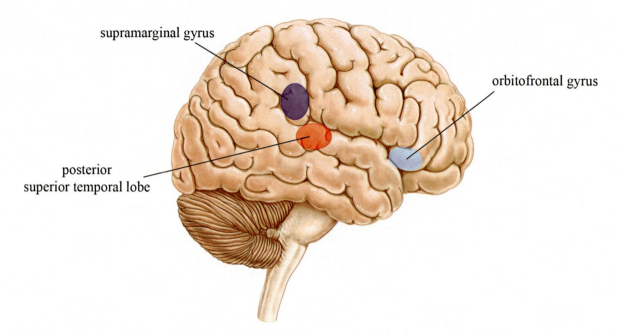

FIGURE 14–7. Right hemisphere regions involved in emotional prosody production (*cool colors*, more dorsal regions) and comprehension (*warm colors*, more ventral regions).

that the RH develops more rapidly immediately after birth, whereas the LH continues to develop over a longer period of time. An example of the nonlinear hemispheric development can be seen in face processing. At birth, infants are RH dominant for face processing. This lateralization disappears around age 5 years (Lochy et al., 2019). Throughout childhood, the RH and LH both have roles in recognition of emotional faces, but eventually this ability becomes lateralized to the right (Kilford et al., 2016; Lochy et al., 2019).

Social development begins with detecting and recognizing others; mimicking their expressions, voices, and behaviors; and developing affiliations with them (Happe & Frith, 2014). RH dominance for face processing has been noted in infancy and in fact may be critical for developing the ability to recognize faces (Le Grand et al., 2003). At approximately 3 months of age, infants more consistently respond to attention-seeking behaviors, such as responding to their name or direct eye contact. These responses involve the medial prefrontal cortex, right inferior frontal gyrus, superior temporal gyrus, amygdala, and fusiform gyrus. Joint attention, which is crucial to socialization, develops between ages 6 and 18 months. Initially, infants begin to respond to joint attention cues; this involves primarily posterior attentional regions such as the posterior superior temporal sulcus, temporoparietal junction, and posterior parietal association areas (Caruana, 2015; Mundy & Newell, 2007). They then develop the ability to initiate joint attention, which involves more anterior attention and social network regions such as the frontal eye fields, prefrontal association areas, dorsal anterior cingulate, dorsomedial and orbitofrontal prefrontal cortex, anterior temporal cortex, and inferior frontal gyrus. There is evidence that the RH is more involved in joint attention than the LH (Caruana, 2015).

The basic theory of mind network is established at approximately age 4 years (Kilford et al., 2016), with continued development through adolescence. The volume of gray matter within this network decreases between adolescence and adulthood, likely due to increasing efficiency of the connections. Processing of emotions involves the amygdala and the dorsolateral and orbital prefrontal cortices (Blakemore & Chourdhury, 2006). The anterior temporal cortex also is involved in integrating social and emotional cues. As with the social networks, the ability to interpret intent or meaning continues to develop through the teenage years.

Lesions and Disorders

Disruptions to the social cognition and mentalizing networks have been implicated in ASDs and schizophrenia

(Sugranyes et al., 2011). Reduced activation or function of areas within the network results in the characteristic symptoms of each of these disorders.

Right hemisphere damage (RHD) is most often caused by stroke, but it also can be a result of a tumor or relatively focal TBI. The resulting deficits are primarily pragmatic in nature and can be characterized by inefficient communication and deficits in understanding intended meaning. Typical communication deficits include disorganized, tangential, and overpersonalized discourse (e.g., stories or conversations); difficulties determining the gist or main idea; difficulties generating inferences and interpreting nonliteral language; poor theory of mind; reduced empathy; and reduced affect and emotional responses. Expressive and/or receptive aprosodia is fairly common after RH strokes, primarily affecting emotional prosody. In addition, cognitive deficits impacting executive function, attention, and memory are common. These are discussed further in the following section on cognition.

With the exception of the anterior–posterior sites for expressive and receptive prosody, there is no clear localization of communicative function within the RH. This means that unlike in the LH, damage to one area of the RH does not provide useful information in predicting what deficits may occur. There also are no clear subtypes of RHD (as there are subtypes of aphasia) or deficits that co-occur on a regular basis. One reason may be that the communication abilities of the RH are controlled by large networks, such as the mentalizing and social cognition networks. The RH has more white matter than the LH, suggesting that it is more highly interconnected.

Cognition

Cognitive functions include executive function, attention, and memory. They underlie communication, including language. Because of this, they are commonly assessed and treated by SLPs and of interest to audiologists.

Executive Functions

Executive functions are novel, context-dependent, and goal-oriented behaviors, controlled predominantly by the prefrontal cortices but with extensive input to and from other cortical areas. Several cognitive functions are encompassed under the umbrella of executive functions. These include inhibition, self-regulation, self-monitoring, cognitive flexibility, and problem-solving. Reasoning, insight, and judgment also can be considered executive functions, or closely related to them. Working memory is necessary to carry out executive functions because it includes short-term memory, mental workspace to manipulate information, and filtering (Figure 14–8).

Daily behaviors are typically a mix of those that are relatively automatic and those that require thought, consideration, and tap into executive functions. For most adults, making coffee or tea in the morning is relatively automatic. But if you have a new coffee maker, or if you find you are out of tea, you will have to engage executive functions for reasoning and problem-solving your way to a solution. Similarly, getting to school or work generally is automatic, but if you get in your car and find your battery has died, or that you have lost your prepaid subway card, you have to consider your goal and determine the best course of action. In relation to communication, effective conversations are dependent on the ability to take another person's perspectives (theory of mind), hold information in short-term memory in order to formulate a response, inhibit immediate reactions, and alter a response to achieve social niceties.

Networks

The prefrontal lobes are extensively connected to nearly all other regions of the cerebrum. They have connections to basal ganglia and thalami, the limbic system, and the other cerebral lobes. There is extensive variety in the specifics of suggested executive function networks as well as their

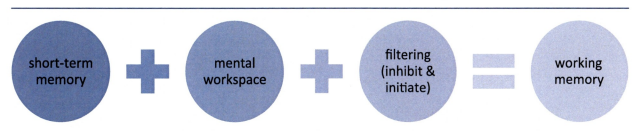

FIGURE 14–8. Conceptualization of working memory.

names (e.g., central executive network, working memory network, cognitive control network, and frontoparietal network). For purposes here, it is sufficient to know that there are extensive frontotemporal and frontoparietal connections and connections with the limbic system. Regarding the latter, the extensive connections between the hypothalamus, limbic system, and frontal lobes are responsible for the fact that internal factors such as pain, hunger, thirst, fear, and fatigue can influence performance on executive function tasks. Recall the last time you were really tired or emotional (either positive or negative) and had to make an important decision or find your way out of a difficult situation. It may have felt like you could not think straight or you could not get your head around all of the factors that had to be considered because your limbic system was interfering with your executive functions. Emotional demands deplete working memory and thus alter our ability to carry out executive functions.

Development

As described in Chapter 4, the prefrontal cortex is the last to develop and the first to decline with typical aging. Executive functions such as inhibitory control, decision-making, selective attention, and working memory continue to develop throughout childhood and into the late teens (Blakemore & Chourdhury, 2006). Evidence from neuropsychology suggests that the prefrontal cortex is susceptible to age-related declines (Daigneault et al., 1992; Daigneault & Braun, 1993). White matter changes account for most typical, age-related changes (Svennerholm et al., 1994; Peters et al., 1996; Salat et al., 1999). In other words, breakdown in myelination and signaling efficiency accounts for declines in working memory, naming, and complex problem-solving.

Lesions and Disorders

The frontal lobes, particularly the prefrontal areas, are commonly damaged in TBI. Thus, it should be no surprise that executive function deficits are some of the most common deficits resulting from TBI. The deficits include disinhibition; poor self-awareness and self-monitoring; and reduced problem-solving, reasoning, organization, and working memory. The severity of the deficits depends on the extent of the brain injury. With mild TBI, some individuals are able to live independently and only notice difficulties when they are in unexpected situations or when they are fatigued or emotional. People with more severe TBIs may not be safe to live alone because they cannot monitor their behaviors or take into account all of the relevant factors needed to make safe, reasonable decisions. Regardless of injury severity, complexity and intensity of task demands, environment, and emotions disrupt working memory and thus alter ability to carry out executive functions. This accounts for discrepancies in performance across contexts with stronger performance under less demands. Most individuals have a threshold for level of demands and once that is eclipsed, they experience across-the-board cuts to available working memory, leading to significant declines in their performance.

Individuals with RHD often are diagnosed with executive function deficits. This could be related to anterior RH strokes that interrupt frontal lobe cognitive processes or to damage to the inputs to the executive function systems.

Although this chapter is not designed to cover assessment of cognition, some insight into the challenges of assessment highlights the nature of executive functions. As described previously, executive functions are context-dependent. Standardized assessments are typically designed to remove extraneous variables and take place in clinical contexts in order to attempt to ensure that the variable being measured is isolated. However, pulling a person out of the complex environment, reducing emotional and social demands, and narrowing the scope of task complexity eliminate the need for good executive functioning. When the person is told to do a specific task in a specific way, given all of the tools needed to complete the task, and stops when they are told to stop, they no longer have to determine how to solve the problem, figure out what to do if they do not have the necessary tools, or monitor time constraints.

In dealing with executive function deficits, there is often a difference between knowing and doing. When presented with a hypothetical problem, a person may be able to explain exactly what to do to solve the problem. However, when put into an actual situation in which that same problem occurs, they may not be able to carry out a logical plan—even the one they provided—because the real situation is more complicated and involves actions, responses, and controlling emotions. Box 14–3 presents an illustration of the concept of knowing versus doing and the problems with hypothetical questions.

Memory

Memory can be classified into different types based on the content of what is stored. **Declarative** memories are

> **Box 14–3.** Bob Knew Better
>
> Bob was a 62-year-old farmer who lived in a remote, rural area. One morning, he began to experience severe chest pain and collapsed on the kitchen floor. His wife and son were present and immediately began CPR after he went into cardiac arrest. Emergency medical services was called and arrived on the scene approximately 15 to 20 minutes after CPR was initiated. Upon admission to a regional medical center, it was clear that along with a myocardial infarction (heart attack), Bob had suffered a diffuse hypoxic brain injury. After rehabilitation, he returned home to his family farm but did not return to working the farm. One morning, while drinking a cup of coffee and looking out the kitchen window, he noticed a couple of his beef cattle were outside of the pasture. This was a clear indication that the electric fence was down.
>
> As a lifelong farmer, Bob knew what to do, and if he had been asked, he would have explained how to begin with fixing the breach and then turning the electric fence back on. But the hypoxic brain injury compromised his ability to use executive functions. What did Bob do in that moment? He jumped on an ATV (which he was no longer allowed to operate) and began to chase after the cattle that left the pasture in an attempt to redirect them back. In the meantime, more cattle began to leave the pasture. Several minutes later, he returned to the farmhouse, not having been successful returning any of the cattle to the pasture. He met a perplexed and concerned son at the door who asked, "What happened?" Demands of the moment clearly eclipsed his capacity to access declarative knowledge and implement it in the moment.

explicit, conscious memories. They can be either **semantic** (fact-based) or **episodic** (experience-based). **Nondeclarative** memories are those that are learned unconsciously and often involve actions or behaviors. **Procedural** memory, or the ability to remember how to do something (even if you can't explain it to someone else), is a type of nondeclarative memory. When people refer to *muscle memory*, they are referring to a form of nondeclarative memory. **Meta-memory** is one's knowledge about their own memory abilities. Knowing that you have a good memory for song titles but not bands is meta-memory. **Prospective** memory is the ability to remember to do something in the future: to mail letters on your way to work or to reschedule your dentist appointment after their office opens are examples of prospective memory. Table 14–3 lists cortical regions associated with these different types of memory.

Networks

Memory can be broken down into four stages: **encoding**, **consolidation**, **storage**, and **retrieval**. Encoding involves thinking about and analyzing the information. It can include visualization, linking the information to previous knowledge or experiences, chunking, or other strategies to increase the likelihood that the information can be retrieved correctly in the future. It is controlled primarily by the frontal lobes with input from other modality-specific areas (temporal lobe for auditory, occipital lobe for visual, and parietal lobe for somatosensory cues). The second stage is consolidation. This is the process of changing short-term memories into long-term memories. Consolidation occurs primarily in the hippocampus in the medial temporal lobes. In the third stage, storage, memories are stored for future retrieval. Storage may occur in the temporal lobes or in modality-specific regions of the cortex. The fourth stage is retrieval. In this stage, the information is accessed from where it is stored. The frontal lobes again play a major role in this stage. Components of executive function, such as self-monitoring and problem-solving, can assist in retrieving and verifying memories.

Development

Episodic memories are a function of the anterior medial temporal lobe. Because they are not fully developed until later in childhood, children younger than age 2 years are unable to store episodic or autobiographical memories. This phenomenon is called infantile amnesia (Lavenex & Lavenex, 2013). For the next 3 to 5 years, children have some ability to form episodic memories, although effective recall does not mature until full, postnatal maturation occurs. Maturation of working memory is positively correlated with development of the prefrontal–parietal networks (Nagy et al., 2004; Olesen et al., 2003). Lateralization of verbal working memory to the LH and visual working memory to the RH is established during adolescence

Table 14–3. Regions Associated With Memory Function

Region	Processes	RH	LH
Hippocampus	Storage, episodic memory	X (especially spatial)	X (especially verbal)
Inferior frontal	Working memory, episodic memory	Recollection, familiarity	
Prefrontal region	Encoding, retrieval (episodic and semantic), working memory	Episodic retrieval, confidence in memory judgments, working memory	Episodic and semantic encoding, semantic retrieval
Parietal lobe	Episodic retrieval, experience of remembering	X	X
Basal ganglia	Working memory, declarative retrieval	X	X
Lingual gyrus	Declarative retrieval		X
Cerebellum	Working memory	X	

Source: From *The Right Hemisphere and Disorders of Cognition and Communication: Theory and Clinical Practice* (p. 195) by Margaret Lehman Blake. Copyright © 2018 Plural Publishing. All rights reserved.

(Nagel, 2013). Prospective memory develops throughout childhood but then stalls at approximately ages 10 to 12 years before improving again into the late teenage years (Blakemore & Chourdhury, 2006).

Lesions and Disorders

Memory disorders are called **amnesias**. **Retrograde amnesia** is the loss of memories prior to a brain injury, whereas **anterograde amnesia** is the inability (or reduced ability) to lay down new memories. Following a TBI, the term **posttraumatic amnesia** (PTA) is used to describe a period of anterograde amnesia after the trauma to the brain. After TBI, most people experience a window of amnesia surrounding the event. They may not remember the minutes or hours prior to the event or the minutes, hours, or days following the event. As the brain heals, sometimes this window shrinks, but for some people there will always be a gap in their memories. This period of amnesia may occur because during the event the encoding systems were dysfunctional and those memories were never encoded.

Box 14–4. What's Your Favorite Video Game?

Tyrone was a 16-year-old male who sustained a severe TBI in a high-speed car crash. When he emerged from his coma, the SLP began asking him orientation questions to monitor his emergence from PTA. Along with questions about his name, where he was, what day it was, and why he was there, the SLP asked a friendly question about what he likes to do. He said, "I like to play video games." Not surprised that a 16-year-old would say that, the SLP asked a follow-up question: "What's your favorite video game?" Tyrone's response was an indicator of the severity of his retrograde amnesia. "Winnie the Pooh is my favorite." Guessing that Pooh was his favorite at age 4 years, that is 12 years of retrograde amnesia. Over time, as orientation and memory recovered, that window of retrograde amnesia decreased markedly.

Memory can be affected by strokes, tumors, and TBI. Damage to either RH or LH and frontal, parietal, or temporal lobes can result in memory deficits. Because memory is dependent on both attention and executive function, deficits to either of those processes can impact memory. In general, LH damage is more likely to impair verbal memory, whereas RH damage is more likely to affect visual memory. Procedural memory is the least likely to be affected by acquired brain injury, whereas prospective memory deficits are quite common.

Attention

Attention is the ability to focus on a stimulus. It is critical for learning and memory, as well as efficient and effective communication. Clinically, attention is classified into several types. Focused attention is the ability to attend to a stimulus when there are no distractions present. Sustained attention is holding that focus over time. Selective attention is when you can focus even when distractions are present, and you ignore or inhibit the distractions. Alternating attention involves switching your focus between two different stimuli or tasks. Divided attention involves splitting attention between two different stimuli or tasks.

> **Box 14–5. Divided Versus Alternating Attention**
>
> True divided attention is possible only when two tasks use different subsystems, such as motor and language, and at least one of the tasks is automatic (requiring very little attention). Carrying on a conversation while driving is possible because the motoric act of driving is so automatic that it takes little attention and the driver can focus on the communication task. When you're driving in an unfamiliar area, or in bad weather, you'll notice that you stop talking or stop listening. This is because driving is no longer automatic. When two tasks share a common subsystem, such as listening in a virtual meeting and reading the comments in the chat box, you'll find that you're actually alternating attention between listening and reading. This is often ineffective because information is missed when your attention is directed elsewhere.

Networks

There are three major bilateral attention networks (Table 14–4) that control focused and sustained attention. Alternating and divided attention additionally engage frontal networks for executive control (dorsolateral prefrontal cortex and anterior cingulate with connections to thalamus, basal ganglia, and cerebellum) and posterior parietal regions involved with shifting attentional focus. The networks have individual functions, but they are interconnected and can influence each other. The **default mode network** is active when someone is at rest, not necessarily thinking of anything specific. It underlies thinking about your past and your future, or just letting your mind drift. It is centered in the frontal lobes, specifically the ventromedial and dorsolateral prefrontal cortices, with connections to the cingulate gyrus and the intraparietal sulcus.

The **dorsal attention network** (DAN) is critical for sustained attention and focused attention directed to the contralateral space. Thus, the LH directs attention to the right side of space and vice versa. The DAN is situated primarily in the dorsal parietal lobes with connections to the frontal eye fields through the superior longitudinal fasciculus. Strategic attention, such as noticing patterns and predicting when stimuli will occur, is controlled by the DAN.

The **ventral attention network** (VAN), although bilateral, is more strongly represented in the RH. The VAN allows you to notice stimuli that have important, distinctive, or relevant features. The VAN includes the middle and inferior frontal gyri, the anterior insula, the superior temporal gyrus and sulcus, the temporoparietal junction, and the ventral supramarginal gyrus. Like the DAN, many of the sites are connected by axons in the superior longitudinal fasciculus.

Finally, there is an attention control network involving the dorsolateral prefrontal cortex and dorsal anterior cingulate with connections to the thalamus, basal ganglia, and cerebellum. This network is involved in alternating and dividing attention as well as controlling responses when there is a conflict between the stimulus and the response (e.g., respond to a green light but not a red light).

Development

Attentional development has been studied primarily in the visual system. The developing attentional system involves three components: alerting, orienting, and attentional executive control (Graziano et al., 2011; Reynolds

Table 14–4. Frontoparietal Attentional Networks

Network	Function	Primary Regions
Default Mode Network	Broad-based activation in the absence of a specific task. Allows stimulus-free thoughts such as autobiographical memory, thinking about the future, or thinking about other people's perspectives.	Bilateral network. Ventromedial and dorsolateral prefrontal cortices. Posterior cingulate gyrus. Intraparietal sulcus.
Dorsal Attention Network	Sustained attention. Top-down attentional processes directed toward the contralateral visual field.	Bilateral network. Frontal eye fields. Dorsal parietal lobes (intraparietal sulcus and superior parietal lobule). Connected by axon tracts within the superior longitudinal fasciculus.
Ventral Attention Network	Attention to unexpected but relevant stimuli. Bottom-up attentional processes for salient, distinctive, or relevant stimuli.	Primarily right hemisphere. Middle and inferior frontal gyri. Anterior insula. Temporoparietal junction. Superior temporal gyrus and sulcus. Ventral supramarginal gyrus. Connected by axon tracts within the superior longitudinal fasciculus.

Source: From *The Right Hemisphere and Disorders of Cognition and Communication: Theory and Clinical Practice* (p. 108) by Margaret Lehman Blake. Copyright © 2018 Plural Publishing. All rights reserved.

Box 14–6. Attentional Processing

A 34-year-old female had an occipital lobe stroke that damaged geniculocalcarine fibers and resulted in a homonymous upper left quadrantanopia. In the weeks after the stroke, she found it difficult to concentrate, especially during reading. Although she quickly learned to shift her eyes in order to read the words that fell within her visual field cut, her comprehension was poor and reading was laborious. An initial guess might be that she had attentional deficits. Another explanation could be that the attention system was not damaged but, rather, overloaded. She was learning a new visual scanning pattern to compensate for her visual field cut and had to pay attention to where her eyes and head were moving. She also had to pay greater attention to the words on the page and the meaning in order to determine if she might have missed something. All of the tasks that used to be automatic now required focused and sustained attention. Because of this, she had less attentional capacity for comprehension processes. Over time, as she adapted to the missing region of her visual field, the compensatory movements became more automatic, and her brain began ignoring the gray splotches in the upper left quadrant of her visual fields, she was able to resume all of her prior activities. Within 5 years of her stroke, she reported that she had fully "recovered" from her stroke, although there had been no repair to the visual fields. The impairment was exactly as bad as it was the day after her stroke, but her recovery was complete because she had fully adapted to the damage and it no longer affected any part of her daily life.

& Romano, 2016; Rueda & Posner, 2013). As previously described for the joint attention network, posterior regions are responsible for automatic orienting and responding, whereas anterior regions control goal-directed attention.

Alerting is present at birth and involves aspects of wakefulness and arousal. This system allows infants to fixate on visual stimuli, but it is primarily reflexive. Within a few weeks, infants begin to develop orienting abilities that allow them to select and track items within their visual field. Orienting is driven by a posterior network that includes the posterior parietal lobe that drives the ability to disengage from one stimulus, the pulvinar, and the frontal eye fields that control voluntary saccades (quick "jumps" of the eye from one fixation point to another).

The anterior executive control network begins developing at approximately age 6 months and continues throughout childhood. This network is responsible for sustained attention and dealing with conflicts of thoughts, feelings, and behaviors. For example, the ability to differentially respond to stimuli (e.g., push a button when you see a green light but do nothing when you see a red light) is linked to the executive control network. At approximately age 4 years (48 months), this network is fairly well established, but increases in the efficiency of attentional control continue through at least age 10 years (Jones et al., 2003; Federico et al., 2017).

Lesions and Disorders

Stroke and TBI commonly cause significant deficits in attention. All of the clinical types (focused, sustained, divided, etc.) can be affected. Because attention to stimuli is necessary for all other cognitive and communication processes, attentional deficits can have wide-ranging effects.

One striking attentional deficit is unilateral neglect, in which a person does not attend to stimuli in one region of space. It most commonly affects visuospatial processing and occurs most often after damage to the RH. Explanations of unilateral neglect implicate both the DAN (reducing the ability to ignore distractors) and the VAN (reduced attention to distinctive features) or the way they impact each other (damage to the right VAN could affect the function of the left DAN).

A person with visuospatial neglect may not read the left page of a book, may not realize someone else is in the room if they are standing to the person's left, may not realize that there is a cup of coffee on the left side of a tray, or may only eat food on the right side of the plate (Figure 14–9). Unilateral neglect is one of the classic deficits associated with RH damage. This is because it is so striking when it occurs, even though other communication deficits are more common than unilateral neglect, particularly beyond the acute phase/first few days of recovery.

Summary

Communication and cognition are core human abilities. They are controlled through multiple complex networks that allow integration of cues from multiple sources to be processed in various areas of the brain. Developmental disorders typically impact multiple cognitive and communication systems, and although gross structural differences are found, it is difficult to directly correlate structural differences with specific cognitive or communication deficits.

Acquired brain injuries, particularly from stroke, result in focal injuries that can impact specific components of communication or cognition.

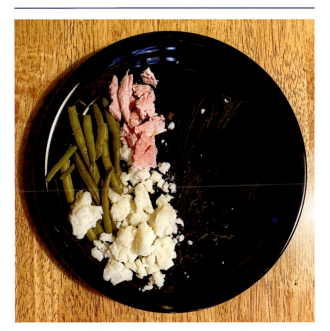

FIGURE 14–9. Consequences of unilateral neglect.

Key Concepts

- Communication involves not only what you say (language) but also how you say it (pragmatics) and how you interact with others (social cognition).
- The dual-stream model of language includes a dorsal stream, responsible for phonological processing (sound characteristics) and motor control, and a ventral stream, responsible for semantic processing (meaning-making) and comprehension.
- Pragmatics and social cognition are controlled by extensive, bilateral networks that extend throughout the frontal, temporal, and parietal lobes.
- The emotional prosody network includes a dorsal, frontal-based stream responsible for production and a ventral, temporoparietal-based region responsible for identification and comprehension.
- Executive function networks are situated primarily in the frontal lobes. Memory networks rely heavily on temporal lobe structures, and attentional networks are dependent on parietal lobe regions.
- Left hemisphere damage can cause aphasia, a disorder of language production and comprehension.
- Right hemisphere damage can cause cognitive–communication deficits that include emotional aprosodia and disorders of pragmatics, social cognition, and attention.
- Traumatic brain injury can affect all aspects of cognition and communication in various ways, depending on the location and extent of damage. Attention, memory, and executive function are most commonly affected.

References and Additional Resources

Abbeduto, L., Chapman, R. S., Fletcher, P., & Miller, J. (2005). Language development in Down syndrome and fragile X syndrome. *Trends in Language Acquisition Research, 4*, 53–72.

Basser, L. S. (1962). Hemiplegia of early onset and the faculty of speech with special reference to the effects of hemispherectomy. *Brain 85*, 427–460.

Bishop, D. V. (2006). What causes specific language impairment in children? *Current Directions in Psychological Science, 15*(5), 217–221.

Blakemore, S. J., & Choudhury, S. (2006). Development of the adolescent brain: Implications for executive function and social cognition. *Journal of Child Psychology and Psychiatry and Allied Disciplines, 47*(3–4), 296–312. https://doi.org/10.1111/j.1469-7610.2006.01611.x

Caruana, N., Brock, J., & Woolgar, A. (2015). A frontotemporoparietal network common to initiating and responding to joint attention bids. *NeuroImage, 108*, 34–46. https://doi.org/10.1016/j.neuroimage.2014.12.041

Chang, E. F., Raygor, K. P., & Berger, M. S. (2015). Contemporary model of language organization: An overview for neurosurgeons. *Journal of Neurosurgery, 122*(2), 250–261.

Chiron, C., Jambaque, I., Nabbout, R., Lounes, R., Syrota, A., & Dulac, O. (1997). The right brain hemisphere is dominant in human infants. *Brain, 120*(6), 1057–1065. https://doi.org/10.1093/brain/120.6.1057

Ciccia, A. H., Lundine, J. P., O'Brien, K. H., Salley, J., Krusen, S., Wilson, B., . . . Haarbauer-Krupa, J. (2021). Understanding cognitive communication needs in pediatric traumatic brain injury: Issues identified at the 2020 International Cognitive-Communication Disorders Conference. *American Journal of Speech-Language Pathology, 30*(2S), 853–862. https://doi.org/10.1044/2020_AJSLP-20-00077

Cornwell, P., Hewetson, R., Blake, M., Johnson, M., Minga, J., & Sheppard, S. (2021). *Mum you have to realise it is NOT dad, not the way he used to be": Exploring the theoretical constructs of social communication impairment after right hemisphere damage (RHD).* Oral Presentation at the 6th Pacific Rim Virtual Conference (INS, ASSBI, CCN), Melbourne Australia.

Crawford, D. C., Acuña, J. M., & Sherman, S. L. (2001). FMR1 and the fragile X syndrome: human genome epidemiology review. *Genetics in Medicine, 3*(5), 359–371.

Daigneault, S., Braun, C. M., & Whitaker, H. A. (1992). Early effects of normal aging on perseverative and non-perseverative prefrontal measures. *Developmental Neuropsychology, 8*(1), 99–114.

Daigneault, S., & Braun, C. M. (1993). Working memory and the self-ordered pointing task: Further evidence of early prefrontal decline in normal aging. *Journal of Clinical and Experimental Neuropsychology, 15*(6), 881–895.

Elahi, F. M., & Miller, B. L. (2017). A clinicopathological approach to the diagnosis of dementia. *Nature Reviews Neurology, 13*(8), 457.

Federico, F., Marotta, A., Martella, D., & Casagrande, M. (2017). Development in attention functions and social processing: Evidence from the Attention Network Test. *British Journal of Developmental Psychology, 35*(2), 169–185. https://doi.org/10.1111/bjdp.12154

Finestack, L. H., Richmond, E. K., & Abbeduto, L. (2009). Language development in individuals with fragile X syndrome. *Topics in Language Disorders, 29*(2), 133.

Fujii, M., Maesawa, S., Ishiai, S., Iwami, K., Futamura, M., & Saito, K. (2016). Neural basis of language: An overview of an evolving model. *Neurologia Medico-Chirurgica, 56*(7), 379–386. https://doi.org/10.2176/nmc.ra.2016-0014

Goodale, M. A., & Milner, A. D. (1992). Separate visual pathways for perception and action. *Trends in Neuroscience, 15*, 20–25.

Graziano, P. A., Calkins, S. D., & Keane, S. P. (2011). Sustained attention development during the toddlerhood to preschool period: Associations with toddlers' emotion regulation strategies and maternal behavior. *Infant and Child Development, 20*, 389–408. https://doi.org/10.1002/icd.731

Grinberg, L. T., & Thal, D. R. (2010). Vascular pathology in the aged human brain. *Acta Neuropathologica, 119*(3), 277–290.

Happé, F., & Frith, U. (2014). Annual research review: Towards a developmental neuroscience of atypical social cognition. *Journal of Child Psychology and Psychiatry and Allied Disciplines, 55*(6), 553–577. https://doi.org/10.1111/jcpp.12162

Herbert, M. R., Zieler, D. A., Makris, N., Filipek, P. A., Kemper, T. L., Normandin, J. J., . . . Caviness, V. S. (2004). Localization of white matter volume increase in autism and developmental language disorder. *Annals of Neurology, 55*, 530–540.

Hickok, G., & Poeppel, D. (2007). The cortical organization of speech processing. *Nature Reviews Neuroscience, 8*(5), 393–402. https://doi.org/10.1038/nrn2113

Huttenlocher, P. R., & Dabholkar, A. S. (1997). Regional differences in synaptogenesis in human cerebral cortex. *Journal of Comparative Neurology, 387*(2), 167–178.

Johnson, M. H. (2011). Interactive specialization: A domain-general framework for human functional brain development? *Developmental Cognitive Neuroscience, 1*(1), 7–21. https://doi.org/10.1016/j.dcn.2010.07.003

Jones, L. B., Rothbart, M. K., & Posner, M. I. (2003). Development of executive attention in preschool children. *Developmental Science, 6*(5), 498–504. https://doi.org/10.1111/1467-7687.00307

Kilford, E. J., Garrett, E., & Blakemore, S. J. (2016). The development of social cognition in adolescence: An integrated perspective. *Neuroscience and Biobehavioral Reviews, 70*, 106–120. https://doi.org/10.1016/j.neubiorev.2016.08.016

Lavenex, P., & Lavenex, P. B. (2013). Building hippocampal circuits to learn and remember: insights into the development of human memory. *Behavioural Brain Research, 254*, 8–21.

Le Grand, R., Mondloch, C. J., Maurer, D., & Brent, H. P. (2003). Expert face processing requires visual input to the right hemisphere during infancy. *Nature Neuroscience, 6*(10), 1108–1112. https://doi.org/10.1038/nn1121

Lenneberg, E. (1967). *Biological foundations of language.* Wiley.

Lochy, A., de Heering, A., & Rossion, B. (2019, March). The nonlinear development of the right hemispheric specialization for human face perception. *Neuropsychologia, 126*, 10–19. https://doi.org/10.1016/j.neuropsychologia.2017.06.029

Lott, I. T. (2012). Neurological phenotypes for Down syndrome across the life span. *Progress in Brain Research, 197*, 101–121.

Lott, I. T., & Dierssen, M. (2010). Cognitive deficits and associated neurological complications in individuals with Down's syndrome. *The Lancet Neurology, 9*(6), 623–633.

Martin, G. E., Klusek, J., Estigarribia, B., & Roberts, J. E. (2009). Language characteristics of individuals with Down syndrome. *Topics in Language Disorders, 29*(2), 112–132. https://doi.org/10.1097/TLD.0b013e3181a71fe1

Minga, J., Sheppard, S., Johnson, M., Hewetson, R., Cornwell, P., & Blake, M. (2021). *Apragmatism: The renewal of a label for communication disorders associated with right hemisphere brain damage.* Presentation at the American Speech-Language-Hearing Convention, Washington DC.

Mundy, P., & Newell, L. (2007). Attention, joint attention, and social cognition. *Current Directions in Psychological Science, 16*(5), 269–274. https://doi.org/10.1111/j.1467-8721.2007.00518.x

Nagel, B. J., Herting, M. M., Maxwell, E. C., Bruno, R., & Fair, D. (2013). Hemispheric lateralization of verbal and spatial working memory during adolescence. *Brain and Cognition, 82*(1), 58–68. https://doi.org/10.1016/j.bandc.2013.02.007

Nagy, Z., Westerberg, H., & Klingberg, T. (2004). Maturation of white matter is associated with the development of cognitive functions during childhood. *Journal of Cognitive Neuroscience, 16*(7), 1227–1233.

Olesen, P. J., Nagy, Z., Westerberg, H., & Klingberg, T. (2003). Combined analysis of DTI and fMRI data reveals a joint maturation of white and grey matter in a fronto-parietal network. *Cognitive Brain Research, 18*(1), 48–57.

Olulade, O. A., Seydell-Greenwald, A., Chambers, C. E., Turkeltaub, P. E., Dromerick, A. W., Berl, M. M., . . . Newport, E. L. (2020). The neural basis of language development: Changes in lateralization over age. *Proceedings of the National Academy of Sciences, 117*(38), 23477–23483.

Peters, A., Rosene, D. L., Moss, M. B., Kemper, T. L., Abraham, C. R., Tigges, J., & Albert, M. S. (1996). Neurobiological bases of age-related cognitive decline in the rhesus monkey. *Journal of Neuropathology & Experimental Neurology, 55*(8), 861–874.

Postema, M. C., Van Rooij, D., Anagnostou, E., Arango, C., Auzias, G., Behrmann, M., . . . Francks, C. (2019). Altered structural brain asymmetry in autism spectrum disorder in a study of 54 datasets. *Nature Communications, 10*(1), 1–12.

Remer, J., Croteau-Chonka, E., Dean, D. C., D'Arpino, S., Dirks, H., Whiley, D., & Deoni, S. C. L. (2017, April). Quantifying cortical development in typically developing toddlers and young children, 1–6 years of age. *NeuroImage, 153*, 246–261. https://doi.org/10.1016/j.neuroimage.2017.04.010

Reynolds, G. D., & Romano, A. C. (2016, March). The development of attention systems and working memory in infancy. *Frontiers in Systems Neuroscience, 10*, 1–12. https://doi.org/10.3389/fnsys.2016.00015

Richards, J. E., Reynolds, G. D., & Courage, M. L. (2010). The neural bases of infant attention. *Current Directions in Psychological Science, 19*(1), 41–46. https://doi.org/10.1177/0963721409360003

Rueda, M. R., & Posner, M. I. (2013). Development of attention networks. In P. D. Zelazo (Ed.), *Oxford library of psychology: The Oxford handbook of developmental psychology* (pp. 683–705). Oxford University Press. https://doi.org/10.4992/pacjpa.74.0_sl005

Salat, D. H., Kaye, J. A., & Janowsky, J. S. (1999). Prefrontal gray and white matter volumes in healthy aging and Alzheimer disease. *Archives of Neurology, 56*(3), 338–344.

Salcedo-Arellano, M. J., Dufour, B., McLennan, Y., Martinez-Cerdeno, V., & Hagerman, R. (2020). Fragile X syndrome and associated disorders: Clinical aspects and pathology. *Neurobiological Disorders, 136*, 1–19. https://doi.org/10.1016/j.nbd.2020.104740

Schirmer, A., & Kotz, S. A. (2006). Beyond the right hemisphere: Brain mechanisms mediating vocal emotional processing. *Trends in Cognitive Sciences, 10*(1), 24–30. https://doi.org/10.1016/j.tics.2005.11.009

Shen, M. D., & Piven, J. (2017). Brain and behavior development in autism from birth through infancy. *Dialogues in Clinical Neuroscience, 19*(4), 325–333. https://doi.org/10.31887/dcns.2017.19.4/mshen

Sugranyes, G., Kyriakopoulos, M., Corrigall, R., Taylor, E., & Frangou, S. (2011). Autism spectrum disorders and schizophrenia: Meta-analysis of the neural correlates of social cognition. *PLoS ONE, 6*(10). https://doi.org/10.1371/journal.pone.0025322

Svennerholm, L., Boström, K., Jungbjer, B., & Olsson, L. (1994). Membrane lipids of adult human brain: Lipid composition of frontal and temporal lobe in subjects of age 20 to 100 years. *Journal of Neurochemistry, 63*(5), 1802–1811.

Szaflarski, J. P., Holland, S. K., Schmithorst, V. J., & Byars, A. W. (2006). fMRI study of language lateralization in children and adults. *Human Brain Mapping, 27*(3), 202–212.

Thatcher, R. W. (1992). Cyclic cortical reorganization during early childhood. *Brain and Cognition, 20*(1), 24–50. https://doi.org/10.1016/0278-2626(92)90060-Y

Thompson, R. A., & Nelson, C. A. (2001). Developmental science and the media: Early brain development. *American Psychologist, 56*(1), 5.

Vargha-Khadem, F., Gadian, D. G., Copp, A., & Mishkin, M. (2005). FOXP2 and the neuroanatomy of speech and language. *Nature Reviews Neuroscience, 6*(2), 131–138.

Zezinka Durfee, A., Sheppard, S. M., Blake, M. L., & Hillis, A. E. (*in press*). Lesion loci of impaired affective prosody: A systematic review of evidence from stroke. *Brain and Cognition.*

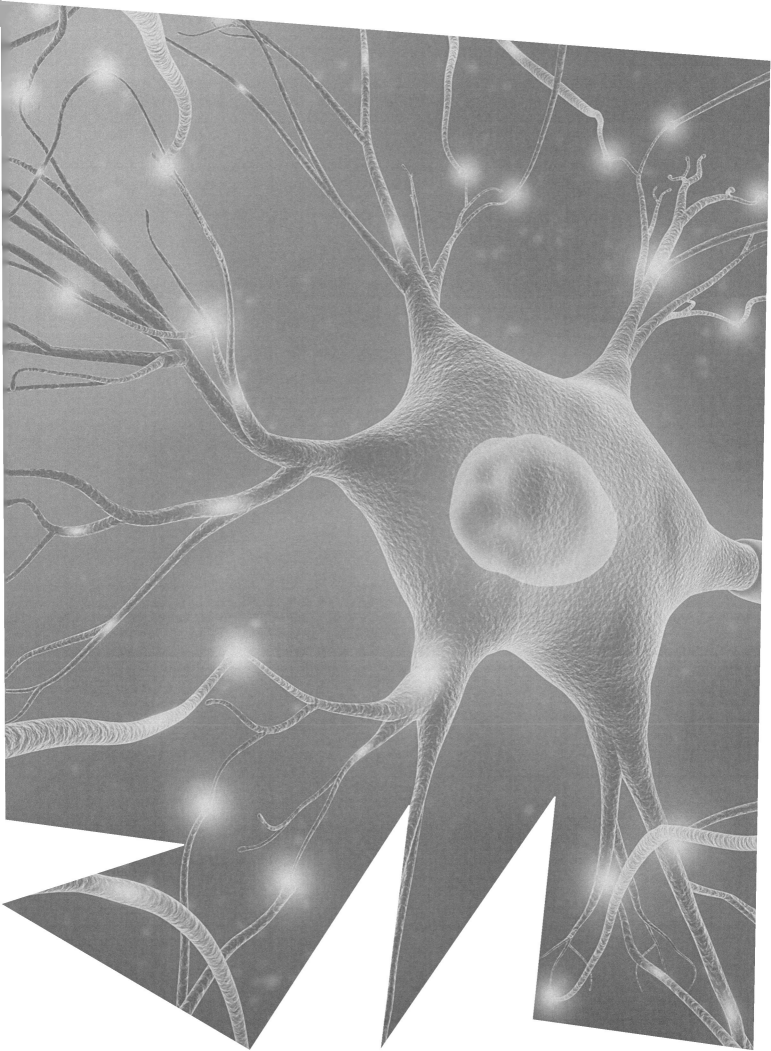

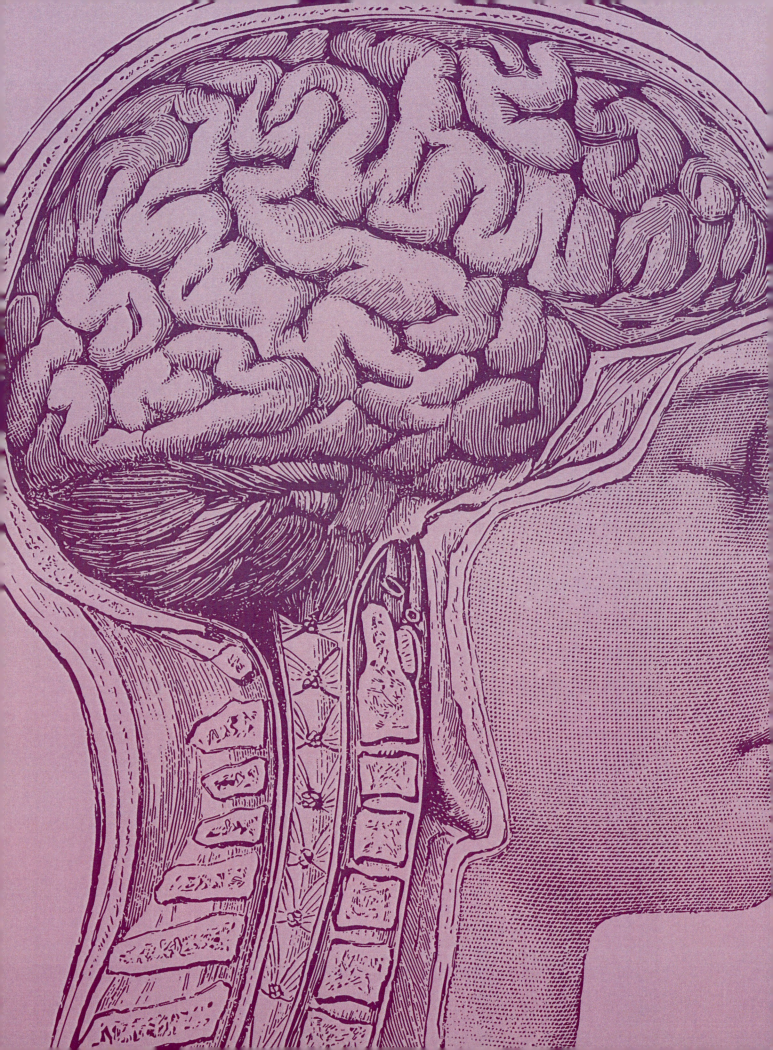

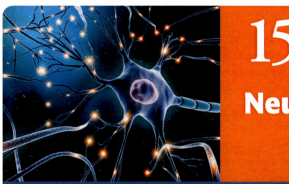

15
Neuroplasticity

CHAPTER OUTLINE

Overview
Neural (Cellular) Plasticity
Behavioral Plasticity
  Intensity and Dosage
  Factors That Contribute to Participation

Functional Reactivation Versus Functional
    Reorganization
Summary
References and Additional Resources

Overview

Neuroplasticity, or the nervous system's ability to change, is a complex construct, and there has been much recent focus on molecular, cellular, and behavioral components. The intent of this chapter is not to address the full breadth of that work but to summarize and highlight pertinent applications of neuroplasticity to the everyday clinical work of speech-language pathologists and audiologists.

There are two main types of plasticity—**neural** and **behavioral**. Other forms of neuroplasticity that relate to recovery after neurological insults are discussed later in this chapter. Neural or microplasticity takes place on the cellular level. Behavioral or macroplasticity relates to changes in function. There is debate as to whether neural (cellular) plasticity drives behavioral plasticity versus behavioral plasticity (changes in participation) driving changes at the cellular level. Regardless of your perspective, understanding a bit about plasticity at both levels is crucial to understanding plasticity's role in development and rehabilitation. Plasticity is highest during development and declines with age, although there are transient increases in plasticity following nervous system injury. However, it is important to recognize that all brains are capable of change due to plasticity. In other words, you do not need to be young or have a lesion for the brain to be able to change. Plasticity has applications to normal development and aging, as much as it does to disrupted development or acquired lesions. In simple terms, we are what we do, or at least a product of what we do, our genes, and the environment in which we live. As we develop, pathways are myelinated and selectively pruned, leading to more efficient signaling. Sensory and motor cortices are pruned soon after birth; association cortices and the corpus callosum follow, and pruning occurs last for the prefrontal cortices (Levitt, 2003). Not all plasticity relates to neural circuitry. Vascular plasticity is also known to have a role in development and post-lesion recovery. Much like neuronal pathways develop and are pruned, vascular supplies develop and prune both pre- and postnatally (Korn & Augustin, 2015) in a process called angiogenesis (Harb et al., 2013).

Neural (Cellular) Plasticity

At the cellular level, the process of increasing neuroplasticity starts with strengthening synapses and networks of synapses. This process is known as **long-term potentiation (LTP)**. Patterns of activity (i.e., doing things consistently over time) lead to patterns of neuron stimulation, which is crucial for a plastic (adaptable) nervous system. Activation of pathways leads to two forms of LTP—early and late LTP (Figure 15–1 provides for a step-by-step depiction of the algorithm for activation and driving neuroplastic

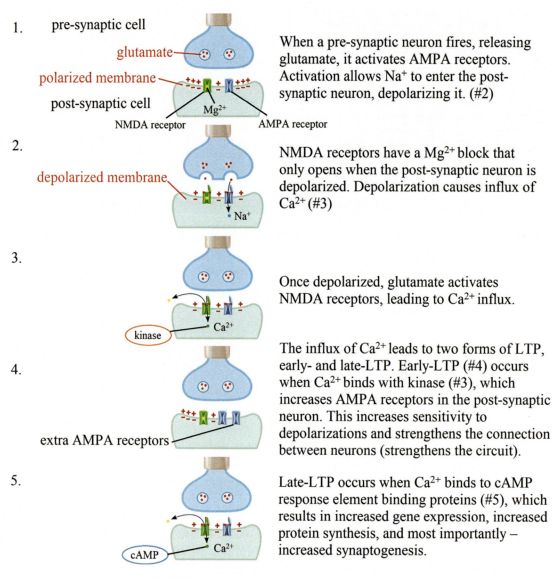

FIGURE 15–1. Process of long-term potentiation (LTP).

change). This process begins with release of glutamate from the presynaptic terminal, activation of α-amino-3-hydroxy-5-methyl-4-isoxazolepropionic acid (AMPA) receptors on the postsynaptic terminal, and, finally, activation of *N*-methyl-D-aspartate (NMDA) receptors on the postsynaptic terminal. When glutamate is released, it activates AMPA receptors first, allowing Na+ to flow into the postsynaptic neuron, depolarizing it, and binding with kinase. This binding leads to early LTP. Early LTP generates more AMPA receptors in the postsynaptic neuron, which increases sensitivity to future depolarizations [excitatory postsynaptic potentials (EPSPs)] and strengthens the connections between neurons (essentially, strengthening the circuit and neural pathways).

NMDA receptor channels only open when the postsynaptic neuron is depolarized. When NMDA receptors are activated, Ca^{2+} enters the postsynaptic neuron and binds to Cyclic adenosine monophosphate (cAMP), which drives late LTP. Late LTP results in increased gene expression, increased protein synthesis, and, most important to plasticity, increased synaptogenesis. Together, these two forms of LTP drive neuroplasticity at the cellular/synaptic level. A common adage in structural, network neuroplasticity is the phrase, *neurons that fire together, wire together.*

The combination of increased AMPA receptors, increased sensitivity to EPSPs, and increased number of synapses creates additional connections between the neurons, analogous to them being "wired together." This process is central to learning and memory. For details about receptors, ions, and proteins, see Box 15–1.

Increases in potentiation can also affect the presynaptic neuron, causing it to release more neurotransmitters. Furthermore, potentiation can be depressed, reducing the activity in a single synapse and eventually the network level. This is called **long-term depression** (depression in this context refers to a decrease in activity, not the emotional state of depression).

Behavioral Plasticity

There is structural (cell or neural network level) and functional imaging evidence of behavioral neuroplasticity in research concerning experience-dependent plasticity, which is correlative to performance on behavioral tasks. Physical and cognitive exercises have been associated with both behavioral and structural or functional imaging change (see Box 15–2).

Experience-dependent neural plasticity has been examined within typical development and aging, developmental disorders, and acquired disorders. Specifically, evidence of cellular regeneration, circuit retraining, and

Box 15–2. Sensorimotor System Plasticity

Nudo and colleagues (1996) trained squirrel monkeys on a motor task that required fine movement of the fingers (digits) but limited movement of the wrist or forearm. Before and after training, they mapped the representation of wrist/forearm and digit muscles in the primary motor area. As can be seen in Figure 15–2, the amount of space controlling digit movements increased after training, at the expense of wrist/forearm control. This indicates that some motor neurons that had been responsible for innervating wrist and forearm muscles were rewired to control digits.

Box 15–1. Pertinent Components of the LTP Process

Glutamate: Recall from Chapter 3 (neuron physiology) that glutamate is one of the primary excitatory neurotransmitters in the nervous system.

AMPA receptors: AMPA receptors are both cation (positive ion: K^+, Na^+, and Ca^{2+}) and glutamate receptors.

NMDA receptors: NMDA receptors are both glutamate and ion channel protein receptors. They are activated when glycine and glutamate bind to them.

Ca^{2+}: Calcium is a cation, integral in cell membrane polarity.

Na^+: Sodium is a cation, integral in cell membrane polarity.

K^+: Potassium is a cation, integral in cell membrane polarity.

Mg^{2+}: Magnesium is a cation, particularly relevant in NMDA pathways because it serves as a block for activation.

Kinase: Kinase is a protein that selectively modifies (catalyzes) other proteins by adding a phosphorus—a process known as phosphorylation.

cAMP: Cyclic adenosine monophosphate (cAMP) is a derivative of adenosine triphosphate and has key roles in intracellular communication.

Synaptic potentiation: This refers to changes at the cell/synapse level; it includes increases in release of neurotransmitters from presynaptic neurons, increases in receptors (e.g., AMPA receptors), and increases in sensitivity to signals.

Structural potentiation: This is changes to networks of neurons, sprouting additional dendrites and dendritic branches or axon collaterals. Structural depression results in a decline in dendrites or axon collaterals, which is called pruning (getting rid of unused neural networks).

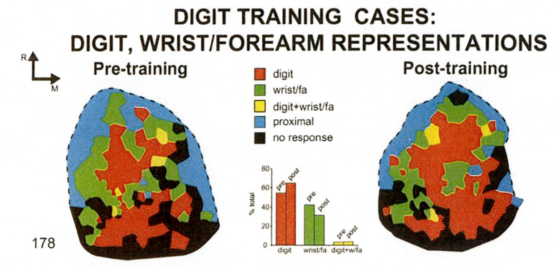

FIGURE 15–2. Primary motor regions pre- and posttraining. *Source:* Reused with permission. Copyright 1996 Society for Neuroscience. Nudo, R. J., Milliken, G. W., Jenkins, W. M., & Merzenich, M. M. (1996). Use-dependent alterations of movement representations in primary motor cortex of adult squirrel monkeys. *Journal of Neuroscience, 16,* 785–807.

cortical reorganization has been correlated with both adaptive and maladaptive behavior changes. Both molecular and behavioral neuroplasticity researchers have identified the need for basic science researchers to collaborate with clinical researchers to address optimal behavior change, the end goal of (re)habilitation. Conversely, researchers within communication sciences and disorders have called for collaboration with neuroplasticity researchers (Ludlow et al., 2008). Cochlear implants represent one example of neuroplastic change within our disciplines (see Box 15–3 for a description).

Two seminal publications on neuroplasticity in communication sciences and disorders were published in 2008. In addition to Ludlow et al. (2008), Kleim and Jones (2008) identified principles of experience-dependent neural plasticity, pertinent to rehabilitation (and habilitation):

- Use it or lose it: Our brains remodel based on the activity we engage in or fail to engage in.
- Use it and improve it: Again, our brains remodel based on the activity we engage in and can improve, assuming we engage accurately. This relates to the old adages of practice makes perfect and practice makes permanent.
- Specificity: Treatment targets must be equivalent or at least as similar as possible to the behavior we hope to change. Thus, it is useful for interventions to be ecologically valid (likely to generalize to everyday activities) and authentic. Furthermore, environment matters because many behavior outcomes are context specific.
- Repetition matters: Errorless repetition = adaptive plasticity. Again, this relates to the adage practice makes permanent. Accurate practice results in adaptive plasticity changes, whereas inaccurate practice can lead to maladaptive plasticity changes.
- Intensity matters: How much intervention is optimal? This relates to the concept of dosage of interventions along the recovery continuum. For instance, low intensity during acute recovery may be best, whereas the need for intensity often increases during subacute recovery.
- Time matters: When is the optimum time for intervention? This relates to the concept of timing of interventions along the recovery continuum. Plasticity is not a single process, and some forms of plasticity function early, whereas others function later. In general, early treatment after brain injury is important.
- Salience matters: This means the more personally relevant an action is, the more impact. This point emphasizes the importance of person-centered interventions and collaborative goal setting. It also

Box 15–3. Deafness, Hearing, and Language

In the disciplines of speech-language pathology and audiology, cochlear implants are a strong example of structural and behavioral neuroplasticity. At birth, the auditory portion of the brain (as with most other regions of the brain) is immature and incomplete, and it develops with auditory input. Children born with severe sensorineural hearing impairments have little or no auditory, sensory input from their environment. If this continues, Heschl gyrus and the auditory pathways will not develop the ability to process auditory information. Thus, timing of interventions, such as cochlear implants, to provide inputs is crucial. Generally, implantation should take place prelingually, in the first 2 to 4 years of life. This enables the brain to learn from signaling processed by the cochlear implant.

Of course, adding auditory input is not the only solution for those with severe hearing impairments. Deaf infants and children exposed to sign language develop communication at rates comparable to those of their hearing peers learning spoken languages. Neural organization reflects the plasticity that occurs: There is generally less white matter in the superior temporal gyrus, possibly due to reduced myelination resulting from limited auditory input (Kumar & Mishra, 2018; Pénicaud et al., 2013). In addition, some studies show greater cortical thickness, which may be a result of lack of pruning of those cortical neurons that normally occurs. The primary visual cortex and fusiform gyrus (involved in face processing) often are more developed, reflecting the visual aspect of sign language and the importance of facial expression in this language. Left hemisphere language regions are critical for language development, regardless of modality, and thus are similarly developed in fluent speakers of signed or oral languages.

relates to motivation and the need to establish relevance and purpose.
- Age matters: Although younger brains are more adaptable, change remains possible across the life span. Furthermore, some damage that occurs at critical points of development may not surface, in terms of behavioral impairments, until a later point in life. For instance, early damage to the frontal lobes may compromise executive functions, but because executive functions are not expected to noticeably emerge until the preteen years, impairments may not surface until that time.
- Transference matters: Plasticity in response to training in one experience can positively influence acquisition of similar behaviors or skills. Generalization depends on authentic intervention in authentic contexts and personally relevant tasks.
- Interference: Plasticity in response to one experience can interfere with acquisition of other behaviors. One experience affects others, and this can be constructive or deconstructive.

Collectively, these principles emphasize the fact that increasing participation produces neuroplastic change. Importantly, not all plasticity is adaptive. Thus, participation must

Box 15–4. Specificity Matters

A good example of the importance of specificity in our discipline relates to nonspeech oral motor exercises. There is a great deal of evidence (Lof & Watson, 2008; McCauley et al., 2009) that nonspeech oral motor exercises do not generalize or transfer to speech behaviors. Although bubble blowing or even isolated oral motor strengthening exercises share some of the physical processes of speech, they are not specific enough to result in improvements to speech. In other words, to improve speech, you have to work on speech.

be contextualized and specific to the behaviors or treatment targets that a given form of practice seeks to improve.

Given evidence of experience-dependent plasticity in animals and human models, interventions designed to increase participation should drive behavioral neuroplasticity. Behavioral interventions that promote such plasticity are complex and should address the following factors: dosing (repetition, intensity, and timing), individualized outcomes (high personal specificity, high personal salience, and ecological validity), effective carryover (treatment adherence, compliance, and therapeutic alliance), intrinsic drive (motivation, self-efficacy, and self-determination), environmental factors (addressing barriers and facilitators, physical environment, and partner environment), and accuracy (errorless productions and treatment fidelity). Figure 15–3 summarizes principles of experience-dependent neuroplasticity applied to (re)habilitation in communication sciences and disorders. Although real-life environments are more difficult to control for the purpose of research design, providing interventions in such context is central to generalizable outcomes in communication and cognition domains. Intervention techniques that seek to enhance access to participation in meaningful contexts should have a positive impact in promoting behavioral plasticity. Figure 15–4 provides for a depiction of the continuum of transference across environments.

There is a conflict between the best environments for research and therapeutic outcomes. In research, the setting is typically controlled and contrived. These settings can be said to have poor ecological validity because they do not closely match the actual settings in which people live. These controlled settings are needed in order to make direct conclusions about the relationship between a treatment and a specific outcome. But the outcomes often do not transfer to daily life. In contrast, authentic and personally relevant environments (good ecological validity) are important for functional outcomes of treatment. However, it is not easy to determine what the "essential ingredients"

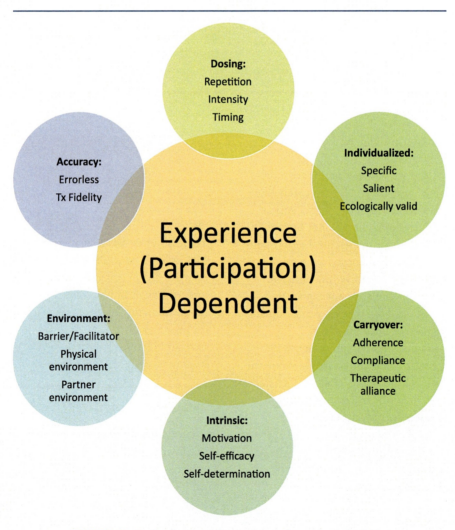

FIGURE 15–3. Applications of experience-dependent plasticity.

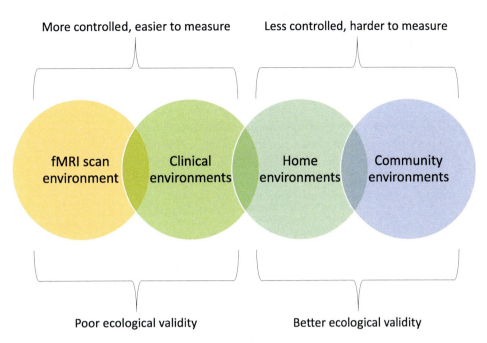

FIGURE 15–4. Continuum of transference across environments. fMRI, functional magnetic resonance imaging.

of a good treatment are when the setting is complex and differs from person to person.

It is also worth noting that correlative measures of activation (functional near-infrared spectroscopy, functional magnetic resonance imaging, positron emission tomography scans, and blood flow) measured in a laboratory may not be equivalent to activation in authentic contexts. Therefore, it is important to recognize limitations of such investigations to generalize within more authentic contexts.

Intensity and Dosage

During approximately the past dozen years, there has been an increasing interest in the most appropriate intensity (total time in therapy sessions and distribution of sessions over time) and dose (teaching episodes per session) for rehabilitation of communication disorders. These factors seem easy enough on the surface, but they quickly become quite complicated.

Intensity refers to the amount of treatment and can be defined in terms of both the total amount of time in therapy sessions and how those sessions are distributed. In massed practice, there are long sessions over a short amount of time, whereas in distributed practice there are many shorter sessions distributed over a longer period of time. Massed practice is like spending 10 hours cramming the night before an exam; distributed practice is like spending 2 hours a day over 5 days.

There is evidence that massed practice, as found in intensive comprehensive aphasia programs (Babbitt et al., 2015; Cherney, Patterson, & Raymer, 2011), may be more effective and more efficient than distributed treatment sessions. In cognitive rehabilitation, evidence suggests that the best intensity depends on the stage of recovery and the rehabilitation goal. In early stages of rehabilitation when clients are learning strategies, distributed practice is more effective. Later, when clients need repeated practice of the strategies in relevant contexts, massed practice is needed (Sohlberg & Turkstra, 2011).

Dosing refers to the number of teaching episodes per session. It is defined as the number of properly administered therapeutic inputs or client acts per session, and it includes not only what the clinician does but also the quality or accuracy of the client's response (Babbitt et al., 2015; Baker, 2012; Harvey et al., 2020). For some treatment targets, such as word repetitions or productions, these are easy to count. For others, such as use of a multistage cognitive strategy, dosage can be difficult to define.

> **Box 15–5.** Not All Plasticity Is Adaptive
>
> Specificity is a crucial element of transference and generalization, as well as in adaptive neuroplastic change. For individuals with spinal cord injuries (complete and incomplete), continuous passive motion machines are often used to keep leg muscles viable/strong while swelling in the spinal cord subsides and function returns. Although there is evidence that this type of intervention can help retain muscle volume and function broadly, spontaneous maladaptive changes are also commonly identified (e.g., spasticity and persistent central pain). Once present, these maladaptive changes can inhibit potential effects of rehabilitation through walking, standing, and swimming (Brown et al., 2011; Hutchinson et al., 2004).
>
> Appropriate afferent input is crucial to adaptive changes. Lack of pressure on the soles of the patient's feet and lack of other environmental stimuli typically associated with walking can result in maladaptive changes. Dietz et al. (2002) observed that fully unloaded (i.e., passive movement of the legs without weight bearing) locomotor training of individuals with complete spinal cord injuries was not effective in inducing leg muscle activation. Conversely, muscle activity can be induced with weight bearing and standing on a treadmill (Dietz et al., 1994). Weight loading, treadmill speed, and kinematic inputs must be tailored to each individual in order to provide appropriate proprioceptive inputs and optimize effects of training (Dietz, 2012). Recently, robot-assisted treadmill training has been used to control proprioceptive and kinematic inputs (Columbo et al., 2000; Field-Fote et al., 2005; Wirz et al., 2005). Although robot-assisted training produces some benefits, manual treadmill training outperforms robot-assisted training (Dietz, 2016; Field-Fote & Roach, 2011; Hornby et al., 2008). This suggests that active participation and sensory awareness are crucial to adaptive change. With the advent of robotic exoskeleton orthotic systems, there is the potential to tailor the level of support to match individual needs. This technology has strong potential.
>
> Intervention and management vary by time post-onset. What is appropriate in chronic recovery may not be appropriate in acute recovery. The nature of sensory input during the acute phase of recovery can also cause maladaptive plasticity changes (Detloff et al., 2014, 2016; Nees et al., 2016). Timing and intensity of acute phase interventions are crucial, as is provision of appropriate sensory inputs (Griesbach et al., 2007; Hansen et al., 2013).
>
> Although this is not a speech, language, hearing, or swallowing example, the concept holds true. Removing context, relevant tasks, and environments can alter the ability to generalize and potentially lead to maladaptive changes. Highly specific (timing, intensity, and task specificity) and individualized interventions are necessary to ensure the likelihood of adaptive changes.

Factors That Contribute to Participation

Several factors are known to contribute to client participation, including therapeutic alliance, motivation, salience, and collaborative goal setting. These factors are crucial to a person-centered approach to intervention. Therapeutic alliance is the degree to which a client agrees with and believes that the approach a therapist is using will result in improvement. Therapeutic alliance has been shown to account for a substantial portion of change in the context of rehabilitation in a variety of settings, including mental health (Horvath & Symonds, 1991), physical therapy (Stenmar & Nordholm, 1994), and brain injury rehabilitation (Darragh et al., 2001). Clients place higher value on interpersonal aspects of care such as communication, empathy, and joint decision-making over physical outcomes (Hush et al, 2011; Rademakers et al., 2011). Schönberger et al. (2006) identified an interaction between therapeutic alliance, patients' compliance, and awareness in the process of brain injury rehabilitation. In a phenomenological study of individuals with traumatic brain injuries, Darragh et al. (2001) identified the central importance of therapeutic alliance. Technical expertise is less of a factor in perceptions than personal characteristics of providers, perceived helpfulness, and practitioner–client relationship (Darragh et al., 2001).

Finally, collaborative goal setting is an essential precursor to ensuring salience and motivation, which are crucial to facilitating neuroplastic change. Clients who are involved in selecting and developing treatment goals are more likely to actively engage in the work to meet those goals, in part because the goals are important to them (Darragh et al., 2001). Collaborative goal setting is also emphasized in developmental contexts, although the collaborator is typically a parent rather than the child (Crais et al., 2006; Forsingdal et al., 2014).

Functional Reactivation Versus Functional Reorganization

Recovery of brain functions after a neurological event or lesion can be attributed to **functional reactivation** or **functional reorganization** (Cappa, 2000; Fridriksson et al., 2009), both of which are forms of neuroplasticity. Functional reactivation refers to recovery of function after some period of latency. Reactivation is a result of both neuronal and vascular plasticity. There is a period of time following stroke and brain injury during which blood flow can be restored to peri-infarct regions through vascular remodeling (new vessels restore blood flow to the peri-infarct region). The degree to which blood flow is restored predicts motor recovery (Williamson et al., 2020). Reperfusion is believed to facilitate behavioral recovery through two mechanisms: (1) recovery of neuronal function (He et al., 2020) and (2) neuronal repair necessary for synaptic remodeling (Clark et al., 2019; Williamson et al., 2020).

Functional reorganization takes place when another brain region takes over functions of a damaged area of the brain. Recovery from aphasia can involve reorganization of the perilesional areas; neurons surrounding the damaged area take over some of those functions. In some people with aphasia due to left hemisphere lesions, there is increased activation of the right hemisphere during language tasks. It is not clear whether this reflects a reorganization of language processes to the right hemisphere (adaptive change) or interference from right hemisphere regions that interrupts left hemisphere language control (maladaptive). It is important to remember that the right hemisphere is responsible for other components of cognition and communication (see Chapter 14), and any reorganization of basic language processes to the right hemisphere would also involve reorganization of the existing communication and cognitive networks.

What is clear is that functional reorganization varies across individuals, lesion location, lesion size, and time after onset (Spielmann et al., 2016). Again, this speaks to the need for individualized interventions with careful attention to timing and dosage.

Summary

Neuroplasticity has relevance to typical and atypical development, recovery from acquired neurogenic disorders, and aging. Whether developing, recovering, or aging, we are a product of what we do and do not do, our genetic makeup, and the environment in which we reside. Our experiences determine how structures change by either strengthening or eliminating neural networks. Parallel to changes in neural architecture are changes to vascular structures. Following onset of strokes or brain injury, there is a period of increased potential for change to both neural and vascular networks. The knowledge that there is potential for adaptive structural and behavioral changes is central to (re)habilitation techniques. Furthermore, knowing that not all plasticity is adaptive challenges us to follow evidence-based practices that result in meaningful change. Those practices should have high specificity and relevance to the individuals we treat.

Key Concepts

- Plasticity is relevant to typical development, aging, and recovery following neurological lesions.
- There are two main types of neuroplasticity—neural (cellular) and behavioral.
- Vascular remodeling is both a developmental process and mechanism of recovery after stroke/brain injury.
- Long-term potentiation is a process of strengthening neural networks through stimulation and is critical for memory and learning.
- Plasticity can be adaptive or maladaptive.
- Several factors are associated with experience-dependent neuroplasticity.
- Personal factors contribute to the degree of engagement and participation, which in turn affect adaptation.
- Reactivation of a brain region following recovery and reorganization via recruitment of another brain region to carry out functions are both mechanisms for neuroplastic change.

References and Additional Resources

Babbitt, E. M., Worrall, L., & Cherney, L. R. (2015). Structure, processes, and retrospective outcomes from an intensive comprehensive aphasia program. *American Journal of Speech-Language Pathology, 24*(4), S854–S863.

Baker, E. (2012). Optimal intervention intensity. *International Journal of Speech-Language Pathology, 14*(5), 401–409. https://doi.org/10.3109/17549507.2012.700323

Bexelius, A., Carlberg, E. B., & Löwing, K. (2018). Quality of goal setting in pediatric rehabilitation—A SMART approach. *Child: Care, Health and Development, 44*(6), 850–856.

Bhogal, S. K., Teasell, R., & Speechley, M. (2003). Intensity of aphasia therapy, impact on recovery. In *Database of Abstracts of Reviews of Effects (DARE): Quality-assessed reviews* [Internet]. Centre for Reviews and Dissemination.

Brown, A. K., Woller, S. A., Moreno, G., Grau, J. W., & Hook, M. A. (2011). Exercise therapy and recovery after SCI: Evidence that shows early intervention improves recovery of function. *Spinal Cord, 49*, 623–628.

Cappa, S. F. (2000). Recovery from aphasia: Why and how? *Brain and Language, 71*(1), 39–41.

Cherney, L. R., Patterson, J. P., & Raymer, A. M. (2011). Intensity of aphasia therapy: Evidence and efficacy. *Current Neurology and Neuroscience Reports, 11*(6), 560.

Clark, T. A., Sullender, C., Jacob, D., Zuo, Y., Dunn, A. K., & Jones, T. A. (2019). Rehabilitative training interacts with ischemia-instigated spine dynamics to promote a lasting population of new synapses in peri-infarct motor cortex. *Journal of Neuroscience, 39*(43), 8471–8483.

Colombo, G., Joerg, M., Schreier, R., & Dietz, V. (2000). Treadmill training of paraplegic patients using a robotic orthosis. *Journal of Rehabilitation Research and Development, 37*(6), 693–700.

Crais, E. R., Roy, V. P., & Free, K. (2006). Parents' and professionals' perceptions of the implementation of family-centered practices in child assessments. *American Journal of Speech-Language Pathology, 15*, 365–377.

Darragh, A. R., Sample, P. L., & Krieger, S. R. (2001). "Tears in my eyes' cause somebody finally understood": Client perceptions of practitioners following brain injury. *American Journal of Occupational Therapy, 55*(2), 191–199.

Darrah, J., Wiart, L., Magill-Evans, J., Ray, L., & Andersen, J. (2012). Are family-centred principles, functional goal setting and transition planning evident in therapy services for children with cerebral palsy? *Child: Care, Health and Development, 38*(1), 41–47.

Davies, K. E., Marshall, J., Brown, L. J., & Goldbart, J. (2017). Co-working: Parents' conception of roles in supporting their children's speech and language development. *Child Language Teaching and Therapy, 33*(2), 171–185.

Detloff, M. R., Quiros-Molina, D., Javia, A. S., Daggubati, L., Nehlsen, A. D., Naqvi, A., . . .Houlé, J. D. (2016). Delayed exercise is ineffective at reversing aberrant nociceptive afferent plasticity or neuropathic pain after spinal cord injury in rats. *Neurorehabilitation and Neural Repair, 30*(7), 685–700.

Detloff, M. R., Smith, E. J., Molina, D. Q., Ganzer, P. D., & Houlé, J. D. (2014). Acute exercise prevents the development of neuropathic pain and the sprouting of non-peptidergic (GDNF- and artemin-responsive) C-fibers after spinal cord injury. *Experimental Neurology, 255*, 38–48.

Dietz, V. (2012). Neuronal plasticity after a human spinal cord injury: Positive and negative effects. *Experimental Neurology, 235*(1), 110–115.

Dietz, V. (2016). Clinical aspects for the application of robotics in locomotor neurorehabilitation. In D. J. Reinkensmeyer & V. Dietz (Eds.), *Neurorehabilitation technology* (pp. 209–222). Springer.

Dietz, V., Colombo, G., & Jensen, L. (1994). Locomotor activity in spinal man. *Lancet, 344*, 1260–1263.

Dietz, V., Müller, R., & Colombo, G. (2002). Locomotor activity in spinal man: Significance of afferent input from joint and load receptors. *Brain, 125*, 2626–2634.

Field-Fote, E. C., Lindley, S. D., & Sherman, A. L. (2005). Locomotor training approaches for individuals with spinal cord injury: A preliminary report of walking-related outcomes. *Journal of Neurologic Physical Therapy, 29*(3), 127–137.

Field-Fote, E. C., & Roach, K. E. (2011). Influence of a locomotor training approach on walking speed and distance in people with chronic spinal cord injury: A randomized clinical trial. *Physical Therapy, 91*(1), 48–60.

Forsingdal, S., St. John, W., Miller, V., Harvey, A., & Wearne, P. (2014). Goal setting with mothers in child development services. *Child: Care Health and Development, 40*(4), 587–596. https://doi.org/10.1111/cch.12075

Fridriksson, J., Baker, J. M., & Moser, D. (2009). Cortical mapping of naming errors in aphasia. *Human Brain Mapping, 30*(8), 2487–2498.

Griesbach, G. S., Gómez-Pinilla, F., & Hovda, D. A. (2007). Time window for voluntary exercise-induced increases in hippocampal neuroplasticity molecules after traumatic brain injury is severity dependent. *Journal of Neurotrauma, 24*(7), 1161–1171.

Hansen, C. N., Fisher, L. C., Deibert, R. J., Jakeman, L. B., Zhang, H., Noble-Haeusslein, L., . . . Basso, D. M. (2013). Elevated MMP-9 in the lumbar cord early after thoracic spinal cord injury impedes motor relearning in mice. *Journal of Neuroscience, 33*, 13101–13111.

Harb, R., Whiteus, C., Freitas, C., & Grutzendler, J. (2013). In vivo imaging of cerebral microvascular plasticity from birth to death. *Journal of Cerebral Blood Flow & Metabolism, 33*(1), 146–156.

Harvey, S. R., Carragher, M., Dickey, M. W., Pierce, J. E., & Rose, M. L. (2020). Treatment dose in post-stroke aphasia: A systematic scoping review. *Neuropsychological Rehabilitation*, 1–32.

He, F., Sullender, C. T., Zhu, H., Williamson, M. R., Li, X., Zhao, Z., . . . Luan, L. (2020). Multimodal mapping of neural activity and cerebral blood flow reveals long-lasting neurovascular dissociations after small-scale strokes. *Science Advances, 6*(21), eaba1933.

Hersh, D., Worrall, L., Howe, T., Sherratt, S., & Davidson, B. (2012). SMARTER goal setting in aphasia rehabilitation. *Aphasiology, 26*(2), 220–233. https://doi.org/10.1080/02687038.2011.640392

Hornby, T. G., Campbell, D. D., Kahn, J. H., Demott, T., Moore, J. L., & Roth, H. R. (2008). Enhanced gait-related improvements after therapist- versus robotic-assisted locomotor training in subjects with chronic stroke: A randomized controlled study. *Stroke, 39*, 1786–1792.

Horvath, A. O., & Symonds, B. D. (1991). Relation between working alliance and outcome in psychotherapy: A meta-analysis. *Journal of Counseling Psychology, 38*(2), 139.

Hush, J. M., Cameron, K., & Mackey, M. (2011). Patient satisfaction with musculoskeletal physical therapy care: A systematic review. *Physical Therapy, 91*(1), 25–36.

Hutchinson, K. J., Gómez-Pinilla, F., Crowe, M. J., Ying, Z., & Basso, D. M. (2004). Three exercise paradigms differentially improve sensory recovery after spinal cord contusion in rats. *Brain, 127*, 1403–1414.

Kleim, J. A., & Jones, T. A. (2008). Principles of experience-dependent neural plasticity: Implications for rehabilitation after brain damage. *Journal of Speech, Language, and Hearing Research, 51*, S225–S239.

Korn, C., & Augustin, H. G. (2015). Mechanisms of vessel pruning and regression. *Developmental Cell, 34*(1), 5–17.

Kumar, U., & Mishra, M. (2018). Pattern of neural divergence in adults with prelingual deafness: Based on structural brain analysis. *Brain Research, 1701*, 58–63. https://doi.org/10.1016/j.brainres.2018.07.02

Levitt, P. (2003). Structural and functional maturation of the developing primate brain. *Journal of Pediatrics, 143*(4), 35–45.

Lof, G. L., & Watson, M. M. (2008). A nationwide survey of nonspeech oral motor exercise use: Implications for evidence-based practice. *Language, Speech, and Hearing Services in Schools, 39*, 397–407.

Ludlow, C. L., Hoit, J., Kent, R., Ramig, L. O., Shrivastav, R., Strand, E., . . . Sapienza, C. M. (2008). Translating principles of neural plasticity into research on speech motor control recovery and rehabilitation. *Journal of Speech, Language, and Hearing Research, 51*(1), S240–S258.

McCauley, R. J., Strand, E., Lof, G. L., Schooling, T., & Frymark, T. (2009). Evidence-based systematic review: Effects of nonspeech oral motor exercises on speech. *American Journal of Speech-Language Pathology, 18*, 343–360.

Nees, T. A., Tappe-Theodor, A., Sliwinski, C., Motsch, M., Rupp, R., Kuner, R., . . . Blesch, A. (2016). Early-onset treadmill training reduces mechanical allodynia and modulates calcitonin gene-related peptide fiber density in lamina III/IV in a mouse model of spinal cord contusion injury. *Pain, 157*, 687–697.

Nudo, R. J., Milliken, G. W., Jenkins, W. M., & Merzenich, M. M. (1996). Use-dependent alterations of movement representations in primary motor cortex of adult squirrel monkeys. *Journal of Neuroscience, 16*, 785–807.

Øien, I., Fallang, B., & Østensjø, S. (2010). Goal-setting in paediatric rehabilitation: Perceptions of parents and professional. *Child: Care, Health and Development, 36*(4), 558–565.

Pénicaud, S., Klein, D., Zatorre, R. J., Chen, J. K., Witcher, P., Hyde, K., & Mayberry, R. I. (2013). Structural brain changes linked to delayed first language acquisition in congenitally deaf individuals. *NeuroImage, 66*, 42–49. https://doi.org/10.1016/j.neuroimage.2012.09.076

Prescott, S., Fleming, J., & Doig, E. (2019). Refining a clinical practice framework to engage clients with brain injury in goal setting. *Australian Occupational Therapy Journal, 66*(3), 313–325.

Rademakers, J., Delnoij, D., & de Boer, D. (2011). Structure, process or outcome: Which contributes most to patients' overall assessment of healthcare quality? *BMJ Quality & Safety, 20*(4), 326–331.

Schönberger, M., Humle, F., & Teasdale, T. W. (2006). The development of the therapeutic working alliance, patients' awareness and their compliance during the process of brain injury rehabilitation. *Brain Injury, 20*(4), 445–454.

Sohlberg, M. M., & Turkstra, L. S. (2011). *Optimizing cognitive rehabilitation: Effective instructional methods.* Guilford Press.

Spielmann, K., Durand, E., Marcotte, K., & Ansaldo, A. I. (2016). Maladaptive plasticity in aphasia: Brain activation maps underlying verb retrieval errors. *Neural Plasticity*, 1–11. https://doi.org/10.1155/2016/4806492

Stenmar, L., & Nordholm, L. A. (1994). Swedish physical therapists' beliefs on what makes therapy work. *Physical Therapy, 74*(11), 1034–1039.

Warren, S. F., Fey, M. E., & Yoder, P. J. (2007). Differential treatment intensity research: A missing link to creating optimally effective communication interventions. *Mental Retardation and Developmental Disabilities Research Reviews, 13*(1), 70–77. https://doi.org/10.1002/mrdd.20139

Williamson, M. R., Franzen, R. L., Fuertes, C. J. A., Dunn, A. K., Drew, M. R., & Jones, T. A. (2020). A window of vascular plasticity coupled to behavioral recovery after stroke. *Journal of Neuroscience, 40*(40), 7651–7667.

Wirz, M., Zemon, D. H., Rupp, R., Scheel, A., Colombo, G., Dietz, V., & Hornby, T. G. (2005). Effectiveness of automated locomotor training in patients with chronic incomplete spinal cord injury: A multicenter trial. *Archives of Physical Medicine and Rehabilitation, 86*, 672–680.

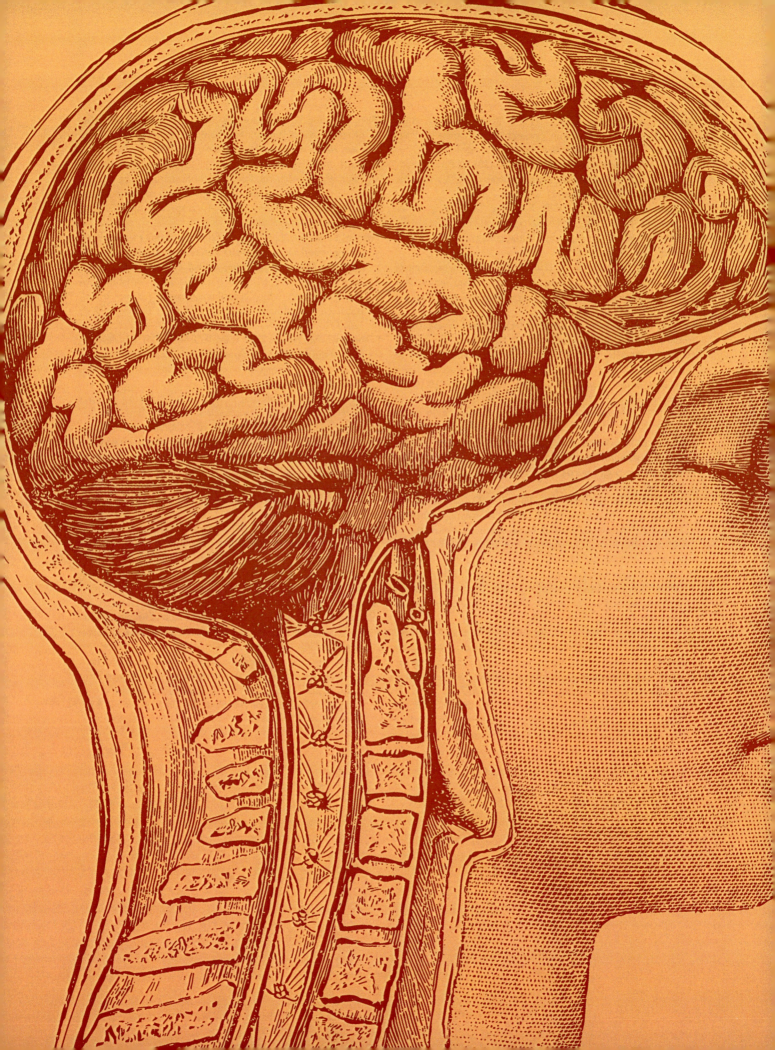

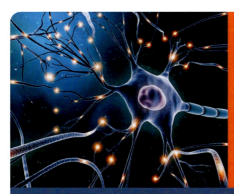

16
Clinical Cases

CHAPTER OUTLINE

Overview
Approach to Solving (Thinking Through) Cases
Section 1: Acquired Cases
   Case 16–1: 48-Year-Old Female With Traumatic Brain Injury
   Case 16–2: 32-Year-Old Male With Postural Headaches and Mixed Upper/Lower Motor Neuron Signs
   Case 16–3: 56-Year-Old Female With Progressive Onset of Dysphagia and Speech Impairments
   Case 16–4: 17-Year-Old Female with Traumatic Brain Injury
   Case 16–5: 63-Year-Old Male With Aphasia and Right Hemiparesis
   Case 16–6: 86-Year-Old Male With Insidious Onset of Cognitive–Communication Changes
   Case 16–7: 45-Year-Old Female With Acute Onset of Confusion and Language Impairment
   Case 16–8: 62-Year-Old Male With Acute Onset of Lethargy and Impaired Attention
   Case 16–9: 52-Year-Old With Acute Onset of "Slurred" Speech and "Drunken" Gait
   Case 16–10: 70-Year-Old Male With Acute Onset of Dysarthria, Vertigo, Nausea, and Double Vision
   Case 16–11: 22-Year-Old Male With Acute Onset of Weakness and Respiratory Distress
   Case 16–12: 62-Year-Old Female With Gradual Onset of Speech and Swallowing Impairments
   Case 16–13: 78-Year-Old Female With Gradual Onset of Speech and Gait Disturbances
   Case 16–14: 52-Year-Old Female With Declining Cognition, Speech, and Swallowing Function
   Case 16–15: 86-Year-Old Female With Memory and Swallowing Difficulties
   Case 16–16: 73-Year-Old Male With Right Facial and Tongue Atrophy
Section 2: Pediatric and Developmental Cases
   Case 16–17: 5-Year-Old Male With Shunt Malfunction
   Case 16–18: 4-Year-Old Male With Fetal Alcohol Syndrome
   Case 16–19: 30-Year-Old Female With Agenesis of the Corpus Callosum
   Case 16–20: 11-Year-Old Male With Brainstem Tumor
   Case 16–21: 11-Year-Old Female with Traumatic Brain Injury
Case Question Answers
Reference

Overview

Damage to neurological structures can alter speech, language, cognition, or swallowing functions, as well as related systems (visual, motor, and sensory). This chapter is intended to help readers integrate knowledge across chapters by applying real cases that cross chapters or disorder-related factors. In real clinical situations, it is common for impairments to involve multiple related systems. In the case of speech-language pathology and audiology, individuals may have concurrent impairments to speech (i.e., articulation, voice, resonance, and fluency), language (e.g., aphasia, pragmatic, and discourse impairments), cognition (i.e., memory, attention, and executive functions), sensory systems (e.g., hearing and vestibular), and swallowing (e.g., dysphagia). In this chapter, these communication impairments are discussed in the context of other impairments that relate to the case. For instance, a case may include unilateral weakness of the arms and legs that may alter self-cares or mobility.

Approach to Solving (Thinking Through) Cases

The purpose of this chapter is to make connections between the real-life case description and anatomical/physiological principles covered in the other chapters of the text. To solve cases, you will need to employ the approaches of **localization** and **differential diagnosis**. Localization is the process of identifying where the damage or impaired development exists within the nervous system. The intention is to help develop one's ability to map symptoms to damage and damage to symptoms. You should be able to work in either direction: If you have information about areas of damage or incomplete development, you should be able to predict what problems/symptoms would exist; if you know what problems/symptoms exist, you should be able to predict areas of damage or incomplete development. Clinically, this is a crucial skill, regardless of the setting in which you work. In a school or pediatric medical context, the problems/symptoms may be developmental or acquired or both. Conversely, in a hospital or health care context, problems tend to be acquired (e.g., through trauma, stroke, or other disease processes), but patients can have pre-existing developmental conditions that will influence the approach to assessment and treatment.

Differential diagnosis is the process of sorting through potential causes/etiologies, eliminating those that do not fit the full profile within the case and narrowing down to the one(s) that fits best. In clinical practice, you typically have case histories, summaries of radiographic imaging findings, reports from other disciplines, and a variety of your own assessment findings to draw upon. Differential diagnosis is a complex skill that takes years of learning and experience to fully develop. It is both a science and an art. At this point in your education, you may not have the requisite knowledge about communication and swallowing disorders to be able to make much more than guesses. That is OK. The purpose of this chapter is to stimulate thinking about neuroanatomy and neurophysiology in relation to clinical practice. This should help solidify why neuroscience is so important for speech-language pathologists (SLPs) and audiologists and will help you further understand the functions of the nervous system.

The cases are intentionally focused on acquired disorders because these best illustrate the relationships between nervous system functions and behavioral impairments. Most of the cases involve adults because they are more susceptible to neurological disorders. Remember, however, that children also can have brain injuries and tumors and even strokes. See Cases 16–17 through 16–21 for application to developmental and acquired disorders in children.

Box 16–1. Localization Is Great, But . . .

Localization is an important skill set and definitely has clinical relevance, but one must recognize that complex functions are not localized to a single region of the brain (e.g., memory is not just processed in the hippocampus, and language expression is not just processed in the Broca area). So, localization helps us make some important connections between lesions (or incomplete development) and symptoms (e.g., communication impairments), but nothing truly happens in isolation, particularly when we consider complex processes such as language and cognition.

Skills you will need to employ:

- Identify and define any terms you do not know or understand. Use this text and other sources to help with this process.
- Identify physical and cognitive–communication signs and symptoms that indicate an impairment, which may manifest/be evident in lesions (damage) or incomplete development of structures.

- Identify probable neurological impairments, given the knowledge you have about areas of damage or incomplete development.
- Map damage location (damage or lesion) to symptoms by comparing a list of brain structure functions to impairments to those functions (i.e., symptoms).
- Map symptoms to damage location—cross-reference symptoms to functional parts of the nervous system.
- Implement steps used in differential diagnosis by identifying a short list of disorders that share features of the case. Begin to eliminate any that do not include key features or those that would not be present given a specific lesion location. Conversely, rule out damage locations that would not be present given symptoms.

For each case, work your way backwards from the diagnosis to make sense of the lesion location in relation to the behavioral status (i.e., cognitive, communication, and swallowing status).

Section 1: Acquired Cases

Case 16–1: 48-Year-Old Female With Traumatic Brain Injury

[Expanded from Box 2–2]

Diagnosis: Epidural hematoma, anterior frontal lobe

Background: A nurse, Penny, was walking briskly to work one morning, crossing the busy road from where she parked toward the hospital. Meanwhile, a 16-year-old boy who recently obtained his driver's license was driving to school. He did not see Penny and struck her with his car, which was traveling at approximately 25 miles per hour, before braking. Penny was propelled over the windshield, then over the roof of the car, and landed behind the car, a bit dazed. As the young man stepped out of the car, she apologized for walking in front of him and said she was fine. The young man pleaded with her to get into the car so he could bring her to the emergency room, which was just around the corner. Moments later, they arrived, and Penny was now unconscious.

1. Given the description above, identify the pertinent information in this case.
2. What medical etiology is your primary concern?
3. What could account for the fact that she was initially alert but then lost consciousness shortly afterward? (Chapters 13 and 14)
4. What aspects of cognition, communication, or swallowing could be affected and why? (Chapters 10, 11, and 14)

She was admitted immediately and sent for a computed tomography scan, which revealed an epidural hematoma.

5. What is a primary concern with this diagnosis and how might it impact cognition or communication?

Quickly, Penny was transferred to surgery for a burr hole procedure (i.e., a neurosurgical intervention whereby a small hole is made in the skull adjacent to a cerebral hematoma; a drain is placed to evacuate bleeding and reduce intracranial pressure). A couple of rough days passed, but the young man's quick thinking and honesty (despite knowing he would be charged with the accident by bringing her to the emergency room) ensured rapid care and a full recovery for this nurse.

Case 16–2: 32-Year-Old Male With Postural Headaches and Mixed Upper/Lower Motor Neuron Signs

[Expanded from Box 2–4]

Diagnosis: Multiple spinal meningeal diverticulum and low-pressure CSF syndrome

Background: A speech-language pathologist developed signs of postural headaches (these occur when standing but subside when lying down) and unrelenting nausea of unknown origin. Physicians could not identify a cause, although it contributed to an initial loss of 40 pounds and substantial restriction in activity level. As the problem progressed, weakness and fasciculations in the feet and calves began to accompany the other symptoms, along with hyperactive reflexes (see Chapter 10 for motor systems).

1. Given the description above, identify the pertinent information in this case.
2. What do the motor signs and symptoms tell you about areas of the CNS (structures and/or pathways) that might be affected? (Chapter 10)
3. What cranial nerve(s) provides sensation to the meninges, pertinent to the painful postural headaches? (Chapter 11)

4. What medical etiology is your primary concern and why?
5. What additional history would you want to know?

A local neurologist suspected the worst, informing his SLP colleague that this was consistent with amyotrophic lateral sclerosis (ALS) and ordering a series of tests to diagnose it. Electromyography (EMG) identified fasciculations and signs similar to but not indicative of ALS (described as "anterior horn cell dysfunction"). That put physicians and the SLP in a "wait and see how it progresses" situation.

6. What areas of communication, swallowing, or cognition would you want to evaluate? (Chapters 11 and 14)

As quickly as it developed, the symptoms resolved and the SLP began to recover. Unfortunately, after a few months passed, the symptoms returned.

7. Does this information change the potential medical etiology?

Eventually, a local neurologist had an epiphany, recalling a rare disease that affects integrity of meningeal tissues (Chapter 2), specifically the dura mater, leading to meningeal diverticula (outpouches). A key symptom is severe postural headaches that resolve upon lying flat. One cisternogram (a radiologic test that involves tracking a radioactive tracer within and outside of the ventricular system) later and the problem was finally identified, lighting up the nerve roots of the spinal cord like an inverted Christmas tree. The diverticula (upwards of 40) were at the junction of the spinal roots and the spinal cord. As they ballooned, the diverticula reached a point where they burst and CSF spilled out of the ventricular system. That led to compression of nerve roots (thus the fasciculations and lower motor neuron signs), and leaks caused the brain to sink down toward the foramen magnum (thus the hyperactive reflexes and upper motor neuron signs). A procedure called an epidural blood patch and eventually several fibrin (clotting elements derived from one's own blood) gluing procedures were used. Essentially, the blood or glue is injected into the epidural space to clot off/glue closed the perforations to the dura mater. After more than 20 epidural blood patch procedures and several fibrin gluing procedures, concerns began to resolve.

Additional information: Medical diagnosis would involve examining the meningeal and CSF systems (Chapter 2). Physicians could conduct physical exams such as looking for pain with bending neck downwards, which can indicate inflammation of the meninges (Brudzinski sign). If headache is present when sitting or standing upright, they can check to see if it resolves when lying in a supine position (postural headache). They could also sample CSF to check opening pressure (below normal pressure would indicate underproduction of CSF or a leak) and check CSF proteins, which can indicate the presence of blood or proteins that help indicate disease processes or trauma.

Case 16–3: 56-Year-Old Female With Progressive Onset of Dysphagia and Speech Impairments

Diagnosis: Bulbar amyotrophic lateral sclerosis

Background: Charmane was a 56-year-old female who experienced gradual onset of dysphagia and speech changes. She was referred to speech-language pathology by her primary care physician to evaluate speech and swallow. An initial examination revealed choking and coughing with solid foods. She tolerated thin liquids without coughing or changes to voice, but sometimes liquids were regurgitated out of her nose. This is consistent with severe oral and pharyngeal dysphagia. Speech was strained, effortful, and hypernasal. An oral mechanism examination revealed moderately slowed diadochokinesis, twitching or fasciculations at the corners of the mouth, nasal emission and moderate hypernasality, hyperactive gag, mild breathiness with laryngeal measures, and mild atrophy and fasciculations along the lateral edges of the tongue blades (some twitching present throughout the tongue blade upon prolonged observation when Charmane was asked to hold tongue at rest with jaw slack for 2 minutes). Charmane also reported a twitching, fluttering sensation in her torso, consistent with fasciculations in the intercostal muscles. She was able to cough on command, although it was weak.

1. Given the description above, identify the pertinent information in this case.
2. What do the characteristics of her speech and swallowing tell you about the articulatory structures affected and the location of damage in the CNS? (Chapters 10 and 11)
3. What medical etiology is your primary concern and why?
4. What additional history would you want to know?

The SLP suspected amyotrophic lateral sclerosis (ALS) and requested a referral to neurology. The neurologic exam revealed mixed upper and lower motor neuron impairments such as hyperactive reflexes, areas of atrophy, and fasciculations. Subsequent electromyography (EMG) and evoked potentials confirmed diffuse degeneration of bulbar and upper spinal motor units.

5. From a diagnostic standpoint, why is the presence of impairments to structures of the face, tongue, pharynx, and larynx important? (Chapters 10 and 11)
6. What do you think will happen to Charmane's speech, swallow, respiration, and mobility as the disease progresses?
7. What kind of education or resources would you provide to the patient?

Case 16–4: 17-Year-Old Female with Traumatic Brain Injury

[Expanded from Box 10–2]

Diagnosis: Acquired cognitive communication disorder

Background: KayLea was a 17-year-old female who was involved in a high-speed motor vehicle crash. She was orally intubated emergently to establish an airway. Given the severity of trauma, the intubation was likely traumatic and may have caused tissue damage in the process. KayLea was airlifted to a regional trauma center where she received neurosurgical intervention, including a bone flap (a portion of skull removed to allow for some brain swelling, typically reinserted subacutely once swelling has resolved) to reduce intracranial pressure. Given the severity of her status, she was sedated and mechanically ventilated. A few days later (as she stabilized), she underwent a tracheostomy and placement of a percutaneous endoscopic gastrostomy (PEG) tube for feeding. The tracheostomy placement allows for a better seal for optimal ventilation and produces less compression/granulations of mucosal linings within the upper airway and vocal folds.

1. Given the description above, identify the pertinent information in this case.
2. What additional history might be useful?

When sedation was reduced, she emerged to a Ranchos level III status (localized responses to external stimuli, in and out of wakeful states, and totally dependent for care), characterized by fairly consistent, differentiated responses to stimuli. This status is indicative of a severe brain injury.

Within days, she was weaned from the ventilator but continued to require non-oral feeding to meet nutritional needs. She continued to emerge from the initial coma and interact with her environment. Attention was severely impaired, which limited oral intake and engagement in interactions. Her oral and pharyngeal swallow onset was moderately delayed, which was greatly a function of her impaired attention and awareness. She made no verbalizations for the first several weeks of her recovery. When she did finally begin to verbalize, it was in the form of a whisper.

3. What does recovery of consciousness tell you about recovery from the accident? (Chapters 12 and 14)
4. What is a possible explanation for the impairments in attention and awareness? (Chapter 15)
5. Discuss the impact of attentional deficits on swallowing and communication. (Chapter 14)
6. What are some potential explanations for her limited vocalizations and whispers? (Chapters 11 and 14)

Gait was marked by severe weakness and ataxic discoordination. Remarkably, over time, she regained speech and language abilities and even returned to college to complete degrees in Spanish and teaching.

7. What could account for the remarkable recovery of her cognitive and communication functions? (Chapters 14 and 15)
8. What kind of education and resources would you provide to the patient?

Case 16–5: 63-Year-Old Male With Aphasia and Right Hemiparesis

[Expanded from Box 13–3]

Diagnosis: Left superior branch of middle cerebral artery (MCA) cerebrovascular accident (CVA)

Background: Darius was a 63-year-old male who was employed as a master plumber prior to this admission. Prior medical history included mild obesity, hypertension, hypercholesterolemia, and borderline diabetes. Hypertension was treated with an angiotensin-converting enzyme (ACE) inhibitor. Hypercholesterolemia was treated with a statin drug. Borderline diabetes was managed through diet. Darius experienced acute onset of right-sided weakness, confusion (disorientation to person, place, and time), and global aphasia.

1. Given the description above, identify the pertinent information in this case.
2. What do the cognitive and communication characteristics tell you about the possible location of damage? (Chapters 1 and 14)
3. What medical etiology is your primary concern and why?

Imaging revealed a large ischemic stroke affecting the left superior branch of the MCA. Etiology was determined to be cardioembolic, secondary to atrial fibrillation. Fibrinolytic therapy [tissue plasminogen activator (tPA)] to dissolve the blood clot was administered. Darius' condition improved over the course of the initial 48 hours of hospitalization. Aphasia began to resolve toward a mild to moderate, nonfluent aphasia. Right hemiparesis persisted with upper extremity weakness worse than lower extremity weakness. Darius was transferred to inpatient rehabilitation, where he stayed for 2 weeks for physical, occupational, and speech-language therapy services. At discharge, he could walk independently with a four-point cane for household ambulation. He was able to dress himself with adaptive equipment from occupational therapy. Mild, nonfluent aphasia persisted at discharge. Atrial fibrillation was managed with an anticoagulant and calcium channel blocker post CVA. The arrhythmia resolved.

4. Explain the relationship between the nonfluent aphasia and the location of the stroke in the superior branch of the left MCA.
5. What kind of education or resources would you provide to the patient and family?

Additional information: Arrhythmias, like atrial fibrillation, contribute to the formation of blood clots as the inefficient and inconsistent movement of blood through vessels leads to stagnancy. Those clots originating the heart can be released as emboli and enter cerebral vasculature (Chapter 13). "Clot busting" medications such as tPA are intended to break down blood clots (emboli or thrombi) that cause occlusions in order to restore blood flow to brain tissues before the effects of ischemia are permanent, causing an infarction and cell death. There is a limited window for application of this type of medication, as the opportunity for saving neurons starved for oxygen decreases over time. Typically, a computed tomography (CT) scan is administered to rule out a cerebral hemorrhage as the underlying etiology because blood thinners and clot busting drugs can exacerbate cerebral hemorrhage. Note that sometimes, despite a clear CT scan, indicating no bleeding, cerebral hemorrhage occurs following administration of tPA. A number of other medications can be used to manage atrial fibrillation (beta blockers and calcium channel blockers) and potential for clotting (anticoagulants).

6. Why is pharmacological management of Darius' atrial fibrillation so important?
7. What is the mechanism of tPA and why did Darius experience substantial improvements in both physical and cognitive functions following administration?

Case 16–6: 86-Year-Old Male With Insidious Onset of Cognitive–Communication Changes

[Expanded from Box 13–4]

Diagnosis: Small vessel disease, vascular dementia

Background: Harold was an 86-year-old male with a history of hypercholesterolemia, hypertension, and diabetes. He presented with severe, bilateral carotid stenosis (narrowing of the artery; 80% occluded on right side and 90% occluded on the left side). Given his age and medical history, it was determined he was not a good candidate for a carotid endarterectomy (a surgical procedure to remove plaque from the artery walls). Harold experienced insidious (slow, gradual) onset of aphasia and confusion. Along with difficulties with word retrieval, comprehension was impaired for conversation-level exchanges. Family noted gradual changes in memory and decision-making as well. This prompted his family to move Harold from an assisted living setting to a skilled nursing facility.

1. Given the description above, identify the pertinent information in this case. (Chapter 13)
2. Given the insidious changes to language and cognition, what brain structures are likely affected? (Chapter 14)

Suspected diagnosis of small vessel ischemic disease was confirmed with magnetic resonance imaging (MRI) with diffusion-weighted MRI and MR angiography. Microemboli (multiple, very tiny emboli) were suspected. Harold was treated pharmacologically with antiplatelet therapy, anticoagulants, and statins, along with dietary restrictions. Donepezil, an acetylcholinesterase (AChE) inhibitor, was also initiated and corresponded with some global improvements in cognition and mobility/self-cares. Harold received physical, occupational, and speech-language therapy services for several weeks, with improvements in communication, memory, decision-making, and activities of daily living in the short term. He remained in the skilled nursing facility following discharge from rehabilitation therapies.

3. Given the diagnosis of small vessel disease, what parts of cerebral vascular territories are likely to be affected?
4. Why would AChE treatment improve cognitive function? (Chapters 3 and 15)

Case 16–7: 45-Year-Old Female With Acute Onset of Confusion and Language Impairment

[Expanded from Box 13–8]

Diagnosis: Burst aneurysm and vasospasm

Background: Marjorie was a 45-year-old female smoker who was otherwise healthy before experiencing acute onset of confusion, severe attention impairments, and language impairments. She had two daughters, who were in their early teens at the time of this event. She was admitted to the hospital with an intracranial hemorrhage due to a large (25-mm) saccular (berry) aneurysm on the circle of Willis, near the junction of the left internal carotid and MCA/ACA branches. The hemorrhage caused cognitive status to deteriorate rapidly upon admission, resulting in a somnolent (sleepy) status as she was taken to surgery.

1. Given the description above, identify the pertinent information in this case. (Chapter 12)
2. What additional history might be useful?
3. What are your expectations for Marjorie's language and cognition? What impairments do you expect to see? (Chapter 14)
4. What risk factors for aneurysm did Marjorie display prior to the incident? (Chapter 13)
5. What are the potential effects of blood in contact with brain tissue? (Chapter 13)

A neurosurgeon evacuated the intracranial hemorrhage and placed a clip on the aneurysm. Initial response to the neurosurgical intervention was good. Marjorie awoke with anomia, somewhat agrammatic spoken language expression, impaired comprehension of spoken language, attention impairments, executive dysfunction, and confusion (including disorientation to place, time, and situation). Over the course of 4 or 5 days, her condition began to stabilize further, and cognitive–communication functions began to improve substantially. Her communication was characterized by anomia, mild nonspecific language impairments, poor attentional control and endurance, and executive dysfunction (characterized by poor inhibition and self-regulation), and she remained disoriented although overall cognitive–communication status was improving. Seven or eight days after initial admission, she was oriented to person, place, time, and situation.

Marjorie was on strict monitoring for intake and output during the first 7 days of her hospitalization. Plans were made to discharge her to home on the eighth day with outpatient physical, occupational, and speech therapy services. Midmorning on the eighth day of hospitalization, she was noted to be more somnolent and disoriented, and her speech was confused. Physicians suspected vasospasm (spasms of the vessels that cause a to-and-fro of blood circulation and compromising perfusion; if diffuse, it can cause widespread cerebral hypoperfusion), and this diagnosis was confirmed through cerebral angiogram. Vasospasm sometimes occurs in conjunction with ruptured aneurysm, but there had been no clinical indications prior to that morning. Physicians and nursing staff did their best to review information about intake and output on the morning of her discharge. As it turns out, a friend came to visit her that morning prior to discharge. Marjorie was a diet cola drinker, so her friend brought her a six-pack of 20-ounce bottles as a get-well present. While sitting alone in her room that morning, she drank all six bottles. Although it is unclear whether this was the primary cause of the vasospasm, she was susceptible as a result of her ruptured aneurysm. The physicians noted that consuming the diet cola resulted in a rapid high-sodium intake (approximately 450 mg). This may have altered her ability to regulate and restore membrane potentials and vessel dilation/constriction. Following the onset of vasospasm, she reverted to a state of lethargy, disorientation, and moderate mixed aphasia (demonstrating impairments to expression and comprehension). Once vasospasm was managed pharmacologically and through diet restrictions, she stabilized and was sent to inpatient rehabilitation to address remaining cognitive–communication impairments (executive dysfunction, poor self-regulation, and anosognosia), self-cares needs (marked by perseverations and poor sequencing), and mobility needs (compromised by poor safety judgment and impulsivity).

6. What are the potential effects of vasospasm on brain function?
7. Given her symptoms (impairments), what brain structures were likely impacted by this incident? (Chapter 14)

8. Draw an image(s) of the brain that accounts for the site(s) of lesions.

Case 16–8: 62-Year-Old Male With Acute Onset of Lethargy and Impaired Attention

[Expanded from Box 13–7]

Diagnosis: Right MCA CVA

Background: Anton was a 62-year-old male with a large circle of friends. He was always willing to lend a hand and was known as a really good listener. One afternoon, his partner became concerned after noticing that Anton was having difficulty focusing on a TV program they were watching and began rambling on about one of the actors. It was difficult to follow him because the story was disorganized, his speech intelligibility was reduced, and he would ramble on, telling long and confusing stories. In addition, Anton complained that he could not find the TV remote even though it was on the table by his left hand. When he got up to get a drink, Anton was able to walk and collided with the left side of the doorway.

1. Given the description above, identify the pertinent information in this case.
2. Given the changes to cognition and communication, what brain structures or networks are likely affected? (Chapter 14)

Anton was diagnosed with a large ischemic stroke of the right MCA. For the first few days, he had a strong gaze preference to the right along with very limited endurance and difficulty maintaining attention to task. When he was alert and eating, he was impulsive, taking large bites and consuming food/liquids at a rapid rate. He needed support to get the spoon to the center of his mouth and tended to miss to the right side without that hand-over-hand support. Residuals remained in his mouth after swallows, particularly in his left cheek (pocketing). After a few minutes of self-feeding, he was exhausted and leaned heavily to the right. At this point, he required maximal assistance to eat, including physical cues/efforts to turn his head toward midline.

3. What physical and cognitive factors likely contributed to his impaired swallow (dysphagia)? (Chapters 11 and 14)

Over the course of several days, Anton's endurance improved markedly and his gaze preference was equal (left/right), except when he was engaged in more complex tasks such as walking and navigating the hospital (right gaze preference returned during those activities). He required moderate assistance to maintain safety when ambulating, even though his balance and gait were fairly functional. For instance, he would still collide with the left side of doorways and lost balance/fell to the left when inattentive or when asked to engage in a task while standing.

4. Why do task complexity and divided attention affect performance? (Chapter 14)

Anton's speech was characterized by mild unilateral upper motor neuron dysarthria, and his communication was marked by rambling and egocentrism (a pervasive tendency to focus on himself). After being home for several weeks, his partner confided that Anton did not seem to care about others the way he used to. Friends who had visited were disturbed by how Anton was focused almost completely on himself and hardly gave them a chance to talk in between his long, confusing stories about his time in the hospital.

5. Explain the changes to communication and brain structures/networks that might be involved.
6. What effects might his communication disorders have on relationships?

Other considerations: Anton's attention across contexts should be evaluated by progressing from basic tasks with few demands to more complex tasks or environments to determine where he begins to break down. This information can be used to address environmental factors in the home (e.g., turning off the TV or radio, limiting the number of visitors, and making sure walking paths are clear of obstructions). Altering the environment to increase his safety—particularly related to eating (given impulsivity) and basic ambulation (in collaboration with other disciplines, specifically physical therapy)—will allow him to live as independently as possible.

Unilateral neglect is likely, because he does not seem to be aware that he is missing out on part of his world, but in order to rule out visual field cuts, a referral to a neuro-ophthalmologist is needed.

Involvement of physical therapy and occupational therapy is important to address the effects of gaze preference and/or unilateral neglect (across other modalities) and how that changes given task complexity/external environmental demands, particularly in determining risk for falls, collisions, etc.

Case 16–9: 52-Year-Old With Acute Onset of "Slurred" Speech and "Drunken" Gait

[Expanded from Box 13–5]

Diagnosis: Cerebellar CVA

Background: Devin was a 52-year-old non-binary person who initially presented with "slurred," confused speech and clumsy, "drunken," gait. They also complained of a severe headache and nausea.

Radiologic findings identified an ischemic stroke in the anterior cerebellar lobe. Devin was somewhat obtunded (lethargic and drowsy) and confused initially but became oriented by the second day of hospitalization. Speech was characterized by ataxic dysarthria, marked by imprecise articulation and irregular qualities. Gait and speech shared features of "drunken" movement, including overshooting and undershooting targets, irregular rate, and timing problems. Gait was unsteady and marked by similar overshoots, such as swinging the right leg across the left leg during attempts to walk a straight line. Devin's eye movements were also disrupted, including the presence of nystagmus (the eyes make rapid twitching movements—either side to side or, in this case, up and down). Cognition improved markedly during the first few days, but speech and gait impairments remained persistent upon discharge.

1. Given the description above, identify the pertinent information in this case.
2. What additional history might be useful?

Additional information: Vascular supply to the cerebellum overlaps with topographical organization in such a manner that the vermis, intermediate, and lateral portions of the cerebellum have mixed blood supply (see Chapter 12). As such, isolated ataxia to only ocular, speech, limb, or trunk is unusual. In this case, Devin demonstrated each of these forms of ataxia. Consider how this information, along with evidence that most symptoms resolved with the exception of speech and gait ataxia, may provide insight into the site of the lesion.

3. What are your expectations for Devin's speech? What impairments would you expect to see?
4. What are your expectations for Devin's swallowing? What impairments would you expect to see? (Chapters 10, 11, and 14)
5. What are your expectations for Devin's cognitive status? What potential impairments would you expect to see? (Chapter 14)
6. Given the site of lesion, paired with the knowledge that cognition improved markedly during the first several days, what types of cognitive difficulties would likely remain? Why? (Chapter 14)
7. Why did the speech and gait impairments persist? How does this relate to the lesion location and size? (Chapters 10, 11, and 12)

Case 16–10: 70-Year-Old Male With Acute Onset of Dysarthria, Vertigo, Nausea, and Double Vision

Diagnosis: Wallenberg syndrome, brainstem stroke

Background: Alando was a 70-year-old male with a history of hypercholesterolemia, hypertension, and smoking (one pack a day for 50 years). Feeling nauseated and fatigued, he told his partner that he must be coming down with a stomach bug, so he was going to take a nap on the sofa. Approximately 2 hours later, his partner woke him to find that his speech was "slurred" and he was unable to stand or walk without assistance. Alando also reported dizziness/vertigo, increased nausea, and diplopia, all of which came and went or were exacerbated by position. His partner helped him to the car and brought him to the emergency room, where he was evaluated through the stroke protocol.

CT scans with and without contrast were negative for any signs of hemorrhage or evidence of hyper- or hypodensities (regions that are more dense than usual are brighter and tissue that is less dense than expected is darker, respectively, with both indicating potential lesions). Nystagmus was present bilaterally, but the reminder of the cerebellar assessment was within normal limits. Nasolabial folds were flattened, and right face, tongue, and velum appeared weak. Along with slow rate and articulatory imprecision, voice quality was harsh and breathy. Moderate to severe oral–pharyngeal dysphagia was present with both liquids and solids. Gait was unsteady and ataxic. Findings were consistent with Wallenberg syndrome (a stroke in the lateral medulla resulting in severe swallowing and voice problems), although they were not confirmed with imaging.

At discharge, he was able to walk with a four-point cane (although ataxia and timing issues remained) and had returned to a regular diet. Moderate to severe dysarthria persisted. Visual symptoms, particularly the nystagmus, and vertigo improved but were present intermittently.

1. Given the description above, identify the pertinent information in this case.
2. What additional history might be useful?
3. Given the case description, what cranial nerves were affected? (Chapter 11)
4. Given the effects to those cranial nerves, draw an image of the brain that accounts for the area of probable lesion.
5. Considering the cranial nerves involved, what are your expectations for Alando's speech? What types of impairments do you expect to see?
6. What are your expectations for Alando's swallow? What impairments do you expect to see? Why are there changes over time?
7. Why did dysphagia and gait improve? Why did his dysarthria persist? (Chapters 11 and 12)

Additional considerations: The distinction that nystagmus was present but cerebellar function was normal was a critical piece for differential diagnosis. Nystagmus and ataxic gait are potentially signs of cerebellar dysfunction, but nystagmus may also relate to cranial nerve VIII damage, and likely relates to damage to cerebellar inputs and outputs, rather than direct damage to the cerebellum.

Case 16–11: 22-Year-Old Male With Acute Onset of Weakness and Respiratory Distress

Diagnosis: Botulinum poisoning and respiratory arrest

Background: Amos was a 22-year-old bachelor in an Amish community. One day, he found something at the top of a jar of canned tomatoes (a ribbon-like, gray-colored growth). Thinking he could just scoop it off, cook it, and everything would be fine, Amos began to enjoy the stewed tomatoes. After consuming the tomatoes, he experienced progressive vision disturbances (diplopia), slurred speech, difficulty swallowing, dry mouth, and eventually respiratory arrest (over the course of 24 hours). The gray growth was botulinum toxin, which paralyzed smooth and striated muscles in his thorax, larynx, pharynx, and oral structures.

1. Given the description above, identify the pertinent information in this case.

Members of his community found help to transport him to a local hospital, where he was intubated (a breathing tube was placed; he eventually received a tracheostomy and PEG tube) and mechanically ventilated until the effects of the toxin began to wear off. Once weaned from the ventilator during daytime hours and pressure support overnight, he began trials of a speaking valve (Figure 16–1) in his tracheostomy for short increments throughout the day. Initially, the goal was to tolerate the speaking valve at rest, but eventually the SLP began to work toward voicing and swallowing functions. His voice was marked by breathiness and poor endurance. He tolerated small sips of thin liquids but struggled with thicker liquids or textures for several weeks (due to severe pharyngeal weakness and poor endurance, thicker liquids and foods resulted in liquid/food residue remaining in the pharynx after the swallow). Oral dysphagia was mild, but pharyngeal dysphagia was moderate to severe. When feasible, clinical evaluation findings are corroborated with a modified barium swallow (MBS; fluoroscopic x-ray examination of swallowing). Barium is

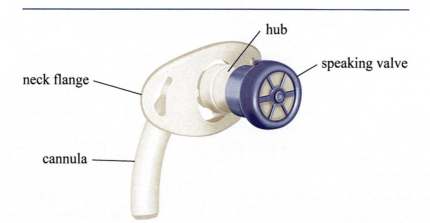

FIGURE 16–1. Tracheostomy tube with speaking valve attached. The speaking valve allows air to enter the tracheostomy tube (and thus the lungs) but does not allow air to pass out of the tube/speaking valve, thus forcing air to pass through the vocal folds and allowing them to vibrate to produce phonation/speech.

radiopaque and thus visible in the video x-ray. Although he could not tolerate an MBS, based on the clinical examination it was assumed that his swallowing impairments were the result of pharyngeal weakness and difficulty achieving closure of the velopharyngeal port and incomplete laryngeal adduction.

2. What structure in what pathway was the botulinum toxin acting on? (Chapter 3)
3. How does this accidental ingestion of tomatoes with the botulinum toxin differ from intentional injection of Botox for limb spasticity or spasmodic dysphonia? (Chapter 3)
4. What neurotransmitter and/or process was disrupted in this incident? (Chapter 3)
5. Given the descriptions from the case, what cranial nerve outputs were clearly affected? (Chapter 11)
6. Given the action of botulinum toxin and the cranial nerves affected, what are your expectations for Amos' speech (specifically, voice/phonation)? What impairments do you expect to see? (Chapter 11)
7. Would you expect oral and laryngeal sensation to be affected? Why or why not?
8. What are your expectations for Amos' swallowing? What impairments do you expect to see? (Chapter 11)
9. Why was mechanical ventilation (a ventilator) necessary? Specifically describe the relevant muscles and neurons/pathways. (Chapter 10)
10. Would you anticipate problems with cognition? Why or why not? (Chapter 14)

Case 16–12: 62-Year-Old Female With Gradual Onset of Speech and Swallowing Impairments

Diagnosis: Myasthenia gravis

Background: Judy was a 62-year-old female who experienced changes to her speech and swallowing function, worsening over time. She was referred for an evaluation, including a modified barium swallow (MBS). Speech was noticeably hypernasal and became more hypernasal and less precise over a short period of time when conversing with the SLP. An initial oral mechanism examination (OME; see Chapter 11) revealed that cranial nerve functions were relatively intact, with the exception of mild velum weakness and associated hypernasality. Swallowing was also characterized by mild oral and pharyngeal symptoms following rest.

1. Given the description above, identify the pertinent information in this case.
2. What additional history might be useful?

At the outset of an MBS study, Judy tolerated thin liquids and initial presentations of purees. Mild nasal penetration was noted, particularly with pureed solids, resulting in a small amount of applesauce coming out of her nose. A banana slice with barium paste was trialed, resulting in moderate pharyngeal stasis (food/barium residues remaining in the pharynx) and nasal penetration of the barium paste. A sip of thin barium was presented, in an attempt to clear the residuals, resulting in nasal regurgitation and laryngeal penetration (liquid noted in the laryngeal vestibule but not into trachea), although the residuals were cleared. Voice became increasingly hypernasal, wet/gurgly, and breathy. A teaspoon of honey-thickened liquids was presented, which resulted in nasal regurgitation and moderate pharyngeal residuals. At this point, Judy had severe hypernasality and required a small sip of thin liquids to clear residuals. Ptosis of both eyelids was now evident as well. The MBS was halted. The SLP suspected myasthenia gravis and requested a referral to a neurologist to confirm the diagnosis.

3. Why was the initial cranial nerves examination essentially normal? (Chapter 11)
4. What structure in what pathway was affected?
5. What neurotransmitter and/or process was disrupted in this situation? (Chapter 3)
6. Explain the significance of increasing weakness over time. (Chapter 3)
7. What are your expectations for Judy's speech? (Chapter 11) What impairments would you expect to see? What would you do to account for limited endurance and decline over time?
8. What are your expectations for Judy's swallow? How would you account for deterioration of swallow over time? What impairments do you expect to see? (Chapters 11 and 14)

Case 16–13: 78-Year-Old Female With Gradual Onset of Speech and Gait Disturbances

Diagnosis: Parkinson disease

Background: Gloria is a 78-year-old female with progressive onset of impairments to speech, swallowing, self-cares/activities of daily living (ADLs), and mobility. She has mild to moderate axial rigidity and postural instability, which results in unsteadiness. Cogwheel rigidity (ratchet-like movement) is present in arms bilaterally. Gait is marked by stooped posture, festinating/shuffling steps (becoming progressively smaller over time), and limited arm swing. Initiation of walking is difficult, and changes in direction result in pedestal turning (short quick steps that result in turning in a tight circle and further unsteadiness). Speech is hypophonic (soft) and includes rapid bursts of mumbled words (festinating speech). Swallowing is marked by occasional coughing or choking episodes prior to swallowing. Gloria has difficulty initiating a complete swallow, and lingual pumping (inefficient back-and-forth movement of the tongue that results in poor bolus control) has been noted in clinical observations and fluoroscopic x-rays of her swallow function. Hyolaryngeal excursion (degree of elevation of hyolaryngeal complex and resultant epiglottic inversion) is reduced. Overall, swallowing is characterized by moderate to severe oral phase dysphagia (swallowing dysfunction) and moderate pharyngeal dysphagia. Other symptoms include hand flapping and pill rolling tremors at rest, masked facies (expressionless, as if cast in stone), and occasional adventitious (extra, involuntary) movements of face muscles. She has difficulty with dressing, sometimes requiring moderate assistance for both upper and lower body dressing.

1. Given the description above, identify the pertinent information in this case.
2. What additional history might be useful?
3. What brain structures are likely to be involved in this case? (Chapter 11)
4. Correlate her physical impairments with brain substrates.
5. Why is she "slow but accurate"?
6. What are your expectations for Gloria's speech? (Chapter 11) What impairments do you expect to see?
7. What are your expectations for Gloria's swallowing? What impairments do you expect to see? (Chapter 11)
8. What are your expectations regarding cognition? (Chapter 14)

Additional information: Parkinson disease is a movement disorder involving dysfunction to structures within the extrapyramidal motor system. In this case, amplitude of movements is overly dampened, resulting in short, quick movements of the gross motor and speech systems. The overall result is hypokinesia (less movement), although shuffling gait is made up of those quick, short movements. Likewise, speech is soft and characterized by "muddled," imprecise articulation because articulators are not moving through their typical or full range of motion. The reduced movement coupled with rigidity results in some weakness within the speech and respiratory mechanism that ultimately extends the effects of the problem. So, a challenge for us to consider is whether to address the underlying movement disorder and/or to address the subsequent "weakness" (noting clearly that this is not a weakness disorder).

Given the characteristics of Parkinson disease, clinicians must develop a rationale for addressing the movement disorder versus weakness. Current evidence-based treatments involve elements that address both movement disorder and subsequent weakness. Consider the Lee Silverman Voice Treatment (LSVT) approach (Ramig, Pawlas, & Countryman, 1995), which encourages speaking loudly—addressing respiratory drive for speech and more amplitude of movements in the speech mechanism. Similar principles apply to dysphagia management.

Case 16–14: 52-Year-Old Female With Declining Cognition, Speech, and Swallowing Function

Diagnosis: Huntington disease

Background: Lucy has adventitious (extra, involuntary) movements of her jaw, shoulders, trunk, and limbs. Her movements are unpredictable and jerky (hyperkinetic). The SLP first sees Lucy in a locked behavioral unit to address swallowing and communication. At first, they are not sure why Lucy is in this unit, given her somewhat muted interactions. Lucy speaks in a slow, harsh, drawn-out manner and frequently struggles to find the right words or how to say things in general. The SLP notes that her language shares characteristics of both anomic and nonfluent aphasia; however, in the context of other cognitive impairments, the SLP is hesitant to call this aphasia. Lucy's swallow is marked by moderate delays in onset of the pharyngeal swallow. She has difficulty coordinating swallowing and breathing, which sometimes leads to severe episodes of choking/coughing. Although she is able to clear her voice following choking episodes, the SLP remains concerned because nursing staff share that she is sometimes even less alert during meals and thus less likely to clear with a strong cough. Lip smacking and extraoral tongue and lip movements are common, further contributing to her impaired bolus (collection of food) control. As she begins to struggle with swallowing and attempts to communicate with the SLP during the swallowing assessment, she becomes very upset. She quickly escalated to an irritable, anxious, and aggressive state. She swings and knocks food from her meal tray onto the floor beside the SLP. Most of this seemed to relate to her struggle in the moment, but two aids quickly came to her room door to check on the SLP. The nurses are concerned with her potential to lash out at staff members.

1. Given the description above, identify the pertinent information in this case.
2. What additional history might be useful?
3. Given the diagnosis and descriptions of impairments, what brain structure(s) is likely affected? (Chapter 10)
4. What does her area of brain damage/dysfunction have to do with her behaviors, and why is she in a locked behavioral unit? (Chapters 10 and 14)

Figure 16–2 illustrates atrophy commonly see in Huntington disease. Motoric symptoms (movement disorders) of Huntington disease are typically unilateral initially, progressing to bilateral as the disease progresses. This means that choreatic movements would impact only one side of the pharynx, one side of the oral structures, and one side of the larynx. Given that Lucy has a fairly recent diagnosis of Huntington disease, consider the likely impact on her speech and swallowing function.

5. What are your expectations for Lucy's speech? What impairments do you expect to see? (Chapter 11)

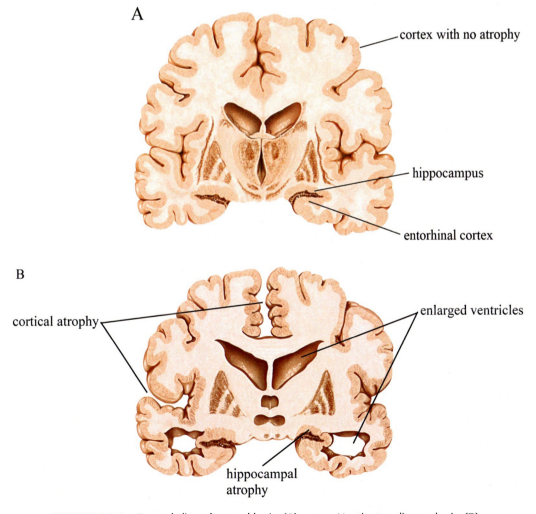

FIGURE 16–2. Coronal slice of normal brain (**A**) versus Huntington disease brain (**B**).

6. What are your expectations for Lucy's swallowing? What impairments do you expect to see? (Chapter 11)

Case 16–15: 86-Year-Old Female With Memory and Swallowing Difficulties

Diagnosis: Dementia, presumed Alzheimer type

Background: Selma is an 86-year-old female with dysphagia and memory problems, admitted initially for rehabilitation following a broken hip and subsequent surgical repair. She was discharged to a skilled nursing facility due to concerns about her ability to live independently. Selma walks with a walker and standby assistance. She enjoys knitting, reading (news, romance novels, and the Bible), and singing. Her vision is impaired, but she can read large print with a magnifying glass. She has a moderate, sensorineural hearing loss but has bilateral hearing aids.

The SLP is asked to see her for a swallowing evaluation. Selma is the classic "fooler" who can talk a good game for a few minutes, but after approximately 10 minutes one begins to recognize substantial repetitions. She is polite but irritable. She refuses assistance and expresses frustration and intolerance of others with dementia (wanderers who invade her room). She is aware that she is in a skilled nursing facility, stating that this is just temporary until her hip heals. She frequently expresses disdain for the physical therapists who "don't know what they're doing."

From a swallowing standpoint, the SLP believes that she could safely swallow thin liquids (would not aspirate or choke) if she would just remember to consistently use a simple strategy: tuck her chin. However, Selma forgets to tuck her chin, eats too fast, and takes large gulps of liquids if someone is not there to remind her. She hates thickened liquids, but she will not allow a certified nurse assistant to sit anywhere near her and remind her to tuck her chin so that she can safely consume thin liquids. In fact, she refuses to eat in the dining room with "all of those senile people." She will consent to dine with residents who she believes are "with it." She will allow someone to sit with her if they sip a cup of coffee and carry on a light conversation. She even allows them to visually cue her to tuck her chin, with a few grumbles here and there.

The SLP notes that in conversations with her, Selma has markedly disordered discourse. The content is impoverished or empty (saying a lot about nothing). She often perseverates on stories the SLP has heard many times by now. Whenever she struggles, the SLP notes that she blames it on external factors—for example, "I'd be fine if it weren't for that stupid wheelchair."

1. Given the description above, identify the pertinent information in this case.
2. What additional history might be useful?
3. What are your expectations for Selma's swallowing? What impairments do you expect? (Chapter 11)
4. What are your expectations about Selma's cognition? What impairments do you expect? (Chapter 14)
5. What impact is Selma's impaired vision and hearing loss likely to have (if any) on her cognition and communication? (Chapters 7, 8, and 14)

Additional information: Along with declines in memory functions, anticipated with Alzheimer disease, a number of other homeostatic mechanisms and brain networks are disrupted. Alzheimer disease is a global, cortical dementia, meaning that over time most cortical regions of the brain will begin to atrophy. Figure 16–3 depicts global cortical atrophy in late-stage Alzheimer disease, and Figure 16–4 is a representation of areas affected in early stage Alzheimer disease. Note that along with hippocampal and medial temporal lobe atrophy initially, there is substantial atrophy to the lateral hypothalamus, resulting in anorexia (loss of appetite). Furthermore, note the swath of atrophy in the lateral parietal and temporal regions, which disrupts the dorsal (where) and ventral (what) streams (see Chapters 7, 12, and 14). Disruptions to the superior, lateral parietal region and dorsal stream result in tactile processing, disorientation to movement, pathfinding/wayfinding problems, and disorientation to place. Likewise, disruptions to the posterior–lateral temporal lobe and ventral stream result in impairments to recognition of colors, shapes, and objects (agnosias—a failure to recognize a sensory stimulus for what it is). Oral agnosias (a failure to recognize food that often results in holding food in mouth, ruminating/perseveratively chewing on food, or spitting food out) are also common in Alzheimer dementia. Damage to the posterior cingulate and fusiform gyri is believed to impair recognition of faces.

6. Given her presumed diagnosis, describe how the patterns of atrophy in Figure 16–4 account for her impairments. (Chapter 14)
7. How might the likely presence of atrophy to the posterior temporal and parietal regions influence swallowing, sensory processing, and cognition? (Hint: Think

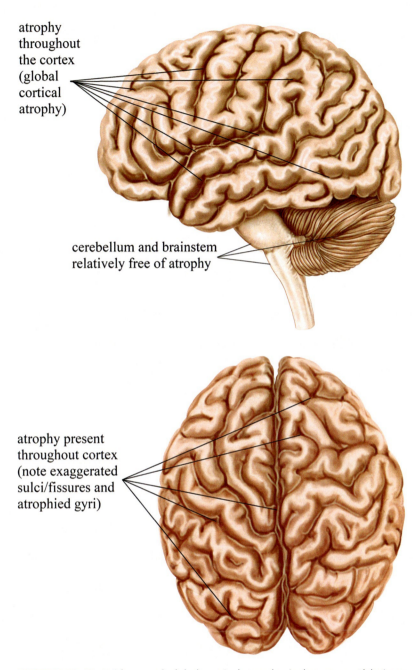

FIGURE 16–3. Evidence of global cortical atrophy in late-stage Alzheimer disease.

about agnosias and the dorsal and ventral streams.) (Chapters 7, 12, and 14)

8. Describe the underlying reasons for her dysphagia. Assuming her speech and voice quality are typical for her age, what does that tell you about the etiology of her dysphagia? (Hint: Think motor versus sensory and cognitive factors.) (Chapters 5, 6, 11, and 14)

9. Why might her interests (knitting, reading, and singing) be helpful in assessing her cognition? (Chapter 15)

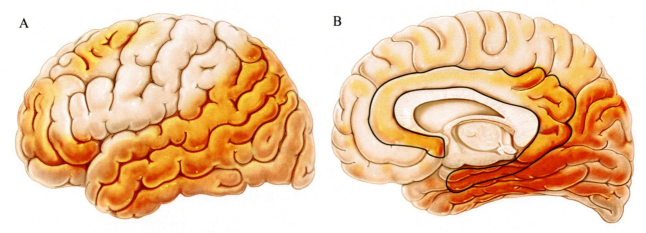

FIGURE 16–4. Medial (**A**) and lateral (**B**) views of Alzheimer pathology in brain. Orange shading represents areas of atrophy in early Alzheimer dementia: Darker shading indicates more atrophy, and lighter shading less atrophy.

Case 16–16: 73-Year-Old Male With Right Facial and Tongue Atrophy

Diagnosis: Acoustic neuroma resection and VII–XII anastamosis

Background: Mordecai is a 73-year-old male who volunteered for a research study on communication. During the evaluation, it was readily apparent that he has asymmetry of the face. The right side has few laugh lines and forehead wrinkles, whereas the left side looks typical for a man of his age (see Chapter 11, Figure 11–9B for an illustration of facial asymmetry). Speech is 100% intelligible despite some mild articulatory imprecision on velars.

An oral motor exam confirms right-sided weakness: limited movement of the lips on the right to create a smile, weak lip seal with air escaping from the right corner of his mouth when asked to sufflate (puff up) his cheeks (Figure 16–5), and limited movement of his right eyebrow. Upon protrusion, his tongue deviated to the right (Figure 16–6). The right side of his tongue was significantly atrophied, which resulted in the median septum being displaced to the right of the midline of the remaining tongue structure.

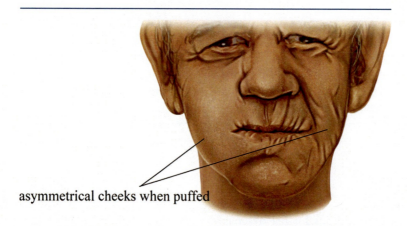

FIGURE 16–5. Mordecai facial asymmetry and inability to create lip seal with cheek sufflation.

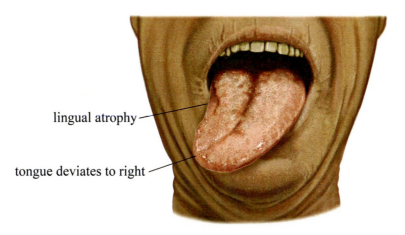

FIGURE 16–6. Mordecai tongue deviation upon protrusion.

Mordecai shares that 40 years prior, he developed hearing loss in his right ear and was subsequently diagnosed with an acoustic neuroma (a benign tumor of the Schwann cell/myelin) on his right auditory nerve (CN VIII). A surgical resection was conducted, which resulted in damage to both the auditory and the facial (CN VII) nerves. Because of this, in addition to the hearing loss, he now also had right facial weakness. In an attempt to resolve the facial weakness, a VII to XII anastomosis was conducted. This procedure involves splitting the healthy hypoglossal nerve and attaching one segment to the facial nerve distal to the surgical damage in order to reinnervate the facial muscles.

In Mordecai's case, the anastomosis did not work well. He continued to have right facial weakness, and in addition he developed right tongue weakness. Upon close examination, however, it was apparent that some of the nerves did reconnect. When producing velar sounds or swallowing, both of which require elevation and retraction of the posterior tongue, Mordecai had twitching of the muscles around his right eye.

1. Given the description above, identify the pertinent information in this case.
2. Why is weakness of both the upper and the lower face an important diagnostic sign? (**Hint:** Is this an indication of UMN or LMN damage?) See Chapter 11, Figure 11–11 for pertinent information.
3. Given lingual atrophy and deviation toward the right, what is the nature of damage?
4. What does the 100% intelligibility tell you about the use of facial and tongue muscles for speech production?
5. What kinds of difficulties with chewing and swallowing would you expect?

Section 2: Pediatric and Developmental Cases

Case 16–17: 5-Year-Old Male With Shunt Malfunction

[Expanded from Box 2–3]

Diagnosis: Exacerbation of hydrocephalus

Background: PJ was a 5-year old boy with severe developmental cognitive delay and progressive hydrocephalus (see Chapter 2) due to Crouzon syndrome. PJ was nonverbal and communicated through vocalizations, some simple switches, and other cues such as joint attention and eye contact. In addition to dealing with feeding and nutrition issues, managing the boy's ventriculoperitoneal shunt [i.e., a surgically placed tube that runs from the ventricles to the gut (peritoneum) to remove excess or obstructed CSF] was a constant battle for his physicians, nurses, and parents. Medical staff and family dealt with shunt revisions and a regular regimen of antibiotics for his infections. As infections arose, the shunt did not function properly and thus did not remove excess CSF from his ventricles. The shunt malfunctions and infections led to increased communication difficulties. His interactions would become muted, and he became lethargic until the infection resolved.

Hydrocephalus also damaged his hypothalamus (see Chapter 5), which compromised his ability to regulate body temperature. During infection, fevers would spike to high levels (e.g., above 105° Fahrenheit), and cooling him down with ice baths was necessary. When infections and malfunctions resolved, previous communicative interactions reemerged. Changes to cognition (alertness levels and communication) likely stemmed from several factors, including buildup of pressure within the ventricles (compressing adjacent brain tissue), inflammation of the meninges (again compressing adjacent structures), and homeostatic impairments due to the hypothalamic damage.

1. Given the description above, identify the pertinent information in this case.
2. What additional history might be useful?
3. What related neurosystems are likely to affect the status of PJ's communication and cognition? (See Chapters 7, 11, and 14)
4. What are your expectations for PJ's communication and cognition? What impairments do you expect to see? (Chapter 14)

Additional information: Crouzon syndrome is a genetic disorder characterized by severe craniofacial anomalies caused by the premature fusion of skull bones (Figure 16–7). Features include external strabismus (due to misalignment of the eyes), exophthalmos (bulging eyes due to small ocular orbits), and maxillary hypoplasia (underdeveloped maxilla). Hydrocephalus is common, and due to the fusing of cranial bones, pressure on the brain causes severe physical and cognitive impairments. Sensorineural hearing loss is also present for some. Craniofacial surgery can be used to address eye orbits and gaze issues, along with maxillary hypoplasia. Note that PJ did not have craniofacial surgery.

5. Consider how vision and gaze issues due to external strabismus would affect PJ's switch access (see Chapter 7). What cranial nerves are likely involved? (Chapter 11) What modifications might the therapy team (occupational, speech, and physical therapy disciplines) need to make to support switch access?
6. Aside from an impaired ability to regulate temperature, what other impairments to homeostasis are possible given hypothalamic dysfunction? (Chapter 5 and 12)
7. How might you distinguish between the acute and chronic (ongoing) impairments to communication, cognition, and swallowing in this case? It might help to consider direct effects of Crouzon syndrome and the effects of shunt malfunction/hydrocephalus.
8. Given the broad description above, what neurosystems were affected in this case? Please address those that were included in the case, mapping evidence for how a structure was affected based on symptoms. Also map those that you believe were likely affected, given the description of PJ's status. (Chapter 2, 5, 12, and 14)

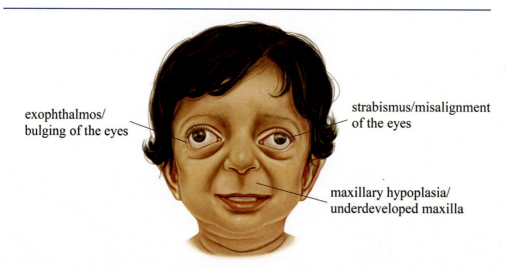

FIGURE 16–7. Craniofacial characteristics of Crouzon syndrome.

Case 16–18: 4-Year-Old Male With Fetal Alcohol Syndrome

Diagnosis: Cognitive impairment

Background: Travis is a 4-year-old male diagnosed with fetal alcohol syndrome (FAS) due to high maternal alcohol consumption during pregnancy. He was born prematurely, at 33 weeks of gestation, with low birth weight (4 pounds). Respiratory function was impaired for the first 2 years of his life but has improved since. At age 4 years, Travis is short in stature (Figure 16–8) and has a small head circumference. His weight is somewhat high for his stature (Figure 16–9). Other characteristics include widely spaced eyes, a flattened philtrum, maxillary and mandibular hypoplasia (i.e., underdevelopment of the mandible, characterized by a small chin; Figure 16–10), cardiac anomalies, and peripheral nerve deformities. Most developmental milestones were delayed, including first words, toileting, crawling, walking, and fine motor functions (e.g., pincer grasp). A recent speech-language evaluation revealed that Travis has a language delay and speech–sound production delays. Cognitive functions are mildly delayed as well, compared with peers.

1. Given the description above, identify the pertinent information in this case.
2. What additional history might be useful?
3. What brain structures and pathways account for Travis' gross and fine motor impairments? (Chapters 10 and 11)
4. What brain structures and pathways account for Travis' speech and language impairments? (Chapter 14)
5. What brain structures and pathways account for Travis' cognitive impairments? (Chapter 14)
6. How might his facial structures impact communication?

Additional information: FAS is developmental disorder caused by alcohol exposure during pregnancy. The degree of damage to the brain depends on the level of alcohol exposure. FAS results in physical symptoms, including low body weight, poor motor coordination, craniofacial anomalies, and cardiac anomalies. Cognitive and behavior symptoms include hyperactivity, attention impairments,

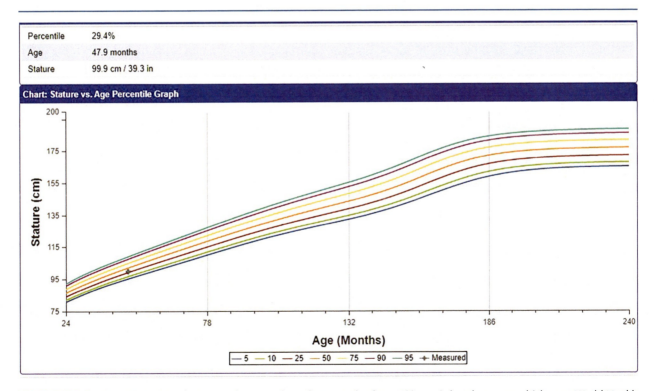

FIGURE 16–8. Growth chart for stature and percentile rank. Created at https://www.infantchart.com which uses World Health Organization metrics for calculation.

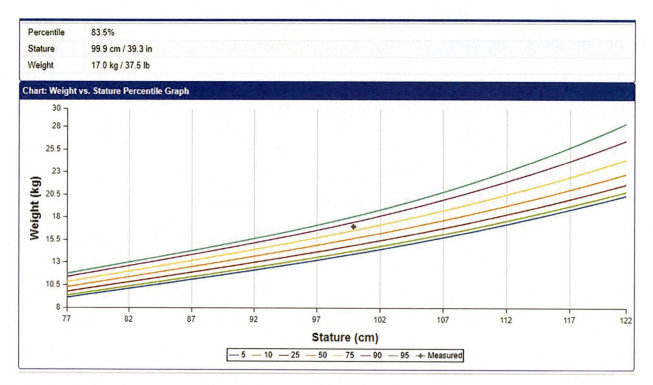

FIGURE 16–9. Growth chart mapping weight versus stature and percentile rank. Created at https://www.infantchart.com which uses World Health Organization metrics for calculation.

memory impairments, learning disabilities, as well as speech and language delays.

Case 16–19: 30-Year-Old Female With Agenesis of the Corpus Callosum

[Expanded from Box 4–1]

Diagnosis: Social cognition impairment

Background: Selika was a 30-year-old female with agenesis of the corpus callosum (ACC). There was a lack of development of the corpus callosum in the medial portion of the brain; however, there was a compensatory commissure anteriorly between the two hemispheres of the prefrontal cortex and posteriorly within the parieto-occipital regions between the two hemispheres. Etiology of Selika's agenesis is unknown; however, disruptions to development of the corpus callosum can include teratogens (medications or environmental toxins) that chemically block the development process or trauma. Note that agenesis literally means "lack of development," but the term actually refers to a continuum of interrupted development from a complete lack of commissural fibers between the hemispheres to a reduction in the number of connecting fibers. Selika had moderate impairments in social communication and pragmatics. She displayed limited empathy for others, minimal theory of mind, and egocentrism. She struggled with social conventions in general, including difficulty producing and understanding figurative language, humor, and sarcasm. One day during a session, she spontaneously shared, "I have a gun in my car." She did not seem to have any malintent by making that statement. She was simply reporting the facts. However, it resulted in an obligatory report to security. Selika's impairments to social cognition and pragmatics frequently led to miscommunication and behavioral incidents.

1. Given the description above, identify the pertinent information in this case.
2. Given the diagnosis, what critical time periods and developmental processes were likely disrupted? (Chapter 4 and 14)
3. What specific brain structures and pathways are likely involved in Selika's social communication impairments, including her difficulties processing figurative

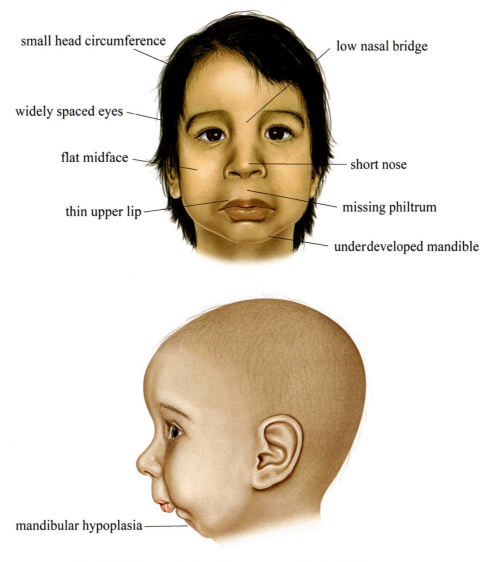

FIGURE 16–10. Craniofacial characteristics of fetal alcohol syndrome.

language, humor, sarcasm, egocentrism, and other pragmatic issues? (Chapter 14)
4. What do the striking impairments in social cognition and pragmatics associated with ACC tell you about the neural control of these complex communicative functions?
5. How might the impairments in social cognition and pragmatics have affected Selika's ability to make and maintain relationships throughout her life?

Additional information: Agenesis of the corpus callosum is a rare disorder that can be inherited as an autosomal or X-linked dominant trait or be due to an infection in the 12th through 22nd week of pregnancy (see Chapter 4 for developmental milestones and timelines) or exposure to alcohol during pregnancy/FAS (see Case 16–18 for characteristics of FAS). It results in a failure of the corpus callosum to connect the cerebral hemispheres. Severity ranges from severe cognitive impairments to mild psychosocial impairments. Craniofacial features vary from no obvious impairments to micro- or macroencephaly (small or large head circumference), bossing forehead, and anomalies to the pinna. Malformations to fingers (specifically lateral bending) are also common. Social communication impairments to figurative language comprehension, humor, social reasoning, and comprehension of facial expression are common in ACC.

Case 16–20: 11-Year-Old Male With Brainstem Tumor

Contributed by Jennifer Lundine and Angela Ciccia

Diagnosis: Medulloblastoma in the posterior fossa, posterior fossa syndrome

Background: Grant was an 11-year-old, typically developing boy with no significant medical history. One day, his parents noted that he had a left-sided facial droop. The following day, he had notable weakness on the left side of his body. They called to schedule an appointment with his pediatrician for the following day, but that night Grant experienced a seizure. His parents called 911, and he was taken by ambulance to a local children's hospital. A CT scan of his brain revealed a large medulloblastoma situated in his posterior fossa. He was scheduled for neurosurgery the following day to resect (i.e., remove) the tumor.

1. Given the description above, identify the pertinent information in this case.
2. What medical etiology is your primary concern?
3. What could account for the fact that Grant was showing no symptoms while surely there was a tumor growing in his brain? What could account for his eventual symptomology?
4. What aspects of cognition, communication, or swallowing could be affected and why?

Within 24 hours after his tumor resection, Grant spoke a few words to his parents but then developed cerebellar mutism (complete inability to speak). This is a fairly common complication following removal of posterior fossa tumors in children, particularly medulloblastomas. He was extremely labile (crying at unexpected times), and he exhibited significant difficulty controlling facial and extremity muscles. He had difficulty controlling his saliva and had limited or no control of oral musculature.

5. What could account for these symptoms after the tumor was removed?

Two weeks later, Grant is beginning to talk in short sentences and is trialing some food by mouth. His speech is characterized by ataxic dysarthria, and his intelligibility is significantly impaired. He is admitted to the inpatient rehabilitation unit, where he will receive intensive occupational therapy, physical therapy, and speech services. Primary speech goals will focus on speech, evaluating cognitive–communication needs in preparation for return to school, and transitioning to a full-oral diet. He will begin chemotherapy and cranial radiation as adjuvant treatment for his cancer.

6. What would be an explanation for Grant's persistent dysarthria?
7. What kind of education would you provide to the parents about his cancer treatments and potential long-term effects to cognition and/or language?

Case 16–21: 11-Year-Old Female with Traumatic Brain Injury

Contributed by Angela Ciccia and Jennifer Lundine

Diagnosis: Diffuse axonal injury, frontotemporal hematoma, diffuse contusions

Background: Maria is a social, typically developing fifth-grade student. In school, she skipped a grade in math and is now taking sixth-grade math. Other than a history of ear infections when she was little, she has no significant medical history. Maria was recently traveling to visit family in another state when her family's vehicle was involved in a head-on motor vehicle crash with a wrong-way driver while traveling approximately 65 miles per hour on the highway. Maria was wearing her seat belt but was found unconscious at the scene. Her mother and father sustained serious traumatic injuries, and the driver of the other car was deceased by the time emergency personnel arrived. Maria was taken emergently to a large children's hospital in a nearby large city. A CT of her brain revealed frontotemporal hematoma and small contusions throughout bifrontal and left temporal lobes. Neurosurgeons determined that no surgical intervention was needed. She was admitted to the intensive care unit (ICU) for initial care. Maria was slow to regain consciousness, and so after 4 days, the medical team requested an MRI of her brain. It showed evidence of diffuse axonal injury (DAI) throughout the frontal, temporal, and parietal lobes.

1. Given the description above, identify the pertinent information in this case.
2. What medical etiology is your primary concern?
3. What aspects of cognition, communication, or swallowing could be affected and why?

After 2 weeks in the ICU, Maria was more responsive and able to be transferred to another floor in the hospital, where she began receiving occupational therapy, physical therapy, and speech services, and an evaluation for inpatient rehabilitation was begun. She was admitted to inpatient rehabilitation 3 weeks from the date of her injury. She remained on the rehab unit for 3 additional weeks. At discharge, she is walking, talking, and able to complete basic activities of daily living (e.g., dressing herself, brushing her teeth, and cleaning herself in the shower). Her language testing reveals that Maria's expressive and receptive language skills are just below the average expected for her age. Neuropsychological testing reveals that Maria's IQ is also just below average and that she shows subtle deficits in memory, processing speed, and attention. The SLP recommends that Maria be evaluated for school services to support her return to the classroom. She has no recommendations for physical therapy or occupational therapy after discharge.

4. What would be the explanation for the recovery that Maria experiences?
5. Considering Maria's language and cognitive testing were just below average, why would the SLP recommend an evaluation at school?
6. What kind of education would you provide to Maria's parents and to her school?
7. Why is it important to ensure that staff at Maria's middle school (grades 6–8) is aware of her history of TBI?

Case Question Answers

Case 16–1

1. Given the description above, identify the pertinent information in this case.
   - Car speed—not too fast, Penny hit and then flipped over the car.
   - Penny was at least partially oriented (she apologized).
   - She lost consciousness soon after the accident.
2. What medical etiology is your primary concern?
   - Traumatic brain injury (TBI)
3. What could account for the fact that she was initially alert but then lost consciousness shortly afterward? (Chapters 13 and 14)
   - Hematoma. The loss of consciousness did not occur until there was enough blood to increase intracranial pressure to the point that it compressed the brainstem and reticular formation.
4. What aspects of cognition, communication, or swallowing could be affected and why? (Chapters 10, 11, and 14)
   - Cognition: executive function, attention, memory—potential damage to frontal lobes and diffuse axonal injury that would affect cognitive processing.
   - Speech production: potential dysarthria due to diffuse axonal injury affecting corticobulbar tracts.
   - Swallowing: potential dysphagia due to diffuse axonal injury affecting corticobulbar tracts.
5. What is a primary concern with this diagnosis and how might it impact cognition or communication?
   - Increased intracranial pressure. Blood in the epidural space cannot reach the surface of the brain, but if it is not removed (evacuated), the excess blood can create pressure within the cranium. The cranium, made up of fused bones, cannot expand to relieve the pressure, causing damage to the soft brain tissue.
   - The pressure can have a generalized effect on cognition, slowing thinking. It also may affect consciousness, respiration, and cardiac function if the pressure results in compression of the brainstem.

Case 16–2

1. Given the description above, identify the pertinent information in this case.
   - Weakness, fasciculations, and hyperactive reflexes
   - Postural headaches

2. What do the motor signs and symptoms tell you about areas of the CNS (structures and/or pathways) that might be affected? (Chapter 10)
   - Lateral corticospinal tract, given UMN and LMN signs in legs
   - Anterior corticospinal tract, given LMN signs in trunk
   - Anterior horn cells, given mixed UMN/LMN signs
3. What cranial nerve(s) provides sensation to the meninges, pertinent to the painful postural headaches? (Chapter 11)
   - CNs V and X
4. What medical etiology is your primary concern and why?
   - Amyotrophic lateral sclerosis—presence of both UMN and LMN signs
5. What additional history would you want to know?
   - Family history of neurologic disorders
6. What areas of communication, swallowing, or cognition would you want to evaluate? (Chapters 11 and 14)
   - Speech and swallowing function. Declines in respiratory drive for speech, phonation quality, and articulation precision could be indications of ALS, along with cough strength to expel potential aspirates and oral–pharyngeal dysphagia. Speech, swallowing, and respiratory assessment are primarily used to identify or rule out bulbar symptoms.
7. Does this information change the potential medical etiology?
   - Mixed UMN and LMN signs in this case indicate that one site of lesion or symptom (in this case) is at the anterior horn cell. In this case, impairments are transitory and partially or mostly resolve with a change in position. In the case of ALS, mixed UMN/LMN signs are progressive—beginning with predominantly UMN signs and moving toward predominantly LMN signs. Furthermore, there is typically early progression to involve speech/phonatory systems and swallowing function.

Case 16–3

1. Given the description above, identify the pertinent information in this case.
   - Gradual onset of difficulties with both speech and swallow

- Weakness of multiple structures innervated by corticobulbar pathways but also corticospinal (intercostal muscle involvement)
2. What do the characteristics of her speech and swallowing tell you about the articulatory structures affected and the location of damage in the CNS? (Chapters 10 and 11)
   - Coughing/choking with solids but not thin liquids—a potential indication of pharyngeal weakness
   - Strained, effortful speech—spasticity in the laryngeal muscles, UMN damage
   - Hypernasality and nasal emission—weakness of the velum, UMN, or LMN
   - Slowed diadochokinesis—possible weakness of oral articulators, UMN, or LMN
   - Fasciculations of the mouth and tongue—weakness and LMN damage
   - Breathiness—weakness of laryngeal muscles, most likely LMN damage
   - Hyperactive gag reflex—UMN damage
   - Weak cough—weakness of laryngeal muscles
3. What medical etiology is your primary concern and why?
   - Amyotrophic lateral sclerosis—presence of both UMN and LMN signs
4. What additional history would you want to know?
   - Family history of neurologic disorders
   - Impact of the speech impairments on daily communication
5. From a diagnostic standpoint, why is the presence of impairments to structures of the face, tongue, pharynx, and larynx important? (Chapters 10 and 11)
   - The presence of mixed UMN and LMN symptoms is important because they are indicative of a small range of diseases. The presence in the speech structures indicates a bulbar presentation of ALS, which has a shorter life span when compared to a spinal onset of ALS.
6. What do you think will happen to Charmane's speech, swallow, respiration, and mobility as the disease progresses?
   - She will eventually become anarthric, losing all usable and intelligible speech.
   - Swallow will further decline, resulting in inability to tolerate any oral intake and inability to manage her own secretions.
   - Respiratory drive for speech and to clear potential penetrates/aspirates in the larynx will be inadequate; eventually mechanical ventilation will be necessary to sustain respiration.
7. What kind of education or resources would you provide to the patient?
   - Referral to SLP for full evaluation and assessment of communicative function
   - Resources such as the ALS foundation and support groups

Case 16–4

1. Given the description above, identify the pertinent information in this case.
   - High-speed motor vehicle crash
   - Increased intracranial pressure, indicating either hemorrhage or brain swelling
   - The need for a ventilator indicates she cannot breathe on her own, suggesting damage to or compression of the brainstem.
2. What additional history might be useful?
   - History of brain injuries
   - Social and educational background: Did she have pre-existing difficulties with socialization or learning?
3. What does recovery of consciousness tell you about recovery from the accident? (Chapters 12 and 14)
   - Pressure or damage to the brainstem is resolving.
4. What is a possible explanation for the impairments in attention and awareness? (Chapter 15)
   - Frontal lobe damage could affect awareness; attentional networks are extensive and could be impacted by focal damage to frontal or parietal lobes or by diffuse axonal injury (DAI).
5. Discuss the impact of attentional deficits on swallowing and communication. (Chapter 14)
   - KayLea is unable to sustain her attention long enough to swallow a mouthful. With such a short attention span, she is unable to hold a meaningful conversation.
6. What are some potential explanations for her limited vocalizations and whispers? (Chapters 11 and 14)
   - Damage to the cranial nerves controlling laryngeal muscles
   - Damage to the vocal folds due to intubation
   - Apraxia of speech affecting motor planning and initiation of speech production
   - Language or cognitive impairments affecting initiation of speech
7. What could account for the remarkable recovery of her cognitive and communication functions? (Chapters 14 and 15)
   - Neural plasticity and rewiring of the brain.

- The initial symptoms were due primarily to swelling of the brain (a temporary condition) rather than damage to neurons and pathways.
8. What kind of education and resources would you provide to the patient?
   - Information about long-term effects of TBI, including the possibility that cognitive deficits may appear when the patient is tired, emotional, or in pain
   - Resources for support groups for survivors of TBI

Case 16–5

1. Given the description above, identify the pertinent information in this case.
   - Past medical history of obesity, diabetes, hypertension, and hypercholesterolemia
   - Pharmacological management of hypertension and hypercholesterolemia
   - Global aphasia, right-sided weakness, and confusion (disorientation)
2. What do the cognitive and communication characteristics tell you about the possible location of damage? (Chapters 1 and 14)
   - Right-sided weakness: left hemisphere motor strip
   - Global aphasia: peri-sylvian region of the left hemisphere
   - Confusion: nonlocalizing
3. What medical etiology is your primary concern and why?
   - Stroke: sudden onset of unilateral weakness and cognitive symptoms
4. Explain the relationship between the nonfluent aphasia and the location of the stroke in the superior branch of the left MCA.
   - Superior branch of MCA supplies language areas and network superior to the sylvian fissure, including Broca area.
5. What kind of education or resources would you provide to the patient and family?
   - Referral to SLP for full evaluation and assessment of communicative function
   - Resources for aphasia organizations (National Aphasia Association, Aphasia Access) and aphasia centers
6. Why is pharmacological management of Darius' atrial fibrillation so important?
   - If the atrial fibrillation is not resolved, clots will likely continue to form and further cardioembolic strokes may occur.
7. What is the mechanism of tPA and why did Darius experience substantial improvements in both physical and cognitive functions following administration?
   - tPA breaks down clots and removes occlusions to blood flow; this can essentially restore perfusion to brain tissue.

Case 16–6

1. Given the description above, identify the pertinent information in this case. (Chapter 13)
   - Severe, bilateral carotid stenosis—restricts perfusion to both hemispheres
   - Past medical history of hypercholesterolemia, hypertension, and diabetes
2. Given the insidious changes to language and cognition, what brain structures are likely affected? (Chapter 14)
   - Word retrieval: left temporal and parietal regions
   - Language comprehension: Wernicke area
   - Discourse comprehension: right hemisphere
   - Memory and decision-making: bilateral prefrontal cortices
3. Given the diagnosis of small vessel disease, what parts of cerebral vascular territories are likely to be affected?
   - Cerebral watershed regions (ACA–MCA and PCA–MCA watershed regions), as this is where the smallest vessels exist cortically.
4. Why would AChE treatment improve cognitive function? (Chapters 3 and 15)
   - This prevents the breakdown of acetylcholine in the brain, particularly in limbic circuits, which can help compensate for the loss of cholinergic neurons. Small vessel disease is thought to break down cholinergic pathways.

Case 16–7

1. Given the description above, identify the pertinent information in this case. (Chapter 12)
   - Social history—specifically smoking
   - She is a female—a higher risk for aneurysm, particularly when combined with smoking
   - Identification of intracranial hemorrhage and the presence of a burst saccular aneurysm on the circle of Willis
2. What additional history might be useful?
   - Any other drugs or medications that increased risk for aneurysm

- Any familial history of aneurysm or other connective tissue disorders
3. What are your expectations for Marjorie's language and cognition? What impairments do you expect to see? (Chapter 14)
    - Deficits in language comprehension—following verbal and written commands, particularly as they become more syntactically complex and lengthy
    - Deficits in language expression—anomia, breakdowns in syntax (particularly in conversation)
    - Impaired orientation which is somewhat better when using supports to reduce language barriers
    - Reduced alertness levels and basic attention to tasks (even how long she can sustain attention to eating, getting dressed, etc.)
    - Anosagnosia—lack of awareness and insight into deficits
    - Executive dysfunction, characterized by poor self-monitoring, reduced self-regulation, behavioral inhibition, and impulsivity. Problems with sequencing complex tasks and perseverations are common.
4. What risk factors for aneurysm did Marjorie display prior to the incident? (Chapter 13)
    - Female, smoker
5. What are the potential effects of blood in contact with brain tissue? (Chapter 13)
    - Increased risk for vasospasm in the region where blood contacted brain tissue.
    - Blood in contact with brain tissue causes edema/swelling, which further reduces perfusion to that region.
    - Blood has cytotoxic, oxidative, and inflammatory effects on brain tissue, essentially killing nearby neurons.
6. What are the potential effects of vasospasm on brain function?
    - The ineffective, to-and-fro of blood leads to poor perfusion and potential for further clotting. Global hypoperfusion leads to hypoxia and potential ischemia if not remedied.
7. Given her symptoms (impairments), what brain structures were likely impacted by this incident? (Chapter 14)
    - Left hemisphere language systems—particularly frontal structures
    - Bilateral prefrontal cortices
8. Draw an image(s) of the brain that accounts for the site(s) of lesions.

Case 16–8

1. Given the description above, identify the pertinent information in this case.
    - Attention impairments
    - Disorganized, confused discourse production
    - Inattention or loss of visual processing on the left side of space
    - Reduced speech intelligibility
2. Given the changes to cognition and communication, what brain structures or networks are likely affected? (Chapter 14)
    - Focusing, responding, and inattention to left side of space: right hemisphere parietal lobe or attentional networks
    - Disorganized, confused discourse: right hemisphere
    - Speech: corticobulbar pathways
3. What physical and cognitive factors likely contributed to his impaired swallow (dysphagia)? (Chapters 11 and 14)
    - Impaired attention
    - Unilateral neglect affecting getting spoon directly into his mouth
    - Limited physical/cognitive endurance
    - Left-sided sensory impairments (oral and pharyngeal), particularly when coupled with attention impairments
    - Left-sided weakness (oral and pharyngeal)
4. Why do task complexity and divided attention affect performance? (Chapter 14)
    - Limited attentional capacity; tasks that used to be automatic now require attention, taxing the attentional system
5. Explain the changes to communication and brain structures/networks that might be involved.
    - Theory of mind deficits—theory of mind or mentalizing network
    - Discourse production disorders—cannot be localized within the right hemisphere due to the large networks
6. What effects might his communication disorders have on relationships?
    - Partner and friends do not feel valued, causing loss of relationships.

Case 16–9

1. Given the description above, identify the pertinent information in this case.

- Speech, limb ataxia—possibly trunkal ataxia
- Altered level of consciousness/alertness
- Disorientation initially
- Nystagmus

2. What additional history might be useful?
   - Nature of disorientation (Person? Place? Time?)
   - Medical history
   - Social history and work history

3. What are your expectations for Devin's speech? What impairments would you expect to see?
   - OME findings: Strength and agility for most structures is probably fine (coordination would be impaired).
   - DDK/AMR findings: You would expect to see inconsistencies in rate and accuracy (perhaps amplitude/volume and coordination of respiration to speech too).
   - Spontaneous speech and reading sampling: You would expect ataxic speech (slurred speech with inconsistencies in rate and coordination).

4. What are your expectations for Devin's swallowing? What impairments would you expect to see? (Chapters 10, 11, and 14)
   - Potential for discoordination and timing given speech deficits—likely oral phase impairments, possibly pharyngeal, may have trouble coordinating respiration and swallow (sometimes aerophagia—swallowing air occurs, resulting in frequent belching)

5. What are your expectations for Devin's cognitive status? What potential impairments would you expect to see? (Chapter 14)
   - Problems with orientation initially/acutely, which likely resolve
   - Attention impairments primarily related to degree of wakefulness, altered level of alertness, and physical/cognitive endurance issues
   - Substantial deficits in working memory acutely/subacutely

6. Given the site of lesion, paired with the knowledge that cognition improved markedly during the first several days, what types of cognitive difficulties would likely remain? Why? (Chapter 14)
   - Working memory deficits—given the role of the cerebellum in working memory

7. Why did the speech and gait impairments persist? How does this relate to the lesion location and size? (Chapters 10, 11, and 12)

- Likely the lesion was primarily in the SCA distribution because limb ataxia, nystagmus, and ataxic dysarthria are the predominant symptoms.
- PICA would likely result in more trunkal ataxia and is often concomitant with symptoms of Wallenberg syndrome/lateral medullary syndrome.
- AICA infarcts are rarer and include more vertigo and hearing dysfunction, facial sensation and motor impairments, and Horner syndrome (decreased pupil size, ptosis, and decreased sweating on affected side of face).

Case 16–10

1. Given the description above, identify the pertinent information in this case.
   - Past medical history of hypercholesterolemia, hypertension, and smoking
   - Nausea, fatigue, ataxia, vertigo, diplopia, and nystagmus, but remaining cerebellar testing was normal
   - Right nasolabial folds flattened, tongue and velum weakness
   - Dysarthria—harsh and breathy voice, articulatory breakdowns
   - Severe dysphagia
   - Wallenberg syndrome (lateral medullary syndrome)

2. What additional history might be useful?
   - Social history, work history

3. Given the case description, what cranial nerves were affected? (Chapter 11)
   - V, VI, VII, VIII, IX, X, XII

4. Given the effects to those cranial nerves, draw an image of the brain that accounts for the area of probable lesion.
   - Lateral medulla, cerebellum PICA distribution

5. Considering the cranial nerves involved, what are your expectations for Alando's speech? What types of impairments do you expect to see?
   - OME findings—impairments to ipsilateral CNs
     i. V (mild weakness of jaw)
     ii. VI (ipsilateral eye—horizontal diplopia)
     iii. VII (flattened nasolabial folds and sensory impairments to ipsilateral face)
     iv. VIII (vestibular signs and nystagmus)
     v. IX (along with V and X—palatal paralysis, nasal regurgitation/hypernasality, and ipsilateral pharyngeal paralysis)

vi. X (pharyngeal and laryngeal paralysis)
vii. XII (tongue weakness/deviation)
- DDK/AMR findings—ataxia and coordination/timing issues, breathiness and related deficits in endurance
- Spontaneous speech and reading sample—breathiness, hypernasality, endurance/phrasing issues, and timing and coordination issues/ataxia

6. What are your expectations for Alando's swallow? What impairments do you expect to see? Why are there changes over time?
   - Overall, profound impairments to most structures of the swallowing mechanism.
   - Increased swelling over time led to increased dysphagia and speech/voice problems.
   - Oral prep/processing issues: strength, sensation, and coordination issues. Problems managing oral secretions.
   - Oral phase: delayed onset of the pharyngeal swallow.
   - Pharyngeal: reduced excursion of the laryngeal mechanism paired with timing issues. Pharyngeal weakness resulting in poor pharyngeal clearance/residuals.
   - Pharyngeal/laryngeal: breathy voice and poor airway protection.
   - Laryngeal/respiratory: impaired cough reflex and potential problems with respiratory drive to clear any potential penetrates/aspirates (food and liquids that enter the larynx and airway)

7. Why did dysphagia and gait improve? Why did his dysarthria persist? (Chapters 11 and 12)
   - Gait changes were more cerebellar; dysphagia was likely a combination of cerebellar (movement control/refinement) and medullary (cranial nerve inputs). Although perfusion to cerebellar blood supply is interrupted early on, given edema, this typically resolves subacutely. Weakness remained, particularly in CN X, XI, and XII distributions, accounting for the persistence of dysarthria. Dysphagia likely remained—just more manageable through diet and compensatory strategies.

Case 16–11

1. Given the description above, identify the pertinent information in this case.
   - Diplopia, dysarthria, and dysphagia
   - Respiratory arrest
   - Botulinum poisoning

2. What structure in what pathway was the botulinum toxin acting on? (Chapter 3)
   - Neuromuscular junction for muscles involved in respiration

3. How does this accidental ingestion of tomatoes with the botulinum toxin differ from intentional injection of Botox for limb spasticity or spasmodic dysphonia? (Chapter 3)
   - Exposure in this case was more systemic, versus focal (local) application within injections.

4. What neurotransmitter and/or process was disrupted in this incident? (Chapter 3)
   - Acetylcholine release from pre-synaptic neuron

5. Given the descriptions from the case, what cranial nerve outputs were clearly affected? (Chapter 11)
   - IX, X for sure; III, IV, and VI appear likely, which means that probably motor outputs (neuromuscular junctions involving cranial and other peripheral motor outputs) from II or III to XII are probably affected.

6. Given the action of botulinum toxin and the cranial nerves affected, what are your expectations for Amos' speech (specifically, voice/phonation)? What impairments do you expect to see? (Chapter 11)
   - OME findings—VII (bilateral facial weakness), IX (along with V and X—velar weakness), X (aphonia/hypophonia and/or problems with closure of the vocal folds), and XII (lingual weakness).
   - Poor respiratory drive and coordination for speech.
   - Speaking valve placement would be necessary to assess voicing and quality of laryngeal closure and respiratory drive for speech/phonation.

7. Would you expect oral and laryngeal sensation to be affected? Why or why not?
   - No, because the botulism affects the neuromuscular junction, so the sensory pathways in the cranial nerves should be preserved.

8. What are your expectations for Amos' swallowing? What impairments do you expect to see? (Chapter 11)
   - Examining voicing and signs of laryngeal closure would be crucial. Placement of the speaking valve would be necessary to examine voicing, which would be breathy/hypophonic or aphonic. This means poor airway protection and risk for aspiration. Although laryngeal sensation is intact,

inadequate laryngeal closure along with poor respiratory drive to clear potential aspirates would be a severe problem.
- Management of oral secretions may also be impaired—sensation should be intact, so he may just expectorate (spit out, typically into a basin or towel).

9. Why was mechanical ventilation (a ventilator) necessary? Specifically describe the relevant muscles and neurons/pathways. (Chapter 10)
   - It is likely that both the diaphragm and accessory muscles of inspiration/expiration (external intercostals, internal intercostals, scalenes, trapezius, etc.) were affected.
   - Botulinum affects signaling at the neuromuscular junction, blocking the release of acetylcholine to activate muscles.

10. Would you anticipate problems with cognition? Why or why not? (Chapter 14)
    - Not necessarily—depends on how quickly breathing/respiration was reestablished and whether there was any hypoxia.

Case 16–12

1. Given the description above, identify the pertinent information in this case.
   - Dysphagia and dysarthria, hypernasality
   - Poor endurance and fatigue of speech/swallowing muscles
   - Rapid onset of weakness, recovery with rest
2. What additional history might be useful?
   - Previous medical history
   - Social history and work history
3. Why was the initial cranial nerves examination essentially normal? (Chapter 11)
   - Muscles innervated by cranial nerves had been "rested"—they had not been activated significantly prior to prompts for OME, speaking, or swallowing.
4. What structure in what pathway was affected?
   - Neuromuscular junction in corticospinal tract
5. What neurotransmitter and/or process was disrupted in this situation? (Chapter 3)
   - Acetylcholine (ACh) and blocked/destroyed ACh receptors
6. Explain the significance of increasing weakness over time. (Chapter 3)
   - Calls for activation of the neuromuscular junction came with every OME, speech, and swallowing task. Acetylcholine was progressively depleted over time, and there was not adequate rest time to recycle and replace acetylcholine stores.
7. What are your expectations for Judy's speech? (Chapter 11) What impairments would you expect to see? What would you do to account for limited endurance and decline over time?
   - OME findings—definite effects to IX (weak velum resulting in hypernasality and nasal regurgitation).
   - DDK/AMR findings—declining over time with fatigue.
   - Spontaneous speech and oral reading sampling—declining over time with fatigue.
   - Differential diagnosis process: An immediate concern with degenerative diseases that affect endurance in the speech mechanism (Parkinson disease, ALS, MS, myasthenia gravis, etc.)—consider differential diagnosis by eliminating those that do not fit by the nature of that fatigue. Recovery with rest eliminates a couple of options (i.e., not ALS or Parkinson disease). The rapid nature of decline and relatively rapid recovery is an important indicator.
8. What are your expectations for Judy's swallow? How would you account for deterioration of swallow over time? What impairments do you expect to see? (Chapters 11 and 14)
   - OME may not be sensitive to weakness initially, so noting changes over time is key.
   - Oral phase: Velar weakness would result in nasal regurgitation but would also reduce pressures in the pharynx, leading to poor pharyngeal clearance.
   - Pharyngeal phase: Pharyngeal weakness, resulting in poor pharyngeal clearance; possibly reduced inversion of the epiglottis, which would reduce airway protection.
   - Pharyngeal/laryngeal: Because food/liquids are not cleared effectively from the pharynx and may enter the laryngeal vestibule, there is a risk for aspiration.
   - Laryngeal/respiratory: Reduced respiratory drive would further compromise ability to clear any potential penetrates or aspirates.

Case 16–13

1. Given the description above, identify the pertinent information in this case.

- Dysarthria, dysphagia
- Troubles with ADLs/self-care and mobility
- Axial rigidity, cogwheel rigidity, postural instability, stooped posture, shuffling/festinating steps, festinating speech

2. What additional history might be useful?
   - Previous medical history
   - Social history and access to supports and living situation

3. What brain structures are likely to be involved in this case? (Chapter 11)
   - Basal ganglia and substantia nigra; reduction of dopaminergic cells in the substantia nigra impacts the functions of both direct and indirect basal ganglia circuits.

4. Correlate her physical impairments with brain substrates.
   - Hypokinesia and bradykinesia relate to dopamine circuits in the basal ganglia and midbrain (although Parkinson disease is not a direct dysfunction of the basal ganglia, reductions in dopamine in the substantia nigra are critical to carrying out functions of the basal ganglia).

5. Why is she "slow but accurate"?
   - Bradyphrenia—an alteration of processing speed

6. What are your expectations for Gloria's speech? (Chapter 11) What impairments do you expect to see?
   - OME findings—festinating speech, hypophonic speech (soft phonation), reduced coordination of respiration and speech, subtle weakness to some oral structures; may see a return of the snout reflex (also known as the orbicularis oris reflex—a pouting-like protrusion elicited by tapping the closed lips, a primitive reflex present in early development which returns with Parkinson disease)
   - DDK/AMR findings—festinating breakdowns over time (increasingly muddled and imprecise over time)
   - Spontaneous speech and oral reading samples—rapid rate of speech, underarticulated, which results in a muddled-imprecise quality, increased breakdowns at the ends of phrases; monoloudness (poor variation in loudness), monopitch (poor variation in pitch), and reductions in stress and timing

7. What are your expectations for Gloria's swallowing? What impairments do you expect to see? (Chapter 11)
   - OME findings—perhaps mild impairments in strength, some problems with coordination of movements (may not be as evident in some isolated tasks)
   - Oral preparatory and oral phase function—extended oral processing time (possibly evidence of lingual pumping—return of a primitive swallowing behavior used in the expression of milk during breastfeeding), impairments in oral clearance (mild residuals remain)
   - Pharyngeal phase—possible occurrence of pharyngeal signs such as changes to voice quality, wet/gurgly voice, coughing, choking, etc.
   - In an instrumental assessment—you could more directly monitor oral processing in MBS or endoscopic exam (FEES), look for lingual pumping, examine oral processing time, look for delays in onset of pharyngeal swallow, and examine pharyngeal clearance.

8. What are your expectations regarding cognition? (Chapter 14)
   - Bradyphrenia (slow thinking) and slow rise time (i.e., performance improves slightly over the course of an interaction).
   - Orientation is likely fine. Attention and processing speed are likely impaired. Working memory is likely impaired.

Case 16–14

1. Given the description above, identify the pertinent information in this case.
   - Hyperkinetic movements
   - Changes to language (aphasia/anomia), cognition, and behavior (inhibition, agitation, and aggression)
   - Dysphagia and dysarthria

2. What additional history might be useful?
   - Previous medical history
   - Social history, level of support, and living situation prior to admission

3. Given the diagnosis and descriptions of impairments, what brain structure(s) is likely affected? (Chapter 10)
   - Caudate nucleus, hippocampus, and frontal cortex

4. What does her area of brain damage/dysfunction have to do with her behaviors, and why is she in a locked behavioral unit? (Chapters 10 and 14)
   - Relates to basal ganglia inputs and outputs to the prefrontal cortex, behavioral inhibition, self-regulation, decision-making, etc.

5. What are your expectations for Lucy's speech? What impairments do you expect to see? (Chapter 11)
   - OME findings—possibly subtle weakness in structures but, more prominently, problems with coordination of movements
   - DDK/AMR findings—unpredictable shifts in volume, pitch, rate, etc.
   - Spontaneous speech and oral reading samples—unpredictable, irregular rate and poor control of volume, pitch, etc. Note that there may be some slow, extended words as Lucy attempts to control her hyperkinetic movements.
6. What are your expectations for Lucy's swallowing? What impairments do you expect to see? (Chapter 11)
   - Oral preparatory and oral phase: Delayed and extended oral processing and problems coordinating timing.
   - Pharyngeal phase: Unilateral effects to the pharynx may further impede swallowing coordination initially but become more bilateral over time.
   - Cognitive impacts on swallowing: Impaired attention and overall awareness, from a cognitive standpoint, is likely to compromise her oral processing and swallowing safety in general.

Case 16–15

1. Given the description above, identify the pertinent information in this case.
   - Dysphagia
   - Memory impairments
2. What additional history might be useful?
   - Previous medical history
   - Previous social and work history, living situation prior to admission
3. What are your expectations for Selma's swallowing? What impairments do you expect? (Chapter 11)
   - Potentially problems with oral processing, may be extended or perseverative
   - Delayed swallow onset
4. What are your expectations about Selma's cognition? What impairments do you expect? (Chapter 14)
   - Memory impairments—episodic and short-term memory/recent memories
   - Disorientation to person, place, and time
   - Pathfinding and navigation problems
   - Difficulty with complex (checkbook, buying groceries) or novel tasks
   - Increasing difficulty with routine, everyday tasks (chores, self-care sequences)
   - Impaired discourse
5. What impact is Selma's impaired vision and hearing loss likely to have (if any) on her cognition and communication? (Chapters 7, 8, and 14)
   - Certainly, both could have an impact. Vision may impact orientation to person, place, and time.
   - Hearing loss is known to co-occur with dementia and further contribute to impairments in cognition and communication.
6. Given her presumed diagnosis, describe how the patterns of atrophy in Figure 16–4 account for her impairments. (Chapter 14)
   - Anterior temporal and hippocampal atrophy account for episodic memory impairments and autobiographical memory impairments.
   - Hypothalamic atrophy accounts for impairments in lack of hunger or interest in eating.
   - Parietal atrophy accounts for disorientation to place, movement, and space.
   - Temporal atrophy accounts for disorientation to person and face recognition.
7. How might the likely presence of atrophy to the posterior temporal and parietal regions influence swallowing, sensory processing, and cognition? (Hint: Think about agnosias and the dorsal and ventral streams.) (Chapters 7, 12, and 14)
   - Disruptions to dorsal stream sending information about orientation to space, movement, etc.
   - Disruptions to ventral stream sending information about orientation to person, face recognition, perhaps object recognition, and color recognition.
   - Agnosias occur with damage to the parietal–temporal swath.
8. Describe the underlying reasons for her dysphagia. Assuming her speech and voice quality are typical for her age, what does that tell you about the etiology of her dysphagia? (Hint: Think motor versus sensory and cognitive factors.) (Chapters 5, 6, 11, and 14)
   - Part of it is cognitive—limited awareness.
   - Part of it is likely sensory/agnosia—oral agnosias are common in Alzheimer disease.
9. Why might her interests (knitting, reading, and singing) be helpful in assessing her cognition? (Chapter 15)
   - Personal relevance/saliency will make her more motivated to participate in activities. Her preserved procedural knowledge will allow her to be successful in these activities.

Case 16–16

1. Given the description above, identify the pertinent information in this case.
   - Right acoustic neuroma resection and VII–XII anastamosis
   - Loss of forehead wrinkles on right
   - Right lingual and facial weakness
2. Why is weakness of both the upper and the lower face an important diagnostic sign? (Hint: Is this an indication of UMN or LMN damage?) See Chapter 11, Figure 11–11 for pertinent information.
   - It helps to distinguish point of lesion is LMN (and not UMN).
3. Given lingual atrophy and deviation toward the right, what is the nature of damage?
   - LMN; damage to both CN VII and CN XII
4. What does the 100% intelligibility tell you about the use of facial and tongue muscles for speech production?
   - There is a great deal of adaptation that can occur. Consider knowledge from prior coursework about the DIVA model of speech production that accounts for feedback, feedforward, and importantly adaptation.
5. What kinds of difficulties with chewing and swallowing would you expect?
   - Problems with oral transfer (anterior-to-posterior bolus propulsion) are likely.
   - Also, problems with oral preparation may occur because of difficulty retrieving masticated food from between teeth or the cheek (buccal) cavity is likely given tongue weakness.
   - Oral preparation problems also relate to facial weakness. Food/liquid may leak out of his lips due to poor labial seal on the weak side, problems retrieving food from utensils, and even problems keeping food out of cheeks.

Case 16–17

1. Given the description above, identify the pertinent information in this case.
   - Hydrocephalus
   - The presence of a ventriculoperitoneal shunt
   - Feeding and nutrition issues
   - Nonverbal
   - Eye gaze issues
   - Uses switches and other augmentative forms of communication
   - Infections and high fevers with recurrent shunt malfunctions, decreased levels of alertness
2. What additional history might be useful?
   - Nature of feeding and nutrition issues, the presence of a feeding tube?
   - The family's social history (Parents? Siblings? School?) and supports (family, friends, and paid support workers); socioeconomic factors
   - Any radiographic imaging reports that would help address brain structure and potential damage by recurrent shunt malfunctions and hydrocephalus
3. What related neurosystems are likely to affect the status of PJ's communication and cognition? (See Chapters 7, 11, and 14)
   - Visuospatial processing impairments, visual acuity and tracking abilities (may need to collaborate with other disciplines to get this information)
   - Tactile–sensory processing for switch access
   - Motor control—gross and fine, including coordinating hand–eye movements
4. What are your expectations for PJ's communication and cognition? What impairments do you expect to see? (Chapter 14)
   - PJ was nonverbal prior to this recent shunt malfunction, so we would expect that to continue. Perhaps nonlinguistic verbalizations would be present (e.g., gurgling, simple cooing, probably not to the level of babbling or reduplicative syllable productions/prelinguistic communication).
   - Given his use of switches and other simple augmentative alternative communication devices, we would anticipate (at least prior to shunt malfunction) that there was a basic comprehension of cause and effect. Obviously, that was altered given the shunt malfunction, and it is unclear whether that would return or how quickly after resolution of the shunt malfunction.
   - It appears that (at least prior to shunt malfunction) PJ had comprehension of some linguistic and nonlinguistic communication, such as orienting responses to stimuli (e.g., joint attention).
   - Following the shunt malfunction, it is evident that compression of tissues had decreased communication and responses to previously established functions.
   - See previous note about orienting responses to stimuli, simple commands (at least prior to the shunt malfunction—altered afterwards).

- Given observational measures of levels of alertness and response to people in the environment (particularly parents and any siblings), it appears that PJ had joint gaze and attention prior to shunt malfunction.
- After the shunt malfunction, compression of brain tissues has reduced the level of alertness (likely due to compression of the reticular activating system, thalamus, and cerebral cortex) and basic attention. This may return if swelling and infection are managed effectively through medical treatment.
- PJ's reliance on motor, tactile, and visual functioning to interact with his world is crucial to understanding these impairments to cognition.

5. Consider how vision and gaze issues due to external strabismus would affect PJ's switch access (see Chapter 7). What cranial nerves are likely involved? (Chapter 11) What modifications might the therapy team (occupational, speech, and physical therapy disciplines) need to make to support switch access?
   - Likely CNs II, III, IV, and VI
   - Determine line of vision and eye–hand coordination for switch activation or perhaps other points of access for switch activation; tactile issues related to switch access
6. Aside from an impaired ability to regulate temperature, what other impairments to homeostasis are possible given hypothalamic dysfunction? (Chapter 5 and 12)
   - Failure to thrive/anorexia (lack of hunger), autonomic regulation
7. How might you distinguish between the acute and chronic (ongoing) impairments to communication, cognition, and swallowing in this case? It might help to consider direct effects of Crouzon syndrome and the effects of shunt malfunction/hydrocephalus.
   - It is important to talk with parents about previous status and distinguish between baseline and current functioning.
8. Given the broad description above, what neurosystems were affected in this case? Please address those that were included in the case, mapping evidence for how a structure was affected based on symptoms. Also map those that you believe were likely affected, given the description of PJ's status. (Chapter 2, 5, 12, and 14)
   - Ventricular, CSF system
   - Hypothalamic system
   - Cognitive systems for regulating levels of alertness —likely effects on the reticular activating system as well as diffuse edema to the cerebrum (particularly periventricular regions)

Case 16–18

1. Given the description above, identify the pertinent information in this case.
   - Prenatal alcohol exposure and FAS
   - Developmental cognitive delays, language delays, delays in meeting physical milestones, and gross and fine motor delays
   - Peripheral nerve deformities
2. What additional history might be useful?
   - Family's social history (parents, siblings, other); socioeconomic factors
   - Mother's medical history; nature of her alcohol and any other drug use
   - Location(s) and nature of the peripheral nerve deformities
3. What brain structures and pathways account for Travis' gross and fine motor impairments? (Chapters 10 and 11)
   - Underdevelopment of motor cortices and pathways
   - Underdevelopment of premotor cortices
   - Peripheral nerve deformities—sensory and motor systems tightly integrated. Loss of sensory information will impact motor control.
4. What brain structures and pathways account for Travis' speech and language impairments? (Chapter 14)
   - Superior temporal gyrus, middle temporal gyrus, Broca area, and Wernicke area
   - Elements of the dorsal (phonological processing) and ventral (semantic processing) streams—arcuate fasciculus, uncinate fasciculus, and superior longitudinal fasciculus
5. What brain structures and pathways account for Travis' cognitive impairments? (Chapter 14)
   - Frontal lobes; executive function and attentional networks
6. How might his facial structures impact communication?
   - Maxillary and mandibular hypoplasia can affect speech production, respiration, and swallowing.

Case 16–19

1. Given the description above, identify the pertinent information in this case.
   - ACC
   - Social communication impairments
2. Given the diagnosis, what critical time periods and developmental processes were likely disrupted? (Chapter 4 and 14)

- Gestational week 6 is crucial for development of the lamina terminalis, a precursor to the corpus callosum. This is followed by a period of neuronal proliferation in weeks 12 to 20.
3. What specific brain structures and pathways are likely involved in Selika's social communication impairments, including her difficulties processing figurative language, humor, sarcasm, egocentrism, and other pragmatic issues? (Chapter 14)
    - Underdevelopment of anterior cerebral structures, particularly prefrontal cortices
    - Perhaps the default mode network or mentalizing network, particularly given the issues of perspective taking, theory of mind, and egocentrism
    - Executive function networks involved in reasoning, such as contemplating consequences of statements one makes
4. What do the striking impairments in social cognition and pragmatics associated with ACC tell you about the neural control of these complex communicative functions?
    - They are not isolated to one hemisphere; disruption of the connections between right and left hemispheres interferes with typical communicative behaviors.
5. How might the impairments in social cognition and pragmatics have affected Selika's ability to make and maintain relationships throughout her life?
    - Reduced empathy and theory of mind make it difficult to make and maintain friends because these are important for showing people you care about them.
    - Difficulties with inferencing and understanding nonliteral language such as sarcasm will cause misinterpretations and communication breakdowns that will further challenge relationships. The inability to use these language forms results in communication that is literal and seems unimaginative. People who have difficulty with these language forms can be judged as boring or cognitively challenged.

Case 16–20

1. Given the description above, identify the pertinent information in this case.
    - Typically developing prior to diagnosis
    - Posterior fossa—ties to brainstem, cerebellum
    - Emergent neurosurgical intervention to resect tumor
2. What medical etiology is your primary concern?
    - Brain tumor/resection
3. What could account for the fact that Grant was showing no symptoms while surely there was a tumor growing in his brain? What could account for his eventual symptomology?
    - The tumor was not yet large enough to elicit any physical/cognitive symptoms.
    - Eventually, the tumor likely began impinging on the brainstem, leading to unilateral weakness and the eventual seizure.
4. What aspects of cognition, communication, or swallowing could be affected and why?
    - Cognition—due to cerebellum's connections to multiple brain areas, executive dysfunction (as part of posterior fossa syndrome) can be expected
    - Communication/speech production—mutism related to posterior fossa syndrome; potential dysarthria related to cerebellar involvement
    - Swallowing—potential dysphagia due to any brainstem involvement; surgical resection
5. What could account for these symptoms after the tumor was removed?
    - Damage from both the tumor and the neurosurgical procedure to remove the tumor could impact motor and cognitive functions. Postsurgical edema likely compressed areas adjacent to resected tumor. Impacts to the brainstem and cerebellum, including downstream effects of impaired fronto-cerebellar communication, could explain motor and affective symptoms.
6. What would be an explanation for Grant's persistent dysarthria?
    - Tumor location/neurosurgical resection affecting the cerebellum and/or brainstem can affect speech.
7. What kind of education would you provide to the parents about his cancer treatments and potential long-term effects to cognition and/or language?
    - Potential for changes to higher level cognitive and language functions as a result of chemotherapy and cranial radiation. Will need to monitor his performance at school, and address needs as they arise/change.

Case 16–21

1. Given the description above, identify the pertinent information in this case.
    - Typically developing prior to injury
    - High-speed motor vehicle collision

- Bifrontal, left temporal lobe involvement
- No surgical intervention needed
- DAI

2. What medical etiology is your primary concern?
   - TBI
   - DAI
3. What aspects of cognition, communication, or swallowing could be affected and why?
   - Cognition—executive functions, memory due to frontal/temporal injury and DAI
   - Language—production and comprehension due to temporal lobe injury and DAI
   - Speech—possible motor involvement due to temporal lobe damage
4. What would be the explanation for the recovery that Maria experiences?
   - Often, physical recovery is faster than cognitive recovery given the complexity and interconnectedness of cognitive processes, as opposed to the relatively discrete sensorimotor processes.
   - Neuroplasticity
5. Considering Maria's language and cognitive testing were just below average, why would the SLP recommend an evaluation at school?
   - Maria was in advanced math classes prior to her injury—it is likely that her current level of function represents a decline from her premorbid level of function and, thus, warrants close monitoring and/or support.
   - Subtle difficulties in language and cognition could impact her ability to keep up with schoolwork at a level she was used to prior to her injury.
6. What kind of education would you provide to Maria's parents and to her school?
   - Maria experienced a severe TBI, and even subtle difficulties may make it difficult for her to perform at school in a way that she is used to.
   - New difficulties may arise once Maria is back in her normal classroom, where there are many distractions and demands.
   - Monitoring for difficulties is essential to address them as soon as possible rather than waiting until Maria is struggling and failing.
7. Why is it important to ensure that staff at Maria's middle school (grades 6–8) is aware of her history of TBI?
   - Because Maria experienced frontal lobe injury, it is expected that new difficulties may arise as she becomes more independent—as executive functions are continuing to develop throughout the teen/early adult years. It is possible that Maria will develop new challenges as her teachers expect her to work more independently—and she may need support to do so successfully.
   - Ongoing monitoring is essential to prevent later-developing difficulties from negatively impacting social and academic performance at school.

Reference

Ramig, L., Pawlas, A., & Countryman, S. (1995). *The Lee Silverman Voice Treatment (LSVT): A practical guide to treating the voice and speech disorders in Parkinson disease.* Iowa City: National Center for Voice and Speech at the University of Iowa.

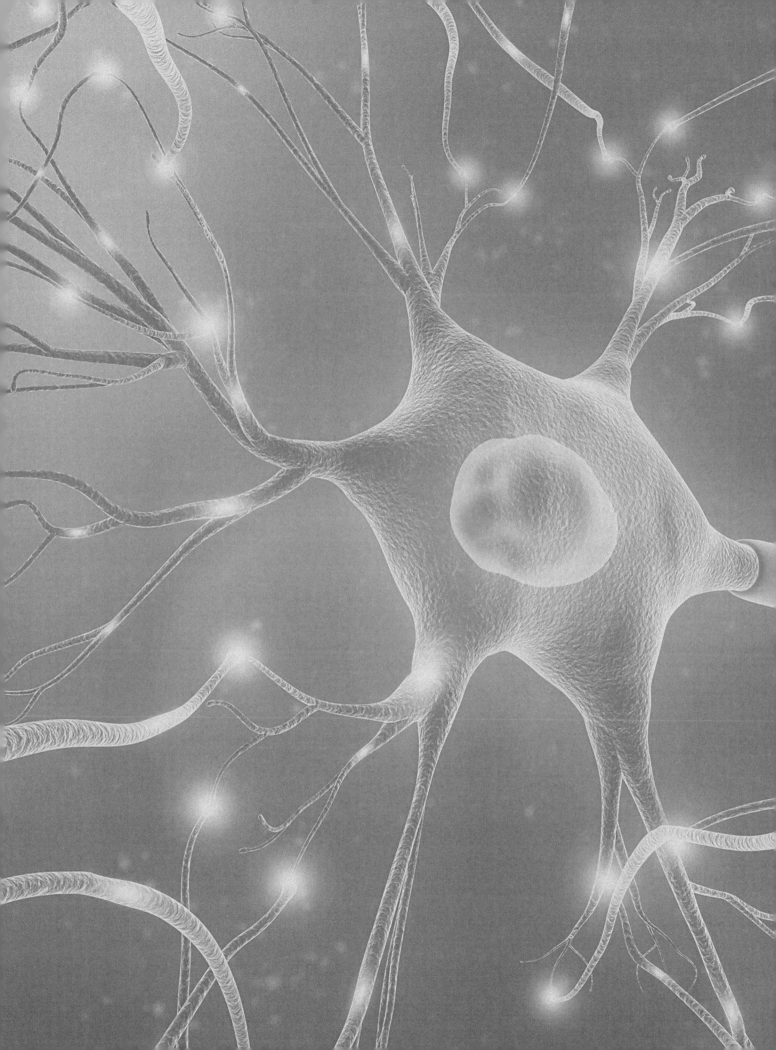

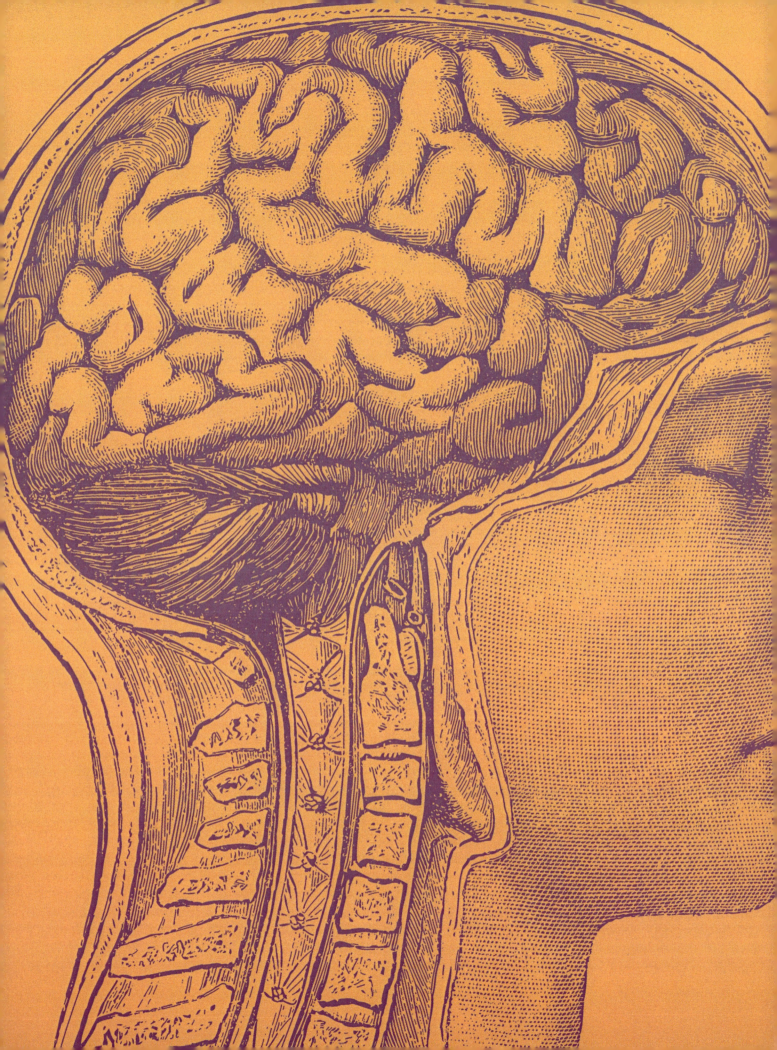

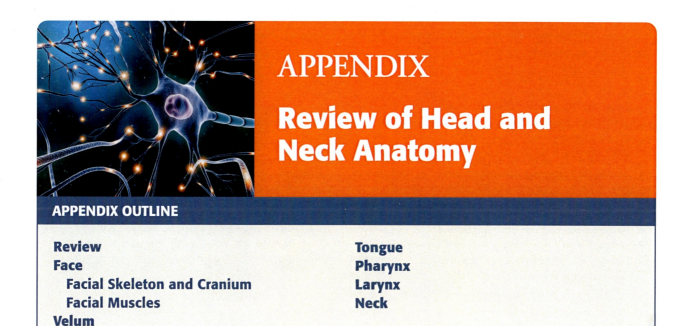

APPENDIX

Review of Head and Neck Anatomy

APPENDIX OUTLINE

Review
Face
    Facial Skeleton and Cranium
    Facial Muscles
Velum

Tongue
Pharynx
Larynx
Neck

Review

This appendix provides a very brief review of the bones, cartilages, and muscles that are involved in speech and swallowing. This will be useful as a reference particularly for Chapter 11.

Face

Facial Skeleton and Cranium

The bones of the facial skeleton (Figures A–1 through A–3) include the frontal bone (forehead), maxilla (upper jaw and midface), zygomatic (cheek bone), and mandible (lower jaw). Internally, the ethmoid, sphenoid, and palatine bones create the borders of the nasal cavity and posterior hard palate. The vomer is the bony portion of the nasal septum, and the nasal bones crate the bridge of the nose. The only moveable joint in the skull is the temporomandibular joint, which allows the mandible to open.

Cranial bones include the frontal, parietal, temporal, and occipital bones. The sphenoid and ethmoid create portions of the floor of the cranium in addition to their structural role in the facial skeleton.

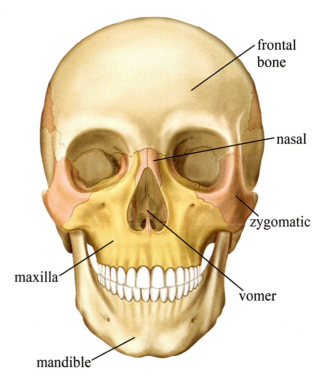

FIGURE A–1. Anterior view of bones of the facial skeleton.

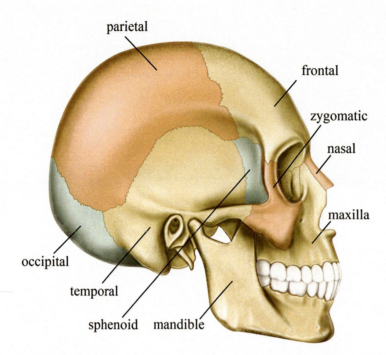

FIGURE A–2. Lateral view of bones of the facial skeleton and cranium.

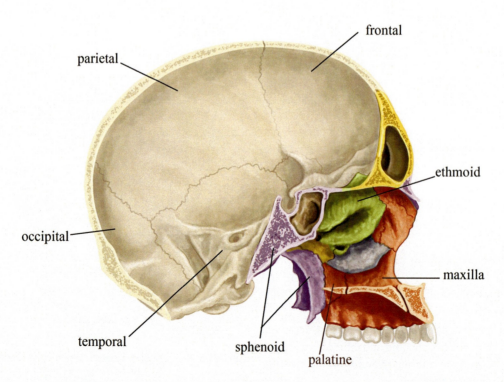

FIGURE A–3. Midsagittal cut showing bones of the facial skeleton and cranium.

Facial Muscles

Facial muscles are divided into two groups: muscles of mastication and muscles of facial expression. Muscles of mastication are those that move the mandible (Figure A–4 and Table A–1). These include the temporalis and masseter muscles, which elevate (close) the jaw; the medial and lateral pterygoids, which protrude the jaw and move it laterally; and the geniohyoid and anterior belly of the digastric muscles, which depress (open) the jaw. These

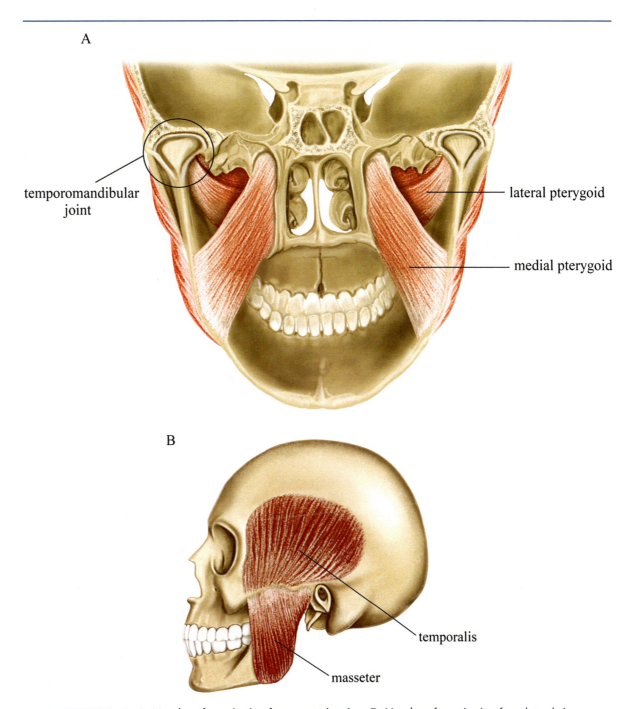

FIGURE A–4. **A.** Muscles of mastication from posterior view. **B.** Muscles of mastication from lateral view.

Table A–1. Facial Muscles

Muscle	Location	Function	Innervation
Masseter	Zygomatic arch to mandibular angle	Elevate (close) jaw	Trigeminal (CN V)
Temporalis	Parietal bone to coronoid process of mandible	Elevate (close) jaw	Trigeminal (CN V)
Lateral pterygoid	Sphenoid bone to condylar process of mandible	Protrude jaw	Trigeminal (CN V)
Medial pterygoid	Sphenoid bone to inner angle of the mandible	Move jaw laterally	Trigeminal (CN V)
Frontalis	Frontal bone	Elevate eyebrows	Facial (CN VII)
Orbicularis oculi	Surround eyes	Open/close eyes	Facial (CN VII)
Nasalis	Frontal bone between eyes to nasal bones	Elevate/wrinkle nose	Facial (CN VII)
Zygomatic major and minor	Zygomatic bone to orbicularis oris	Elevate corner of upper lip (smile)	Facial (CN VII)
Orbicularis oris	Surrounds and forms lips	Pucker and close lips	Facial (CN VII)
Levator labii	Anterior maxilla to orbicularis oris	Elevate upper lip (create snear)	Facial (CN VII)
Levator labii superioris alaeque nasi	Superior frontal portion of maxilla to lateral nose and orbicularis oris	Elevate upper lip	Facial (CN VII)
Levator anguli oris	Zygomatic to corner of mouth	Elevate and retract corner of lips (smile)	Facial (CN VII)
Depressor labii	Anterior mandible to orbicularis oris	Depress lower lip	Facial (CN VII)
Depressor anguli oris	Anterior mandible to orbicularis oris	Pull corners of the mouth down (frown)	Facial (CN VII)
Mentalis	Anterior mandible to orbicularis oris	Protrude lower lip (pout)	Facial (CN VII)
Risorius	Lateral fascia of cheeks to lateral orbicularis oris	Draws the corners of the lips laterally and upward	Facial (CN VII)
Buccinator	Anterior maxilla and mandible and temporomandibular joint to orbicularis oris	Tenses and flattens cheeks	Facial (CN VII)

muscles are innervated by cranial nerve (CN) V, the trigeminal nerve.

Muscles of facial expression include all of the muscles of the face that move the lips and nose, open/close the eye, and elevate the eyebrows (see Table A–1 and Figure A–5). All muscles of facial expression are innervated by the facial nerve, CN VII.

Velum

In the oral cavity, the velum (soft palate) is formed by several muscles that elevate and tense the velum in order to close off the oral cavity from the nasal cavity (Table A–2 and Figure A–6). This region is known as the velopharyngeal port.

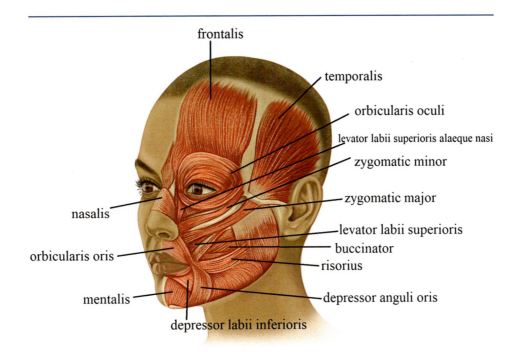

FIGURE A–5. Muscles of facial expression. The zygomatic muscles attach into the orbicularis oris. Here they are shown deviated toward the nose in order to show all of the muscles that attach into the superior orbicularis oris.

Table A–2. Muscles of the Velum

Muscle	Location	Function	Innervation
Musculus uvula	Posterior hard palate to uvulae aponeurosis	Provides tissue bulk for velopharyngeal closure	Vagus (CN X)
Levator veli palatini	Temporal bone to palatal aponeurosis	Elevates the velum (soft palate)	Vagus (CN X)
Tensor veli palatini	Sphenoid to palatal aponeurosis	Tenses the velum (soft palate)	Trigeminal (CN V)
Palatoglossus	Palatal aponeurosis to posterior–lateral tongue	Either elevates the base of the tongue or depresses the velum	Vagus (CN X)

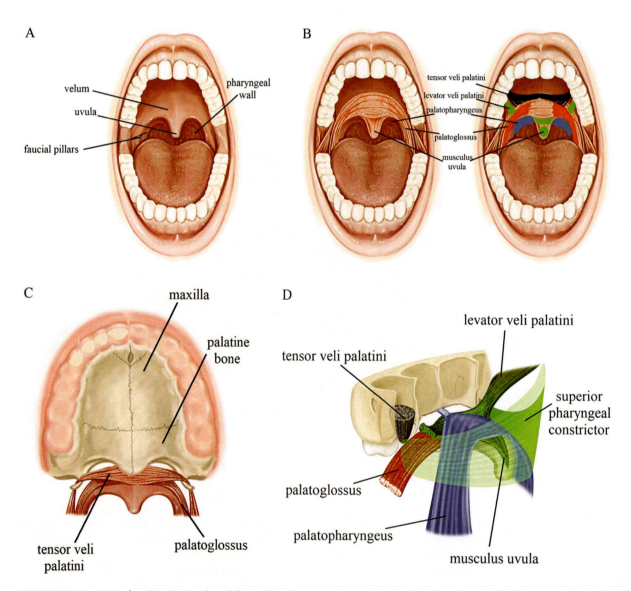

FIGURE A–6. **A.** Oral cavity. **B.** Muscles of the velum from an anterior view. **C.** Muscles of the velum contextualized with hard palate. **D.** Muscles of the velum from a superior–lateral view.

Tongue

The tongue is made up of intrinsic and extrinsic muscles (Table A–3 and Figure A–7). Intrinsic muscles exist completely within the tongue. These muscles create fine movement and change the shape of the tongue. Extrinsic muscles originate outside of the tongue and insert into the tongue. These are responsible for gross movements of the tongue.

Pharynx

The pharynx is made up of a series of muscles that form the posterior wall of the oral cavity (throat): the superior, middle, and inferior constrictors (Figure A–8). These function primarily in swallowing by constricting in a superior–inferior quasi-peristaltic pattern to move food down toward the esophagus. Importantly, as the superior constrictor contracts (aiding closure of the velopharyngeal port), it relaxes the middle constrictor (increasing volume and decreasing pressure to help the bolus move downward). Likewise, as the middle constrictor contracts, it relaxes the inferior constrictor (again increasing volume in that space and decreasing pressure in order to draw bolus toward the esophagus). The superior constrictor muscle also works along with the velar muscles to close off the velopharyngeal port during both swallowing and production of oral speech sounds.

Larynx

The larynx is made up of several cartilages and sits on the superior extent of the trachea. It is connected through tissues to the hyoid bone. The thyroid cartilage articulates with the cricoid cartilage, which sits upon the superior-most ring of the trachea. On the posterior cricoid are two pyramidal-shaped arytenoid muscles. The vocal folds are muscles (and vocal ligaments) covered in several layers of tissue that extend from the inner thyroid cartilage anteriorly and attach to the arytenoid cartilages posteriorly.

Table A–3. Extrinsic and Intrinsic Tongue Muscles

Muscle	Location	Function	Innervation
Extrinsic			
Genioglossus	Inner surface of anterior mandible to body of the tongue	Retract and protrude tongue	Hypoglossal (CN XII)
Hyoglossus	Hyoid bone to body of the tongue	Depress tongue	Hypoglossal (CN XII)
Palatoglossus	Soft palate to posterior and lateral tongue	Elevate posterior tongue	Vagus (CN X)
Styloglossus	Styloid process of the temporal bone to lateral tongue	Elevate and retract posterior tongue	Hypoglossal (CN XII)
Intrinsic			
Superior longitudinal	Tip of tongue to root of tongue along superior surface	Elevate tongue tip	Hypoglossal (CN XII)
Inferior longitudinal	Tip of tongue to root of tongue along inferior surface	Depress tongue tip	Hypoglossal (CN XII)
Transverse	Extends horizontally from left to right edges of tongue	Thicken and round tongue	Hypoglossal (CN XII)
Vertical	Extends vertically from inferior to superior tongue	Flatten tongue	Hypoglossal (CN XII)

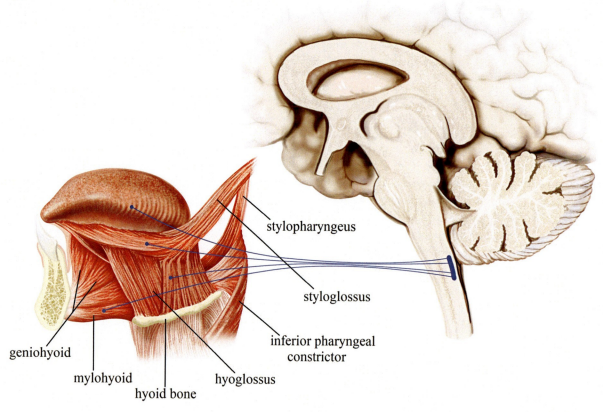

FIGURE A–7. A. Lateral view of extrinsic tongue muscles. **B.** Cross section of intrinsic tongue muscles.

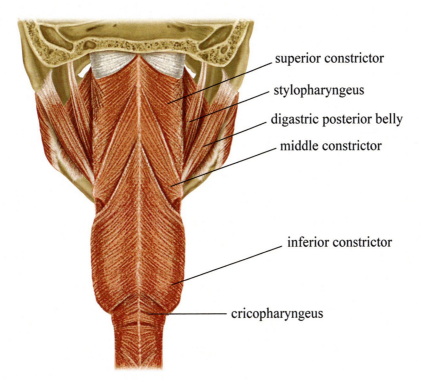

FIGURE A–8. Posterior view of pharyngeal constrictor muscles.

Movement of the arytenoids will adduct (close) and abduct (open) the vocal folds. Intrinsic muscles of the larynx are those that exist entirely within the larynx. Their function is to tense, lengthen, and adduct/abduct the vocal folds. These muscles are listed in Table A–4 and shown in Figure A–9. Extrinsic laryngeal muscles have one insertion point in the larynx and the other outside the larynx. Their function is to elevate or depress the larynx, and they work primarily during swallowing to move the larynx anteriorly and superiorly to aid in movement of food and liquid into the esophagus. Suprahyoid and supralaryngeal muscles such as the thyrohyoid, geniohyoid, and stylohyoid muscles attach to a structure superior to the larynx. Their function is to elevate the larynx. Infrahyoid muscles such as the sternothyroid and sternohyoid muscles will depress or pull the larynx down because of their connection to structures inferior to the larynx.

Neck

Two additional neck muscles deserve a quick note. The sternocleidomastoid muscle originates from the mastoid process of the temporal bone directly posterior to the external ear and attaches to both the clavicle and the sternum. Its function is to pull the head down or to the side. The trapezius muscle on the back has attachments to the occipital lobe and bones in the shoulder (scapula and clavicle) and upper rib cage. It can pull the head back or elevate the shoulders and rib cage. These muscles are shown in Figure A–10.

Table A–4. Intrinsic Laryngeal Muscles

Muscle	Location	Function	Innervation
Cricothyroid	Anterior cricoid to inferior anterior/lateral thyroid	Pull thyroid down, lengthening vocal folds to increase pitch	Extrinsic laryngeal branch of superior laryngeal nerve of the vagus (CN X)
Posterior cricoarytenoid	Posterior cricoid to arytenoid	Abduct vocal folds	Recurrent laryngeal nerve of the vagus (CN X)
Lateral cricoarytenoid	Superior surface of lateral cricoid to arytenoid	Adduct vocal folds	Recurrent laryngeal nerve of the vagus (CN X)
Transverse and oblique arytenoid	Posterior surface of one arytenoid to posterior surface of the other arytenoid	Adduct vocal folds	Recurrent laryngeal nerve of the vagus (CN X)
Thyroarytenoid (vocalis)	Inner surface of anterior thyroid to arytenoid	Tense and relax vocal folds	Recurrent laryngeal nerve of the vagus (CN X)

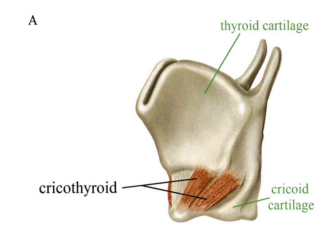
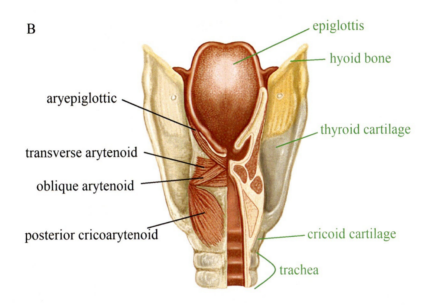
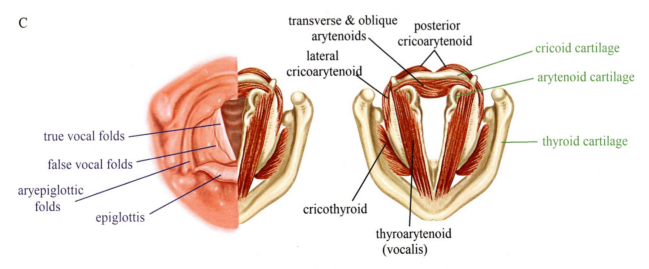

FIGURE A–9. **A.** Lateral view of intrinsic laryngeal muscles. **B.** Posterior view of intrinsic laryngeal muscles. **C.** Superior view of intrinsic laryngeal muscles and tissues. Black labels, muscles; green labels, cartilage/bone; blue labels, tissues.

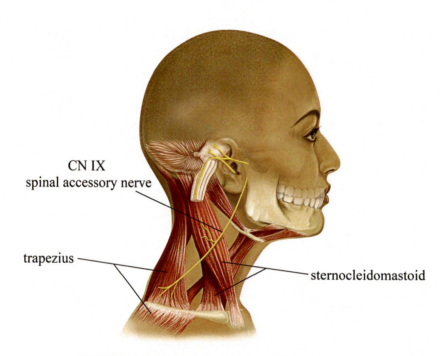

FIGURE A–10. Sternocleidomastoid and trapezius muscles.

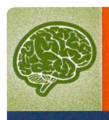

Index

Note: Page numbers in **bold** reference non-text material.

A

α-amino-3- hydroxy-5-methyl-4-isoxazolepropionic acid (AMPA) receptors, 264–265, **264**, **265**
Abasia, 169, 170
Abducens Nerve (CN VI), 134, 173, **176**, **177**, 179–182, **180**
Absolute refractory period, 52–53, **52**
Abulia, 88, 151
ACA. see Anterior Cerebral Artery (ACA)
ACoA. see Anterior communicating artery
Agenesis of the corpus callosum (ACC), 68–69, **69**, 74, 76, 294–295
Acetylcholine (ACh), 57, **58**, 163, 167–168, 300, 303–304
　ACh receptors, 62–63, 167–168, 304
　enzymatic destruction of, 64
Acetylcholinesterase (AChE), 59, 168, 280
　inhibitors, 64
Achromatopsia, 117
Acoustic energy, 121–122
Acoustic impedance, 122
Acoustic neuroma, 132, 290–291, 307
Action or intention tremor, 169, **169**
Action potential, 47, 49–56, **53**, **55**, 59, 64, 84, 132, 134, 141, 154, 165. *See also* Nerve impulses
Active transport, 50, 64
Active zones, 55, 57
AD. *See* Alzheimer disease
Adaptation rate, **92**, 93
Adenosine triphosphate (ATP), 50, 52, 64, **141**, 144, **145**
Ageusia, 146, 147
Agnathia-astomia, 76
Agnosia, **96**, 116–117, **147**, 288–289, 306
　anosognosia, 116, 281
　autotopagnosia, **96**
　apperceptive, 116
　associative, 116
　finger, **96**
　oral, **147**, 288
　prosopagnosia, 116, **117**
　visual, 117

AICA. see Anterior Inferior Cerebellar Artery
Akinetopsia, 117
Alar (sensory) plate, 72, **73**
Alexia without agraphia, 117, **118**
Allodynia, 103
Alzheimer disease (AD), 14, 34, 57, 58, 61, 64, 116, 143, 147, 202, 288, 289, 306
　cortical atrophy, **289**
Amacrine cells, 108, **108**, 109
Amines, 57–59, **58**, 65
Amino acids, 57–59, **58**, **145**, 231
AMPA receptors, 264–265
Ampulla, 134
Amygdala, 84, 142, **143**, 187, 199–206, **201**, **205**, **206**, **208**, 209, 210, 213, 248, 250
Amyotrophic lateral sclerosis (ALS), 61, 78, 167, 240, 278, 298–299, 304
　bulbar-onset, 167, 278
　spinal-onset, 167
Anastomosis (anastomoses), 218–219, 290–291, 307
Anatomical position and terms of direction, **10**, **11**
Anaxonic, 46
Androstenedione, 200
Anencephaly, 72
Aneurysm, 35, **36**, 232, 233–234, **233**, 281, 300–301
Angiogenesis, 263
Angiotensin II, 40
Angular gyrus, 24, **96**, **242**, **243**, 246
Anosmia, 142–143, 147
Anoxia, 231, 240
Anterior cerebral artery (ACA), 219, 222–224, **222**, **223**, **224**, 226–227, **226**, **227**, **233**, 281, 300
Anterior communicating artery (ACoA), 219–220, **220**, **221**
Anterior (ventral) corticospinal tract. *See* Corticospinal tract
Anterior inferior cerebellar artery (AICA), 226–228, **228**, 229, **230**, 302
　distribution, 227, 229
　infarcts, 227, 302
Anterior nuclear complex, 84–85, **85**

325

Anterograde amnesia, 205–206, 254. *See also* Memory
Anterolateral spinothalamic tract. *See* Spinothalamic tract
Anticholinergic drugs, 63
Antidiuretic hormone (ADH), 200, 202
Anton syndrome, 116. *See also* Visual anosognosia
Aphasia, **96**, **117**, **118**, 133, 217, **224**, **226**, **242**, **244**, 246, **247**, **251**, 258, 269, 271, 279–280, 281, 286, 300, 305
  thalamic, 88, **88**
Apraxia of speech, 165–166, 170, 246, 299
Aprosencephaly, 76
Aprosodia, 133, 251, 258
Arachnoid layer, 34, 36
  granulations, 36, 37, 40
  trabeculae, 36
Arcuate fasciculus (AF), 243–244, **244**, 308
Arrhythmias, 232, 280
Arteriovenous malformations (AVM), 234
Articulators, 62, 63, 105, 150, 162, 166, 168, 192, 286, 299
Aspiration, **63**, 188, 189, 196, 303–304
Association areas, 7, 24, **85**, 95, 114, 117, 133, 250
Association tract, **11**
Astrocytes, 16–17, **16**, 167, 239
Atasia, 169–170
Ataxia, 169-170, 211, 228, 229, 283
  Friedreich, 238
  gait, 227–229, 283
  hemi-ataxia, 88
  limb, 227, 283
  speech, 227, 283
Ataxic dysarthria, 169, 227, **228**, 283
Atelencephaly, 76
Atherosclerosis, 232, 241
Atropine, 63, 167
Attention, 255
  alternating, 255
  deficit, 88, 257
  divided, 255, 282
  focused, 255
  networks, 255, **256**, 257
    default mode network. 255, **256**, 309
    dorsal attention network (DAN), **245**, 255, **256**, 257
    executive control network, 257
    ventral attention network (VAN), **245**, 255, **256**, 257
  orienting, 255, 257, 307
  processing, 21, 256
  selective attention, 252
  sustained attention, 255–256
Attention-deficit disorder, 212
Auditory assessment, 194, **195**
  Rinne test, 194
  Weber test, 194

Auditory system, 7, 48, 121, **122**, 125, 128–129, 131–132, 134–136. *See also* Cochlea
  hair cells, **126**
  hydraulic energy, 122-123
  localization, 128, 129, 131, 136
  outer hair cells (OHCs), 125
  phase locking, 129–130, **130**
  place coding, 123
  pathway, 73, 86, 121, **127**, 130–131
  primary auditory cortex (A1), 64, 128–129, **127**, **128**, 224
  spiral ganglion, 126–127
  stereocilia, 125
Auditory-vestibular nerve (CN VIII), **124**, **126**, 128, 132, 134, 136, 174, **176**, **177**, 186, 194, 291
Autism spectrum disorder (ASD), 238–239, 249, 250
Autonomic nervous system, 2, 40, 46, 72, 87
Autotopagnosia. *See* Agnosia
Axons, 2, **11**, 14–15, 19, 28, 29, 45–46, **46**, 47, **48**, **49**, 50–51, 53–54, **53**, 59, 62, 64, **98**, **100**, **101**, 111. *See also* motor and sensory pathways
  collaterals, 14, 54, 59, 84, 156, 165, 265
  hillock, 14, 50–51, 53
  myelinated, **17**, 19, 54, **55**
  terminal, 14, 47–50, **49**, 54–55, **55**, **56**, **58**, 59, 63, 64
  unmyelinated, 54, 94

B

Barium, 196, 284–285
Basal (motor) plate, 72, **73**
Basal ganglia, 26–29, 62, **75**, 76, 84, **85**, 87, 89, 149, **150**, 151–155, **153**, **154**, 162, 168–169, 204, 205, **205**, 207, **207**, 210, 226, **226**, **227**, 239, **242**, **246**, 248, 251, **254**, 255, 305
Basilar artery, 218–219, **220**, 228, 229, **230**
Basilar membrane, 123–125, **123**, **124**, 128–129, **128**,132. *See also* Auditory system
Benzodiazepines, 64
Bipolar neurons, **46**, **46**, 108–109, **108**, 125, 127, 134
Bite strength, 193
Blepherospasm (eye twitching), 169
Blind spot, 109
Blindness, 115–118, 133
Blood patch, 42, 278
Blood perfusion, 231–232, 234
Blood pressure, 40, **58**, 187, 200, 229
Blood supply to the brain, 217-234, **223**, **226**, **227**, **229**, **230**
  basal ganglia, **223**, **226**, **227**
  cerebellum, 226–228 **228**
  thalamus, **223**, **226**, **227**
  brainstem, 228-230, **229**, **230**
  spinal cord, 228-230, **229**, **230**

Blood vessels, 230–232
  damage to, 35
Blood–brain barrier (BBB), 17, 40, 63, 217, 230–231, 234, 241
Body schema, **96**, 135–136
Bony labyrinth, 122
Botulinum toxin (Botox), 63, 167, 285
  poisoning, 284-285, 303–304
Brachial arch, 175
Bradykinesia, 62, 305
Bradyphrenia, 62, 209
Brain, 1
  cells, 7, 12, 40
  development, 76, 79, 259–260
  injury rehabilitation, 270, 273
  tissue, 34, 42, 72, 232
Brainstem, 2-5, 12, 14, 26, 28-29, 31-32, 34, 36-37, 57-58, 67, 72, 74, 79, 83-86, 89, 97-99, 101, 103, 125, 127, 132-133, 181-182, 185, 187, 189, 201, 209, 217, 228-230, 242, 283
  stroke, 283
Brodmann areas, 6–7, **8**
  area 4, 150, 246
  area 6, 246
  area 17, 114
  area 22, 131
  area 41, 128–129
  area 42, 131
Brown-Séquard syndrome, 102, **104**
Buccal cavity, 190, 307
Bulbar, 158, 167, 184, 278–279, 298–299

C

C-shaped development, 68, 76–77, 79
C-shaped structures, **77**
C-SLIMA, 128
Cacosmia, 142
Calcarine sulcus, 19, **21**, 26, 113–114
Calcium (Ca^{2+}), 49, 56, 265. *See also* Ions
  channel, 48, 54, 56, 134
Caloric test, 135
cAMP, see Cyclic Adenosine Monophosphate
Cardiac arrhythmias, 232
Cardiac ischemia, 234.*See also* Myocardial infarction
Carotid arteries, 218, **177**, 178, **226**, 280, 281, 300
  external, 218, **219**
  internal, 218, **219**, **220**, **221**, 222, **233**, 281
Caudate nucleus, 26, **27**, 57, 151, **153**, 154, **154**, 224, **227**, 238, 239, 305
  degeneration of, 168
Cebocephly, **76**
Cell membranes and ion channels, **48**

Cellular organization, 6–7. *See also* Brodmann areas
Cellular regeneration, 139, 265
Central nervous system (CNS), 1–2, 5, **4**, **5**, 7, 12, 29, 31, 43, 47, **48**, 57, **58**, 65, 67, 72, **74**, **75**, 125, 129, 149, 231, 277, 278, 298, 299
Central pain disorder, 103. *See also* Thalamic pain syndrome
Central sulcus, 18, **19**, 21, 95, 224
Cephaloceles, **72**
Cerebellum, 1, 26, 28, 29, 32, 34, 35, 36, 37, 57, 58, 67, 72, 74, 75, 84, 85, 86, 101, 102, 105, 127, 135, 149, 150, 154-158, **157**, 169, 170, 204, 205, 207, 229, 242, 254, 255
  blood supply, 226, 227, 283
  climbing fibers, 156, **157**
  coordination, 155
  damage, 246, 284
  developmental language disorders, 238, 239
  granule cells, 156, **157**
  infarcts, 227, 283
  mossy fibers, 156, **157**
  mutism, 296
  parallel fibers, 56, **157**
  peduncles, 28
  Purkinje cells, 46, 156-157, **157**
  vascular distributions, **228**
Cerebral amyloid angiopathy, 241
Cerebral angiography, 232, 234
Cerebral aqueduct, 37, **38**
Cerebral arteries, 86, 218, 220, **222**, 223–224.*See also specific arteries*
Cerebral blood supply, 217–218, **218**, 222–225, **222**, **223**, **224**, **225**, 226
Cerebral palsy (CP), 78, 238
Cerebrocerebellum, 155–156
Cerebrospinal fluid (CSF), 2, 16, 31, 32, 34, 36, 37–42, **41**, **42**, 43, 239, 240, 277–278, 291, 308
  path, 37
Cerebrovascular accident (CVA), **224**, 234, 279–280, 282, 283, *See also* Stroke
Cerebrum, 1, 6, 28, 31, **33**, 34, 36, 37, 39, 68, **68**, 72–73, 76–77, 79, 135, **160**, 211, 218, 222–224, 308
Cervical spinal cord, 31
Cervicomedullary junction, 31 *See also* Cervical spinal cord
Cheek sufflation, 193
Chiari malformation, 72
Chloride (Cl$^-$), 40, **49**, **50**, 56, 64, 141 *See also* ions
Choroid plexus, 37, **39**
Chronic fatigue, 212
Cilia
  ependymal cells, 16
  auditory system, **48**, 125, 132, 136
  vestibular system, 134, 136. *See also* Stereocilia
  olfactory system, 139–141

Ciliary muscles, 107
Cingulate gyrus, 18–19, 76, 84–85, **85**, 95, 199, **201**, 205–206, 207, 211, 214, 224, 239, 248, 250, 255, **256**
Circadian rhythms, 87, 113, 202, 212
Circle of Willis, 34, 218–**220**, **221**, 233, 234, 241, 281
Circumventricular organs, 40
Cisternogram, 41, 278
Cleft lip and palate, 76
Climbing fibers. See Cerebellum
Clinical bedside swallow examination (CBSE), 196–197
Clinoid processes, **33**, 34–35
"Clot busting" drug, see Tissue Plasminogen Activator (tPA) 224, 280
Cochlea, 34, 122–125, **123**, **124**, 131–134, **135**, **177**, 186
    oval window, 122–123, 125, 186
    scala media, 123, **123**
    scala tympani, 123, **123**, 125
    scala vestibuli, 123, **123**, 125
Cochlear implants, 266–267
Cognitive deficit/impairment, 57–58, 88, 240, 259
    developmental, 74
    rehabilitation, 269
Collaborative goal setting, 266, 270–271
Coma, 88, 212, 214, 229, 254, 279
Commissure, **11**, **69**, 142, 294
    commissural tract (fibers), **11**, 19, **69**
Common carotid arteries. See Carotid artery
Communicating arteries, 86, 218, **220**. See also Anastomoses
Communication between neurons. See Synapses
Computed tomography (CT), 232, 280
Concentration gradient, 14–15, 47–48, 51, 141
Cones. See Photoreceptors
Contralateral cortical control, 118
Contrecoup injury, 240
Contusions (bruises), 240
Conus medullaris, 38
Cornea, 107–108, **108**, 115, 118, **182**, 186
Corona radiata, **98**, **100**, 159, 160, **160**, 162, 166, 179
Coronal (frontal) section, **9**, 12, **13**, **20**, **27**, **151**, **153**, 223, **287**
Corpus callosum, 19, 68–69, **69**, 72, 117, 294
Cortex, 2, 6, 7, 11, 37, 57, **58**
    layers and connections, **7**
Cortical blindness, 116, 118, 133
Cortical damage, 91, 104–105, 107, 116, 133
Cortical deafness, 133
Cortico-basal-thalamo-cortical circuits, **154**
Corticobulbar tract/pathways, 149, 158, 162, 173–174, **174**, 179
Corticospinal tracts, 46, **104**, 149, 158–160, **160**, 162, 170, **230**, 299, 304
    anterior (ventral), 159–161, **161**, 170, 298

    lateral, 159–160, **159**, 162, 170, **230**, 298
Coup injury, 240
COVID-19, 146–147
Cranial fossae, 32, **33**, 34, 36, 182, 296
Cranial Nerves. See also specific nerves.
    agenesis of, 74
    functional Classifications, **117–178**
    damage to, 179
    mnemonics, **176**
    nuclei, **175**
Cranium, 1–2, **2**, 28, 29, 31, 32, 34, 35, 39, 42, 43, 140, 143, 218, 240, 313, 314
Cribriform plate, 34, 140, **140**, **141**, 143
Crista galli, 32, 34, 35, **140**
Crouzon syndrome, 291–292, **292**
CSF. See Cerebrospinal fluid
Cupula, 134. See also Vestibular system
Curare, 63, 167
Cyclic Adenosine Monophosphate (cAMP), 264–265
Cyclopia, 76

D

DCML, See Dorsal column-medial lemniscus
Deafness, 133, 229, 267, 273
Declarative. See Memory
Decussate, 32, 97, 101, 179
Default mode network. See Attention
Dementia, 117, 241, **242**
    Alzheimer, 147
    frontotemporal dementia, 241
    lewy body, 241–241
    mixed, 241
    prion-related dementia, 241
    proteinopathies, 241
    small vessel disease (SVD), 225, **226**, 241, 280–281, 300
    spongiform encephalopathy, 231
    vascular, 226, 240–241, 280
Dendrites, 14–15, **14**, 45–46, **46**, 50, 91, **98**, **100**, **101**, 134, 156, **157**, 265
Depolarization, 47–54, **47**, **48**, **49**, **50**, **52**, **53**, 56–57, **56**, 64, 109, 125, 126, **128**, 134, 141, **145**, 163
Dermatomes, 102–103, **103**
Developmental disorders, 237–238
    language (DLD), 238
    neurologic, 238
Developmental stressors, 213
Diadochokinesis, 169, 278
    laryngeal diadochokinetic (DDK) rate, 196
    oral diadochokinetic (DDK) rate, 196
Dichotomy of motor and sensory systems, 67, **68**, 72, 76
Diencephalon, 5–6, 73, 75–76, 83, **84**, 87–89, 204–205
Differential diagnosis, 170, 246, 276–277

Diffuse axonal injury (DAI), 240, 296, 298
Diplophonia, 189
Diplopia, 181–182, 193, 229, 283, 284
Direct motor system, 149–150, **150**
Distributed practice, 269
Diuresis, 202
DNA, 14
Donezepil (Aricept), 64
Dopamine, 57-58, 62, 168, 208, 210, 231
    pathways, **208**, **210**
Dorsal attention network (DAN). *See* Attention
Dorsal cochlear nuclei, 127. *See also* Auditory system
Dorsal column-medial lemniscus (DCML), 91, 97–99, **98–99**, 102, 104–105, 165
Dorsal induction, 70, 72, **72**, 79
    anomalies of, 72
Dorsolateral prefrontal cortex, 21, **22**, 77, 248, 250, 255, **256**
Double vision, 62, 118, 193. *See also* Diplopia
Down syndrome (DS), 238-239
Dual-stream model. *See* Language
Dura mater, 34–36, **35**, **41**, 182, 278
Dural venous sinuses, 36
Dysarthria, 88, 105, 166
    ataxic, 169, 227
    flaccid, 167
    hypokinetic, 168
    spastic, 166–167, 233
Dysdiadochokinesis, 169
Dysesthesia, 103
Dysgeusia, 146
Dysmetria, 169-170
Dysosmia, 142
Dysphagia, 165-166, 196, 200, 229, 276-289
Dystonia, 169

E

Ectoderm, 70, **70**, **75**, 79
Edema, 32, 34, 42, 232, 234, 240
Edinger-Westphal nuclei, **175**, 181
Electrical gradient, 47, 125
Electrical signal, 14, 15, 46–47, 54, 64, 231. *See also* Synapse
Electromyography (EMG), 167, 278-279
Embolus, 232
Embryo, 70, 75
Embryologic (embryonic) development, 68, 69, 175
    precursors and roles at maturity, **70**
Emotion, 206
    facial expression, 187
    networks, 248
    processing, 248, 260
    prosody network, 258

prosody production, 248, 250
    regulation, 40, 77–78, 199, 206, 211, 213
Empathy network, 248
Endocrine system, 40, 86, 89
Endoderm, 70, **70**
Endolymph, 123, **123**, 134
Endorphins, 57, 87
Enkephalins, 57, **58**
Entorhinal cortex, 142, **143**, **199**, **201**, 203, **203**, 206–207, 211, 213, **242**
Enzymatic destruction, 63, 64
Ependymal cells, 16, **16**, 37
Epidural, 34, 37, 42, 277–278, 298
    blood patch, 42, 278
    hematoma, 34, **37**, 277
    space, 34, 42, 298
Epilepsy, 57
Episodic memory. *See* Memory
Epithalamus, 83, 86, 89
EPSP, see Excitatory Postsynaptic Potentials
Esophageal phase. *See* Swallowing
Ethmocephaly, 76
Ethmoid bone, 34–35, **140**, 143
Eustachian tube, **122**, 184
Excitatory Postsynaptic Potentials (EPSPs), 49, 50, 51, **52**, 54, , 56–57, 59, 61, 64, 264, 265
Excitatory signals, 49–50, 61, 95, 154–155, 168, 239
Excitotoxicity, 57
Executive functions, 21, 34, 67, 68, 77, 211, 224, 251–252, 253, 267, 276
    deficits, 252
Exencephaly, 72, **73**
Experience-dependent neural plasticity. *See* Plasticity
External auditory meatus, 121, **122**, 132, 182, **182**, 185
External laryngeal nerve. *See* Vagus nerve
Extralinguistic, 248
Extraocular
    cranial nerve, 193
    movements, 173, 193
Extrapyramidal tracts, 150, **150**, 158, 162–163, 170, 286

F

Face processing, 250, 259, 267
Facial nerve (CN VII), 132, 144, 159, 162, 174, 185-187, **185**, **186**, 192, 193, 197, 291, 317
Facial expression, 193, 197
Facial muscles, 63, 185–186, 192, 239, 291, 315, **316**
Facial sensations, 193
Facial skeleton, 2, 313–314, **313**, **314**
Falx cerebelli, 35–36, **36**
Falx cerebri, 34–36, **36**
FAS. *See* Fetal alcohol syndrome

Fasciculus cuneatus, **97**, 98, **98**, **230**
Fasciculus gracilis, **97**, 98, **98**, **230**
Faucial pillars, 192, 194
Festination, 62, 286, 305
Fetal alcohol syndrome (FAS), 238, 293, **295**
Fibrillations, 167
Finger agnosia. *See* Agnosia
First-order neurons, 46, 97, **98**, **100**, 101, **101**, 102–103, 105, 139–141, 179, 182, 184, 185, 187
Fissure, 11, 24
Flaccid dysarthria, 167. *See also* dysarthria
Flaccid paresis, 179
Flexible Endoscopic Evaluation of Swallowing (FEES), 197
fMRI, see functional magnetic resonance imaging
fMR1 gene, 239
Folia, 28
Foliate, 144
Foramen, 1, 28, 31–32, 34, 37, 43, 72
　magnum, 1, 31, **32**, 34, 72
　Luschka, 37, **38**
　Magendie, 37, **38**
　Monro, 37, **38**
Fornix, 76, 199, 205–207, **206**, **207**, 214
　damage to, 206
Fovea, 108–109, **108**
Fragile X syndrome, 239
Frontal aslant tract (FAT), 244
Frontal lobe, 9, 21, **22**, **23**, 32, 77, 78, **85**, 95, 239, 240, 252, 277, 299, 308, 310
　attention, 255
　Broca area, 217, 224, **243**, 244, **276**
　cognition, 10, 21, **22**, 62, 251, 252
　language, 244
　memory, 142, 253
　motor, **9**, 21, **23**, 26, 149, 150–151, 156
　pragmatics/social cognition, 241
Frontal operculum, 145, 147, 248
Frontalis muscle, 185
Frontotemporal dementias. *See* Dementia
Functional magnetic resonance imaging (fMRI), 245, 269
Functional organization, 7, 207, **207**, 217, 234
　reactivation, 263, 271
　reorganization, 271
Fungiform papillae. *See* Taste
Fusiform gyrus, 24, **25**, 115, 239, 267. *See also* Occipitotemporal gyrus

G

G protein, 55-56, 141, 144-145
　G protein-coupled receptors (GPCRs), 55-56, 141, 144-145

Gamma-aminobutyric acid (GABA), 57–58, 64, 153, 156, 208
　agonist drugs, 57
Ganglion, 11, 26
Ganglion cells, 108–109, 128. *See also* Visual system
General somatic afferent (GSA), **177–178**, 179
　glossopharyngeal nerve, 187
General visceral afferent (GVA), **177–178**, 179
　glossopharyngeal nerve, 187
　superior laryngeal nerve, 188
General somatic efferent (GSE), **177–178**
General visceral efferent (GVE), **177–178**
　facial nerve, 185
　vagus nerve, 187
Geniculocalcarine fibers, **111**, **112**, 113, 256. *See also* Visual system
Gerstmann syndrome, **96**
Gerstmann-Straussler-Scheinker Disease (GSS), **242**
Gestation, 67–68, 72–74, 76, 293
Glabrous (non-hairy) skin, **92**, 94
Glial cells, 12, 15–16, **16**, 29, 54, 57, 73, 86, 139, 217, 241. *See also specific cell types*
Globus pallidus, 26, 28, 151, 153–154, **153**, **154**, 224, **227**, **242**
　external, 26, **153**, **154**
　internal, 26, 28, **153**, **154**
Glomeruli, 141, **141**
Glossopharyngeal nerve (CN IX), 144, **176**, **177**, 184, 187, **189**, **191**, 192
Glutamate, 17, 57–58, 109, 125, 134, 144, 264–265
　reuptake, 57
Golgi tendon organs (GTOs), 94–95, **94**
Golgi type I, 46
Golgi type II, 46
Gonadal systems, 86
Gonadotropin-releasing hormone, 40
Gradients, 47–48, 52, 54, 64
Granule cells, 156. *See also* Cerebellum.
Graphesthesia, 96
Gray matter, 1, **2**, 6, **11**, 15, 28, 67, 72, 77, 83, 154, 165, 210, 239, **242**, 249, 250
Growth chart
　stature, **293**
　weight versus stature, **294**
Guillain-Barré syndrome, 39
Gustation, 139, 141, 144, 146–147, 193, 199, 203. *See also* Taste.
　gustatory cortex, 145–146
　gustatory nucleus, **145**, 185
　gustatory stimulation, 147
　impairments, 139, 146
Gyrus, **11**

H

Habenulus (habenulae), 86
Hamstring, 165
Hearing loss, 125, 228, 238, 267, 291 *See also* Auditory system
    conductive, 121, 132, 136, 142-143
    sensorineural, 121, 132, 136, 142, 288, 292
Heart, 36, 178, 187, 218–219, 232, 234, 280
    attack, see myocardial infarction
    heartbeat, 58, 210
    rate, 5, 58, 200, 213, 214
Helicotrema, 123
Hematoma, 34–35, 277, 296
    epidural, 34, 37
    subdural, 34
Hemianopsia, **115**, 116
    bitemporal heteronymous hemianopsia, **115**
    heteronymous, **115**
    homonymous hemianopsia, **116**
    nasal hemianopsia, **116**
Hemidystonia, 88
Hemiparesis, 88, 104, 224, 279-280
Hemisensory loss, **104**, 104, 105
Hemispheric development, 249, 250
Hemorrhage, 34–37, **35**, 39, 202, 232-234, 241, 280, 281, 283. *See also* Stroke
Herniation, 32, 34, 72
Heschl gyrus, 24, 127–129, 131, 133, 224, 243, 267. *See also* Auditory System
Heteromodal areas, 7, **7**, 199
Hippocampus, 24, 57-58, 74, 84-85, 142-143, 199, 201, 204-208, 210, 213, 242, 253-254, 276
Holoprosencephaly, 76
Holotelencephaly, 76
Homeostasis, 5, 40, 199-203, 213, 292, 308
    homeostatic mechanisms, 199, 202, 288
Homonymous, 115–116
Homonymous quadrantanopsia, 116
Homunculus, 7, 95–96, 150, 159
Horizontal cells, 108. *See also* Visual system
Hormonal systems, 28, 87
    regulation, 36
Horner syndrome, 228, 302
HPA axis. *See* Hypothalamic-pituitary-adrenal axis, 3
Huntington disease (HD), 57, 58, **168**, 286–287
Hydraulic energy, 122-123. *See also* Auditory system
Hydrocephalus, 31, 34, 39–42, **41**, **42**, 76, 291–292
    communicating, 42
    non-communicating, 40
    normal pressure, 42
    progressive, 40, 291

Hyperactive reflexes, 41, 165-167, 277–279
Hyperalgesia, 103
Hyperkinetic, 168, 286, 305, 306. *See also* Dysarthria
Hypernasality, 63, 167–168, 188, 194, 278, 285, 299, 302, 303, 304
Hyperpolarization, 47, 49–50, 51–52, 53–54, 64, 125, 134, 136
Hypertonia, 166, 167
Hypoactive or absent reflexes, 165, 167
Hypoglossal nerve (CN XII), 173, **176**, **177**, 178, 190, **191**, 192, 291, 319
Hypoglossal nucleus, 179, 190, **242**
Hypokinesia, 62, 286
Hypokinetic dysarthria, 168
Hyponatremia, 202
Hyposmia, 142
Hypothalamic-pituitary-adrenal (HPA) axis, 213
Hypothalamus, 40, 72, 73, 75, 83, 84, 87, **87**, 89, 113, 142, 143, 145, 147, 185, 187, 199, 200, 201, 202, 206, 209, 212, 213, 252, 288
    damage to, 202, 292
Hypotonia, 169
Hypoxia, 231, 234, 240

I

Immune cells, 16
Incus, 122
Indirect (extrapyramidal) motor systems, 150, **150**
Induction, 70, 72, **72**, **76**, 79
Infantile amnesia, 253. *See also* Memory
Infarct (infarction), 232, 227, 229, **231**, 232, 241, 271, 280, 302
Inferior colliculus, 73, **85**, 86, 127–128, **127**, **128**, 131
Inferior fronto-occipital fasciculus (IFOF), 243–244, **244**
Inferior oblique muscle, 179–181, **180**
Inferior rectus muscle, 179–181, **180**
Inferior sagittal sinus, 36. *See also* Dural venous sinus
Infratentorial space, 36
Infundibulum. *See* Pituitary
Inhibitory Postsynaptic Potentials (IPSPs), 49–50, **50**, 56, 59, 64
Inhibitory signals, 45, 49–50, **50**, 57, 59, 62, 64, 95, 104, **154**, 155, 158, 165, 168, 239
Inner ear, 59, 121–123, **122**, **123**, 128, **135**, 229
Inner hair cells (IHCs), **124**, 125, **125**, **126**, 128
Interference. *See* Plasticity
Internal auditory meatus, 127, 132, 134
Internal capsule, 159, 160, **160**, **161**, 166, 224, **227**. *See also* Motor and sensory tracts
Internal carotid artery. *See* Carotid arteries
Internal laryngeal nerve. *See* Vagus (X) cranial nerve

Internal medullary lamina, 83
Interneurons, 46, 59–60, 95, 141, 156
Interventricular foramen, 37, **38**
Intracranial pressure, 32, 34–35, 37, 39, 277, 279
Intralaminar nuclei of the thalamus, **85**, 86
Intraoperative monitoring, 61
Intraparietal sulcus, 21, **24**, 255, **256**
Ions, 14–15, 47–53, **48**, **53**, 54, **55**, **56**, 64, 125
    calcium (Ca^{2+}), 40, 48, **48**, **49**, 54–55, 56, **56**, 57, 64, 125, 134, 141, 224, **265**, 280
    chloride (Cl^-), 40, 49, **49**, **50**, 56, 64, 141
    magnesium (Mg^{2+}), **265**
    potassium (K^+), 14, 17, 40, **47**, 48–49, **49**, 50–52, **52**, 53, 56, 64, 123, 125, 134, **265**
    sodium (Na^+), 14, 40, **47**, **48**, 48–49, **49**, 50, 51, 52, **52**, 53, **54**, **54**, **56**, 57, 64, 123, 141, **202**, **265**, 281
    channels, 14–15, **15**, 47–48, 50–51, 54–56, 125, 144–145
    pumps, **15**, **47**, 50, **52**, 57
Ionic osmolality, 40
Ionotropic channels, 48, **48**, 55
    receptors, 56
IPSP. *See* Inhibitory Postsynaptic Potentials
Iris, 107–108, **108**, 181
Ischemia, 229, 231–232, **231**, **232**, 234, 241, 280, 301

J

Jaw movements, 193
Jaw-jerk reflex, 193
Joint attention network, 257
Joint position. *See* Proprioception), 95
Joint receptors, 94
Jugular vein, 36

K

Kinase, 264-265
Kinocilium, 125, 134
Korbinian Brodmann, 6

L

Labial seal, 192–193
Labyrinthitis, 135
Lacrimal glands, 177, 185
Lamina terminalis, 67–68, 72, 75–76, 79
Language, 6, 7, 9, 21, **23**, 24, 29, 64, 67, 69, 83, 84, **85**, 86, 88, **88**, 121, 151, 156, **207**, 217, 232, **233**, 241, 243-251, **255**, 258, **267**, 271, **276**, 279, 280, 281, 286, 293, 294–295, 296, 297, 299, 300–301, 305, 308, 309, 310
    development, 78, 245, 267
    developmental disorders, 238, 239–240
    body language, 45, 241, 248
    morphology, 241, 248
    processing networks, 248
        dorsal stream, 205, 243, **245**, 248, 288
        dual-stream model, 243, 248, 258
        ventral stream, 243, **245**, 248, 258
Laryngeal function, 194
    adductor reflex, 192
    laryngeal diadochokinesis, 196
Laryngeal branches of the vagus nerve. *See* Vagus (X) Nerve.
Lateral corticospinal tract. *See* Corticospinal tract
Lateral dorsal nucleus of the thalamus (LD), 85-86, **85**
Lateral Geniculate Nucleus (LGN) of the thalamus, 85-86, **85**, 111, 113, 175
Lateral inhibition, 59-61
Lateral lemniscus, 127–128
Lateral nuclear complex of the thalamus, **85**, 86
Lateral posterior (LP) nucleus of the thalamus, **85**, 86
Lateral rectus muscle, 179–182
Lens, 107–108, 111, 177, 179
Leptin hormones, 200
Levator veli palatini muscle, 187, 194, 317
Lewy body dementia, 241–242
Ligand-gated, 48, **48**, 56
Limbic system 19, **58**, 84, **85**, 86, 87, **143**, 145, 147, 151, 185, 187, 199–211, 213, **199**, **209**, 251, 252, 300
    memory, 204
    inputs and outputs, **201**
    reward circuits, **209**
    structures, **200**
Lingual motor functions, 194
Linguistic, 246, 248, 307
Localization, 276
    of damage, 217
    cortical localization of functions, 251, **276**, 276
    of nerve signals, 61, 93, 200
    of sound, 128–129, 131, 136
Long-term depression (neural plasticity), 265
Long-term potentiation (LTP), **263**, 263–264, 271
Low-pressure CSF syndrome, 41, 277
Lower motor neuron (LMN), 41, **158**, 158–160, 162-163, 165, 174, 179, 181-182, 184-187, 189-190, 197
    damage, 165, **167**, 170, 179, 184, 186-187, 193-194, 197, 291
Lumbar puncture procedure, 39, **39**
    opening pressure, 39, 278

M

Macrophages, 16, 58
Macroplasticity. *See* plasticity
Macula, 134

Magnetic resonance imaging (MRI), 69, 76, 226, 232, 234, 280, 296
Malleus, 122
Mammillary bodies, 199, 201, 205-206
Mandibular branch (V3). *See* Trigeminal nerve (CN V)
Massed practice, 269
Mastication, 31, 193
   muscles of, 162, 176-177, 182, 184–185, 191, 315
Masticator palsy, 185
Maxillary branch. *See* Trigeminal nerve (CN V)
Mechanical energy, 121–123
Mechanically gated ion channels, 48
Mechanoreceptors, 59, 61, 91–94, **92**, 98
   mechanosensitive nociceptors, 94
   mechanoreceptive neurons, 59
Medial geniculate nucleus (MGN) of the thalamus, 85–86, **85**, 127–128
Medial lemniscus, 97–99, 105, 165, 230
Medial rectus muscle, 179–181
Mediodorsal (MD) nuclear complex of the thalamus, 84, **85**
Medulla oblongata, 28, 31, 32, 72, **75**, 98, **98**, 102, **104**, 144, 150, 158, 159, 160, **160**, 162, 163, 170, 179, 182, 187, 189, 190, 200, 210, 211, 229, **229**, **230**, **242**, 283, 302
   medulloblastoma, 296
Membranous labyrinth, 122–123, 134–135
Memory, 21, 58, 68, 77, 83-85, 199, 201-204, **205**, 208, 213, 251-253, 255, 258, 265, 271, 276
   auditory short-term, 243, 246
   autobiographical, 256
   consolidation, 24, 205, 253
   declarative, 78, 199,204–205, 252, 253, 254
   disorders, 207, 254
   encoding, 253–254
   episodic, 205-206, 253–254
   impairments, 62, 88, 202, 207, 209, 226, 255, 276, 280-281, 288, 294, 297
   meta-memory, 253
   non-declarative, 253
   procedural, 253, 255
   prospective, 253–254
   retrieval, 253
   retrograde amnesia, 254
   semantic, 204, 244, 253
   short-term, 251
   storage, 204, 253-254
   verbal, 206-207
   visual, 239
   working memory, 34, 78, 204, 224, 240, **251**, 252-254
Meninges, 2-3, 31, 34, **35**, 37, 43, 177, 182, 240, 277
   meningeal arteries, 34
   damage, 31, 42
   diverticula, 41
   dural sinuses, **36**
   extensions, **36**
   herniation, 72
   veins, 36
Meningitis, 31, 34, 38, 40, 42, 135, 278, 292
   mechanical, 42
Mental health, 270
Mentalizing network, **248**, 250
Mesencephalic flexure, 74
Mesencephalon, 72, **72**, 75
   mesencephalic nucleus, 182, 184
Mesocortical pathway, 210
Mesoderm, 70, **70**
Mesolimbic pathway, 210, **210**
Metastatic tumors, 234
Metencephalon, **72**, 75
Microfilaments, 14
Microglia, 16
Microneurons, **46**
Microtubules, 14
Midbrain, **28**, 62, 72, 74-75, 83, 86, 111, 127, 134, 151, 158-159, 162, 181-182, 200, 209, 227-230
Middle Cerebral Artery (MCA) **217**, 217-219, 222-227, 232
   distribution, 223–224
   perfusion, restrictions to, 217, 232-233, 279-282
Middle ear, 34, 122, 125, 132, 177, 184–185, 187
Midsagittal slice, 12–13, 84, 314
Mirror neurons, 150
Modified barium swallow (MBS), 196, 284–285
Monocular blindness, 115
Monosynaptic, **158**, 162, 179, 197
Mossy fibers. *See* Cerebellum
Motor system, 26, 28, 29, 46, 57-58, 86-87, 91, 101, 104-105, 121, 135, 149-151, 155-156, 158, 160, 170, 192
   control, 26, 83, 149, 150, 162, 169, 226, 258
   cortices, 21, 162, 263
   damage, 165, 166, 169, 238, 286
   deficits, 57-58, 62, 88, 239
   end plate, 163
   homunculus, 159
   innervation, 175–176, 183, 197, 224
   learning, 155–156, 205
   pathways, 158, 165–166, 179, 211
   strip, 21, 149–150, 158-162, 185, 224
MRI, see magnetic resonance imaging
Multiple sclerosis, 39, 61-62, 166-167, 240
Multiple spinal meningeal diverticulum, 41, 277
Multipolar neurons, 46, **46**, 95
Muscles
   damage to, 170
   eye, 173, 176, 179-181, **180**

Muscles *(continued)*
  facial, 31, 162, 173, 176, 185, 191, 193
  muscle memory, 253
  paralysis of, 63
  spasticity, 62
  weakness, 62, 202
Muscle spindle afferents, 94–95
Myasthenia Gravis, 45, 58, 61–62, 65, 167–168
Mydriasis, 181, **181**
Myelencephalon, **72**, 75
Myelin, 11, 15, 17–18, 53, 54, 59, 68, 72, 167. *See also* Schwann cells
  diseases of, 62, 167, 240, 241, 291
  myelinated axons, 15, 53, 54, 55
  myelination, 15, 19, 25, 68, 69, 74, 76–78, 245, 252, 267
Myocardial infarction, 234, 253
Myotomes, 102, 160

N

N-methyl-D-aspartate (NMDA) receptors, 264-265
Nasal cavity, 34, 122, 139, 142, 146, 197
Nasal fields. *See* Visual system
Nasal regurgitation, 188, 285
Nasolabial folds, 283
Nasopharynx, 122, 176
Nerves
  fibers, 32, 80
  impulses. *See* Action potentials
Neural plasticity. *See* plasticity
Neural architecture, 156
Neural development. *See* Neuroembryology
Neuroactive hormones, 38
Neuroembryology, 67, 69, 73, 75, 77, 79
  neural crest cells, 72
  neural plate, 70, 72
  neural tube, 67, 69-75, **73**, 79
  primary neurulation, 72
Neurofilaments, 14
Neurohormones, 40
Neuromuscular junction, 63–64, **154**, 163, 167
Neuron, 8, 12, 14, **16**
  adaptation of, 93
  cerebral, 46, 68
  circuits, **60**
  neuronal death, 35, 61–62, 239
  migration, 17
  precursors, 73
  membrane, **15**
  migration, 73–74
Neuronal pathways, 38, 74, 263
Neuroplasticity. *See* Plasticity

Neurotransmitters, 46, 50, 57, 59
  norepinephrine (NE), 57–58
  receptors, 15
NMDA receptor. *See* N-methyl-D-aspartate receptor
Nociception, **58**, 61
  nociceptors, 61, 93, 94
  pain perception, 86
Nodes of Ranvier, 15, 54–55
Non-declarative memory. *See* Memory, 253
Nonverbal communication, 193
Norepinephrine (NE), 57–58. *See also* Neurotransmitters
Notochord, 70, 72
Noxious stimuli, 40
Nucleus, 11, 14
Nucleus accumbens, 200, 208
Nucleus cuneatus, 98
Nucleus gracilis, 98
Nystagmus, 135, 169

O

Occipital bone, 28, 189
Occipital cortex, 117
Occipital lobe, 24, 28, 78, 113, 116
  pole, 26
  occipitotemporal gyrus, 24
Oculomotor nerve (CN III), 134, 154, **176**, **177**, 179, **180**, 181, **242**
Odorants, 139, 141–142, 146
Olfaction, 139, 142, 199, 202, 204
  impairments of, 142
Olfactory nerve (CN I), 140, **142**, 143, **143**, **176**, 192–193
Olfactory system
  bulbs, 139, 143, 201–204, **203**
  cortices, 199, 213
  epithelium, 139–140, 146
  neurons, 34, 139, 141–143, 146
  pathway, 139, 147
  receptors, 139, 141, 143, 146
Oligodendrocytes, 17–18, 62
Opening pressure. *See* Lumbar puncture
Ophthalmic branch (V1). *See* Trigeminal nerve (CN V)
Optic nerve (CN II), 76, **76**, **85**, 86, 109, 111, **111**, 115, **115**, **176**
Optic pathways. *See also* Visual system pathway
  chiasm, 34, 111, **111**, 113, **113**, 115–116, **115**, 118
  geniculocalcarine fibers, **111**, 113, **256**
  nerve. *See* Optic Nerve (CN II)
  radiation, **111**, 113, 116
  tract, 83, 111, **111**, 113, 116
Oral mechanism exam (OME), 187, 192–197, 285
Oral preparatory phase. *See* Swallowing
Orbicularis oris muscle, 185, 193

Orexin, 200
Organ of corti, 123–**124**, 136
Organelles, 14
Orienting. *See* Attention
Oromandibular dystonia, 169
Ossicles, 122–123, 125, 132
Otoconia. *See* Vestibular system
Otolith organs. *See* Vestibular system
Ototoxicity, 125
Outer ear, 121
Outer hair cells (OHCs), 125. *See also* Auditory system
Oval window. *See* Cochlea

P

Pacinian corpuscle, **92**, 93, 94–95
Pain, 86, 88, **92**, 94, 95, 98, **100**, 102–103, **102**, **104**, 105. *See also* Nociception
  thalamic pain syndrome, 88, 103–104.
Papillae, 144
Parahippocampal gyrus, 24, 201, 203, 207
Paralinguistic, 248
Parallel fibers. *See* Cerebellum
Parasympathetic nervous system (PNS), 5, **5**, **177–178**, 181, 192
Paresthesias, 167
Parietal lobes, 18, 21, **24**, 26, 86, 96, **96**, 114, 116, 135, 150, 296, 299, 301
  attention, 255, **256**, **257**
  blood supply, 224
  memory, **254**
  pragmatics/social cognition, 241, 248
  somatosensory, 95
Parkinson disease (PD), 57, **58**, 61, 143, 150, 168, 231, 240, **242**, 285–286, 304–305
Parosmia, 142
Pars compacta, 151, 154
Pars reticulata, 151
Passive transport, 48–49, 64
Patellar tendon stretch reflex, 95, 163, 165
PCA. *See* Posterior cerebral artery
PCoA. *See* Posterior communicating artery
Peduncles, 28, 156
Penumbra, 232
Peptides, 57–59, 65
Peri-sylvian region, 243, **243**, 245, 246, 248, 300
Perilymph, 123, 125
Peripheral nervous system (PNS), 1, 2, 5, **5**, 17, 29, 47, **48**, 54, 57, **58**, 65, **98**, **100**, **101**, 173, 174, 211
Peritoneum, 40, 42, 291
Phantosmia, 142
Pharmacological, 63, 78, 232, 280, 300
Pharyngeal branch of the Vagus. *See* Vagus nerve (CN X)

Pharyngeal phase of swallowing. *See* Swallowing
Pharyngeal plexus, 173, 189, **189**, 192, 194. *See also* Glossopharyngeal nerve (CN IX) and Vagus nerve (CN X)
Phase locking. *See* Auditory system
Phonemic paraphasia, 88, 246
Phonology, 241
Photoreceptors, 108–109, **108**, 118
  cones, 108–109, **108**, **109**, 117, 118
  rods, 108–109, **108**, **109**, 118
Pia mater, 31, 34, 36–37
PICA, *See* Posterior inferior cerebellar artery
Pineal gland, 86–87, **87**
Pinna, 121, **122**, 131, 177, 185, 194
Piriform cortex, 142–143, 199, 201, 203
Pituitary fossa, 34
Pituitary gland, 34, 76, 87, 200
  stalk (infundibulum), 87
  tumors, 88
Place coding. *See* Auditory system
Planum temporale, 24, 131
Plasticity, 263-269, 271–273
  behavioral, 263, 265–268
  dosing, 267–269, **268**
  effective carryover, 268
  experience-dependent, 265, **268**
  interference, 267, 271
  macroplasticity, 263
  neural, 263
  synaptic, 239
  vascular, 263, 271
PNS. *See* Peripheral nervous system
Polarization, 47, 50–51, 53
Pons, 28, 72, 75, 150, 158-159, 162-163, **164**, 182, 184, 229
  corticobulbar tract, 158
  reticular activating system, 211
  reticulospinal tract, 163, **164**
  rubrospinal tract, 162
Postcentral gyrus, 21, 95, 98
Posterior cerebral artery (PCA), 219, 222–224, 228
Posterior communicating artery (PCoA), 219
Posterior inferior cerebellar artery (PICA), 226–227, 229
Postnatal development, 69, 74
Postsynaptic neurons, 49–51
Posttraumatic amnesia (PTA), 254
Postural headaches, 41–42, 275, 277–278
Postural instability, 211, 285
Potassium (K+). *See* Ions
Pragmatics, 241, 248, 258
  networks, 248
Pre-dorsal premotor area, 150
Prenatal environmental stressors, 213

Prenatal genetic testing, 240
Presbycusis, 132
Presynaptic neurons, 47, 265
Primary auditory cortex (A1). See Auditory system
Primary motor strip (M1). See Motor system 21, 149–150, 158
Primary sensory strip (S1). See Somatosensory system. 84, 86, 95, 97–98, 174, 179, 185
Primary somatosensory cortex (S1), 95
Primary visual cortex (V1), 113
Principal sensory nucleus, 182
Prion-related dementia. See Dementia
Procedural memory. See Memory
Progressive bulbar palsy, 167
Projection tract, 11
Propagation, 53–54
Proprioception, 91, 95, **98**, 101, **102**, 104, 105, 155, **156**, 175, 184, 193
   joint position, 95
   proprioceptive input, 98, 101, **102**, 105, **270**
   sensory receptors, 91, 94, **101**
   unconscious, 101
Prosencephalon, 72–73, 75–76, 83
Prosopagnosia, 116–117
Prospective memory. See Memory
Prostigmine (neostigmine), 168
Proteinopathies. See Dementia
Pruning (synaptic), 67–68, 78, 265
Pseudounipolar neuron, 46, 98
Ptosis, 181, 228
Pulvinar, **85**, 86, 257
Pupil, 107–108, 181
   dilation, 200
Pure word deafness, 133
Purkinje cells. See Cerebellum
Putamen, 26, 151, **153**, **154**, 224, **227**, 239, **242**
Pyramidal decussation, 160, **160**, **166**, **230**
Pyramidal motor neurons. See Upper Motor Neurons
Pyramidal system, 149–150, 170
   pyramidal tracts, 149, 158, 162
Pyridostigmine (Mestinon), 62-64

Q

Quadrantanopsia, 115, **115**. See also Visual system

R

Radial migration, 73
Rapidly adapting receptors, 93
RAS. See Reticular activating system
Reciprocal connections, 84, 202–203, 205–206
Reciprocal inhibition, 165
Recurrent laryngeal nerve (RLN). See Vagus nerve (CN X)
Reflex arc, **165**
Refractory period, 52-53
Reissner membrane, 123
Repolarization, 47, 52–53
Respiratory system, 105, 218
Resting membrane potential, 47, 50–53, 64
Reticular Activating System (RAS), 199, 211–212, **211**
   caudal projections, 211
Reticular formation, 199, 202, 209, 211
Reticulospinal tract, 149, 163, 211
Retina, 107–109, 114–115. See also Visual system
Retrograde amnesia. See Memory
Reuptake (endocytosis), 57, 59, 62–63
Reverberating circuits, 59
Reward circuit, 208
RHD. See Right hemisphere damage
Rhombencephalon, 72, 74–75
Right hemisphere damage (RHD), 251, 252
Right-left confusion, 96
Rinne test. See Auditory system assessment
Risorius muscle, 193
Rods. See Photoreceptprs
Rubrospinal tract, 149, 162, 230
Ruffini endings, **92**, 93, 94

S

Saccule, 134
Sagittal slice, 12
Sagittal sulcus, 18, 35–36, 160
Salience, 266, 268, 270
Salivary gland, 185
Saltatory conduction, 54
SCA. See Superior cerebellar artery
Scala media. See Cochlea
Scala tympani. See Cochlea
Scala vestibule. See Cochlea
Scarpa ganglion. See Vestibular system
Schizophrenia, 57, 210, 214, 250
Schwann cells, 17, 72, 239
Secretory granules, 57-58
Selective attention. See Attention
Selective serotonin reuptake inhibitors (SSRIs), 63
Semantic memory. See Memory
Semantic processing, 243, 258
Semantics, 241
Semicircular canals, 122, 133–134. See also Vestibular system
Sensory homunculus. See Somatosensory system, 95–96
Sensory innervation, 91, 102, 183, 197
Sensory inputs, 14, 214, 270

Sensory neurons, 46
Sensory pathways, 97, 179
Septo-optic dysplasia, **76**
Septum pellucidum, 19, **76**
    agenesis, **76**
Serotonin (5-HT), 57, 63–64, 78
Sex hormones, 200
Shingles virus, 102
Shuffling gait, 62, 168
Sign language, 267
Sinus, 36, 193
Skeletal muscles, 2, 158, 160, 162
Sleep disorders, 212
Slowed thinking. *See* Bradyphrenia
SMA. *See* Supplementary motor area
Small vessel disease (SVD). *See* Dementia
Social cognition, 241, 248, 258
Social cognition networks, 251
Sodium (Na^+). *See* Ions
Sodium ion channels, 54
Solitary tract, 144, 185, 230
Somatic muscles, 175
Somatic nervous system, 2
Somatic systems, 175
Somatoparaphrenia, 96
Somatosensory system, 46, 59, 91, 95, 107
    assessment, 102
    homunculus, 95–96
    neurons, 61, 85
    receptors, 91–93, 105
    primary somatosensory strip (S1), 59, 104, 217
    somatotopy, 7, 160
Sound waves, 125
Spasmodic dysphonia (SD), 63, 169
Spastic dysarthria, 166–167, 233
Spasticity, 166–167, 270
Spatial summation, 50, 64
Special Somatic Afferent (SSA), **177–178**
Special Visceral Afferent (SVA), **177–178**, 179, 185
    facial nerve, 185
    glossopharyngeal nerve, 187
Special Visceral Efferent (SVE), **177–178**, 185
    external laryngeal nerve, 188
    facial nerve, 185
    glossopharyngeal nerve, 187
    oculomotor nerve, 181
    recurrent laryngeal nerve, 188
    spinal accessory nerve, 189
Sphenoid bone, 31, 34
Spina bifida, 72
Spinal accessory nerve (CN XI), 173, 176, **176**, **177**, 178, 189–190, **190**, 194

Spinal canal, 1, 16
Spinal cord
    ascending sensory tracts, **97**
    hemisection, 102
    injury 91, 102, 270, 272
Spinal dysraphism, 72
Spinal meningitis, 135
Spinal muscular atrophy, 167
Spinal nerves, 158
Spinal trigeminal nucleus, 182
Spindle afferents. *See* Muscle spindle afferents
Spinocerebellar tract, 102
Spinocerebellum, 155
Spinothalamic tract, 86, 97, 98–99, **101**, **102**, 103, **104**, 211, **230**
    anterior, 98–99, **100**, 104
    lateral, 98–99
Spiral ganglion neurons. *See* Auditory system
Spongiform encephalopathy. *See* Dementia, 231
Stapedial reflex, 186
Stapedius muscle, 185–186
Stapes. *See* Ossicles
Stereocilia. *See* Auditory system
Sternocleidomastoid (SCM) muscle, 189
Strabismus, 181–182, 292
Stretching, 92, 165–166
    resistance to, 166
Stria medullaris, 86
Stria terminalis, 199, 201, 209
Stria vascularis, 123
Striatum, 151, 153–155, 201, 210, 242
Stroke, 231, 257
    cardioembolic, 118
    cerebellar, 227
    hemorrhagic, 232–233
    pathophysiology of, 228
    prenatal, 238
    thalamic, 88
Subarachnoid space, 36–37, 239
Subarachnoid hemorrhage, 37
Subclavian arteries, 218
Subdural hematomas, 34
Substance P, 57–58
Substantia nigra, 26, 61, 87, 151, 168
Subthalamic nucleus (nuclei), 26, 87, 151, 154–155
Subthalamus, 83, 87
Subthreshold signals, 50
Sulci, 18-19, 28–29, 73
Sulcus, 11
Sulcus limitans, 67, 72, 74, 79
Summation, 50–51, **51**, 64
    temporal, 50, **51**, 64

Summation *(continued)*
  spatial, 50, **51**, 64
Superior cerebellar artery (SCA), 226
Superior laryngeal nerve (SLN). *See* Vagus nerve (CN X)
Superior longitudinal fasciculus (SLF), 243–244
Superior oblique muscle, 179–181
Superior olivary complex (SOC), 127–128, 131
Superior rectus muscle, 179–180
Superior sagittal sinus, 36. *See also* Dural venous sinus
Supplementary motor area (SMA), 150-151
Suprachiasmatic nucleus, 202, 212
Suprahyoid muscles, 192
Supramarginal gyrus, 115, 255–256
Supranuclear region, 175
Supratentorial space, 36
Sustained attention. *See* Attention
SVA components. *See* Special Visceral Afferent
SVE components. *See* Special Visceral Efferent
Swallowing
  esophageal phase, 196
  instrumental assessment, 173, 196–197
  oral preparatory phase, 196, 286
  pharyngeal phase, 197
  safety, 194, 306
Sylvian aqueduct, 37
Sylvian fissure, 18, 20, 24, 131
Sympathetic nervous system, 2–3, 5, **58**, 187, 192, 200, 211, 214
Synapses, 47, 48, 50, 54, **56**
  chemical, 54
  electrical, 54
Synaptic cleft (gap), 47, 55–56, 59, 62-64, 163
Synaptic potentiation, 265
Synaptic vesicle, 55, 59
Synaptogenesis, 239, 245, 259, 264
Syndrome of inappropriate antidiuretic hormone (SIADH), 202
Syntax, 241, 244, 246

T

Tangential migration, 73
Tastants, 144–145
Taste, 139, 147, 185 *See also* Gustation
  fungiform papillae, 144
  first order afferents, **144**
  pathways, **145**
  perception, 139, 146
  vallate papillae, 144
Tau protein, 14
Tears, 34, 185, 272
Tectorial membrane, 125
Tectospinal tract, 149, 162

Tectum, 28, 72, 162
Tegmentum, 28, 208–211, 242
Telencephalon, 73, 76, 79
Temperature regulation, 202
Temporal bone, 31, 34–35, 134, 185
Temporal lobe 24, **25**, 34, 206, 239, **242**, 288, 296, 310
  blood supply, 223, **223**, 224
  emotions, 206
  face processing, 115, 117
  hearing, 128
  Heschel gyrus, 128, **128**
  language processing, 133, 243, **243**, 244
  memory, 24, **202**, 204, **205**, 207, 253
  prosodic processing, 133, 248, **250**
  theory of mind, **249**
  visual processing, 114
  Wernicke area, 24
Tensor veli palatini muscle, 194
Tentorium cerebelli, 35, 182. *See also* Meninges
Teratogens, 67, 78
Testosterone, 87, 200
Tetrodotoxin, 54
Thalamus, 28, 83–84
  anterior, 199, 205–206
  aphasia, 88
  adhesion, 83
  cortical connections, 6
  damage, 91, 103
  nuclei, 83-85, **85**, 91, 95, 205
  pain syndrome, 88, 103
  stroke, 88, 104
  syndrome, 88
  ventral nuclear complex, 86
  ventral posterolateral (VPL) nucleus, 86, 95, 97–99
  ventral posteromedial (VPM) nucleus, 86, 135
  ventroanterior (VA) nucleus, 86
  ventrolateral (VL) nucleus, 86
  ventroposterolateral (VPL) nucleus, 84, 95
Theory of mind, 69, 248–251
  affective, 248
  cognitive, 248
Therapeutic alliance, 268, 270
Thermoreceptors, 61, 91, 200
Thrombus, 232. *See also* Stroke
Thyrovocalis muscle, 63
Tissue Plasminogen Activator (tPA) **224**, 280, 300
Tonotopy, 128–130
Torticollis, 169
Toxins, 54, 67
tPA. *See* Tissue Plasminogen Activator
Tracheostomy tube, **284**
Transverse sinuses, 36. *See also* Dural venous sinus
Transverse temporal gyrus, 24